AF342148

SHINTO BENGI OSHIGATA

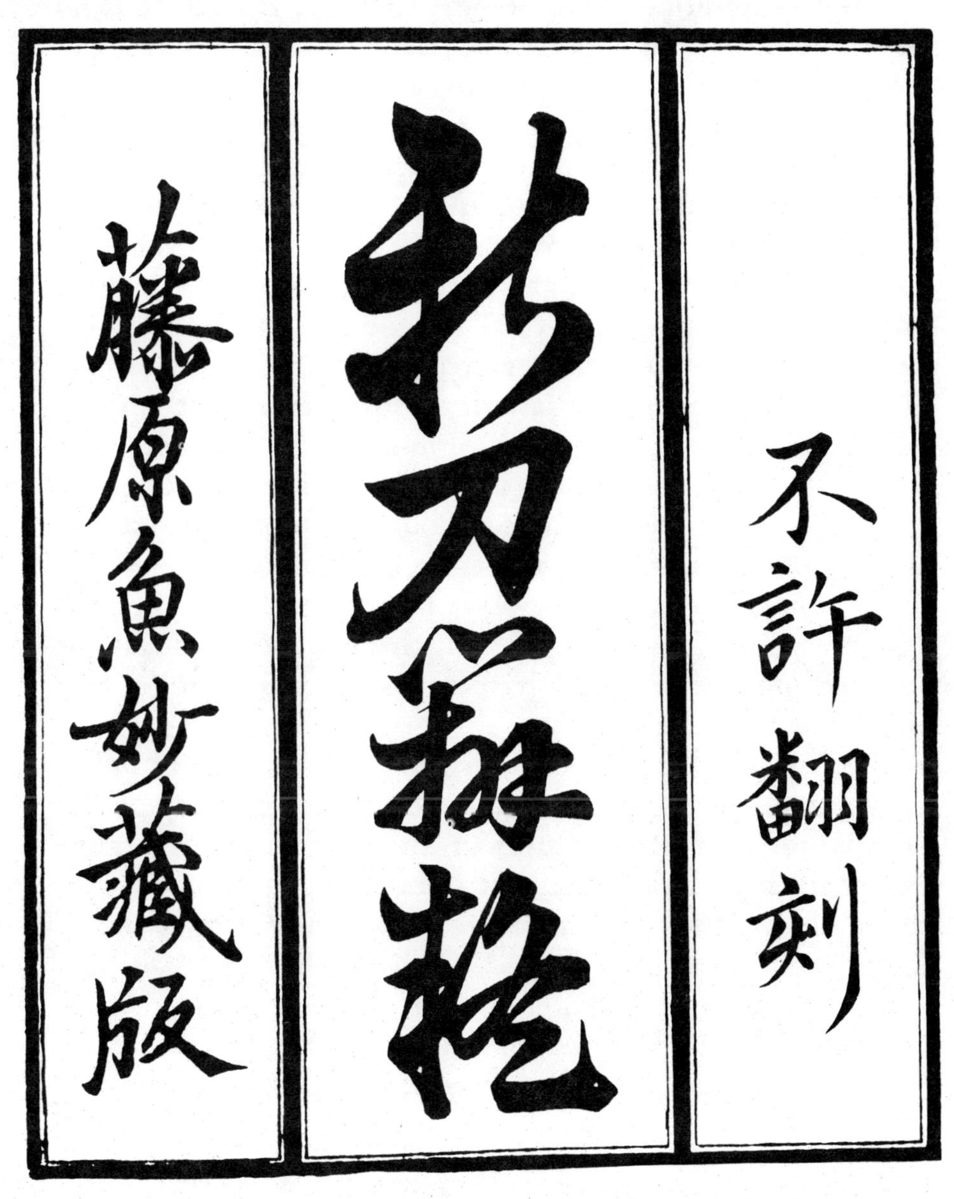

Among the thousands of books published in Japan on their famous swords, relatively few are available to Western collectors. Especially those produced before Meiji in the old wood-block printing, have become so scarce that there is no hope of owning one. A few, such as the Koson Oshigata and Umetada Meikan and now the first half of the Shinto Meijin are reprinted but the originals being hand drawn are not accurate enough to use for checking for forgeries,

Of the hundreds of modern books, excellently produced by photography from the swords themselves or from rubbings emphasis is always on the great masters and we find the same swords shown over and over. These are fine for checking for forgeries which, unfortunately constitute 90% of the swords found in the Western world today. However, almost entirely lacking are the run-of the-mill Shinto smiths that form the bulk of most of our collections. While these signatures are seldom forgeries, (faking these would be unprofitable) we still lack research material to seperate the generations.

The Shinto Bengi however is an exception to the rule, not only including a lot of lesser smiths, but the reproductions are suprisingly accurate and have details of chisel strokes that enable checking for forgeries.

The years from about 1590 to 1779 the date of publication take it from the end of Koto to the beginning of the Shinshinto era with a number of the later smiths still alive and producing. This means that the rubbings (oshigata) were taken from almost new unrusted tangs giving very clear reproductions.

In the present work, only the oshigata are reproduced rearranged and keyed by number to my Japanese Swordsmiths which see for additional information such as dates, places, etc.

W. M. Hawley
8200 Gould Avenue, Hollywood, Cal. 90046

SHINTO BENGI OSHIGATA

Akifusa AK 20	Amainu AM 7	Bokuden BO 3	Bokusen BO 4

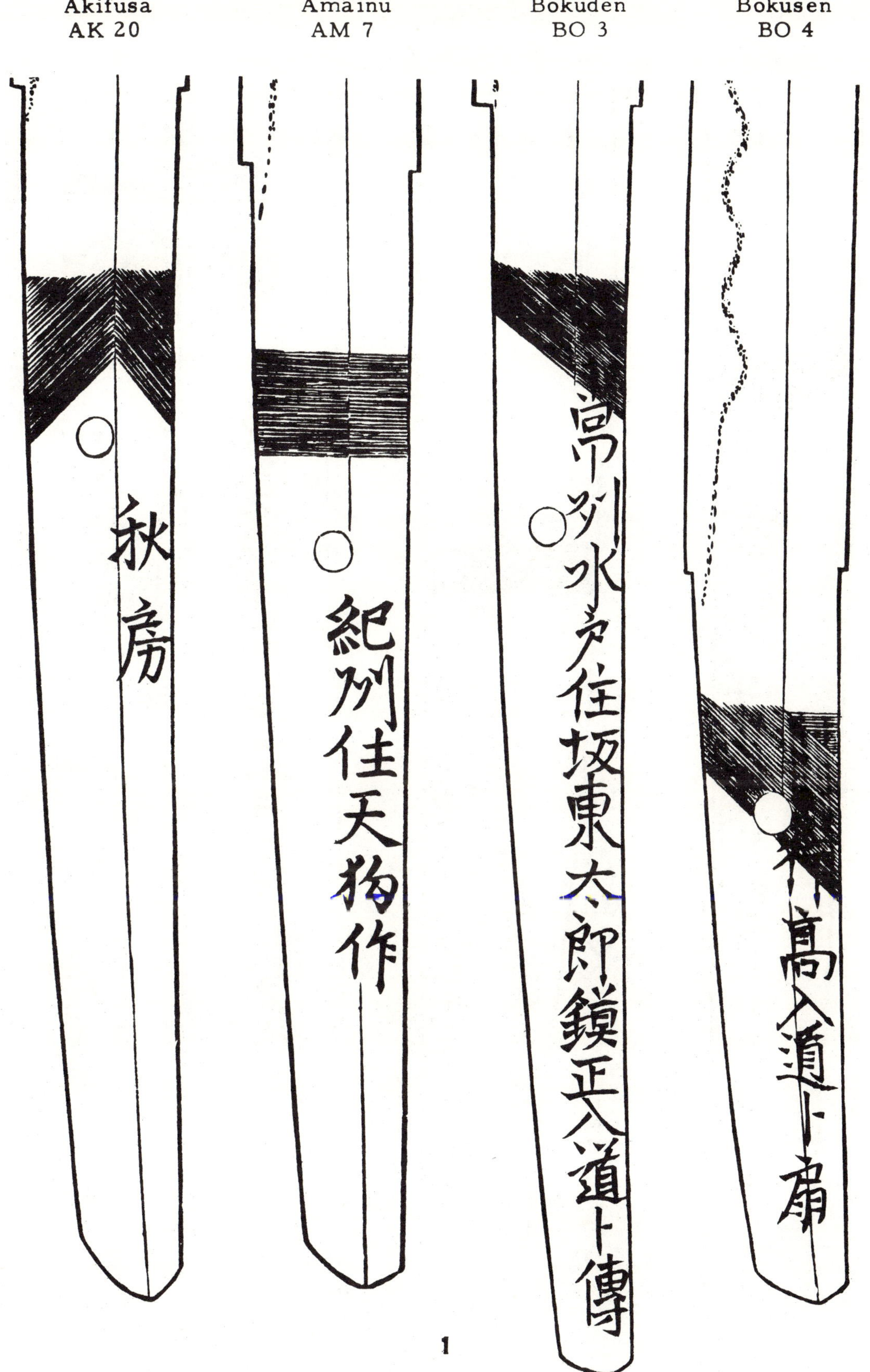

SHINTO BENGI OSHIGATA

Daiminkin
DA 26

Fuyutsura
FU 108

Haruhisa HA 71aa

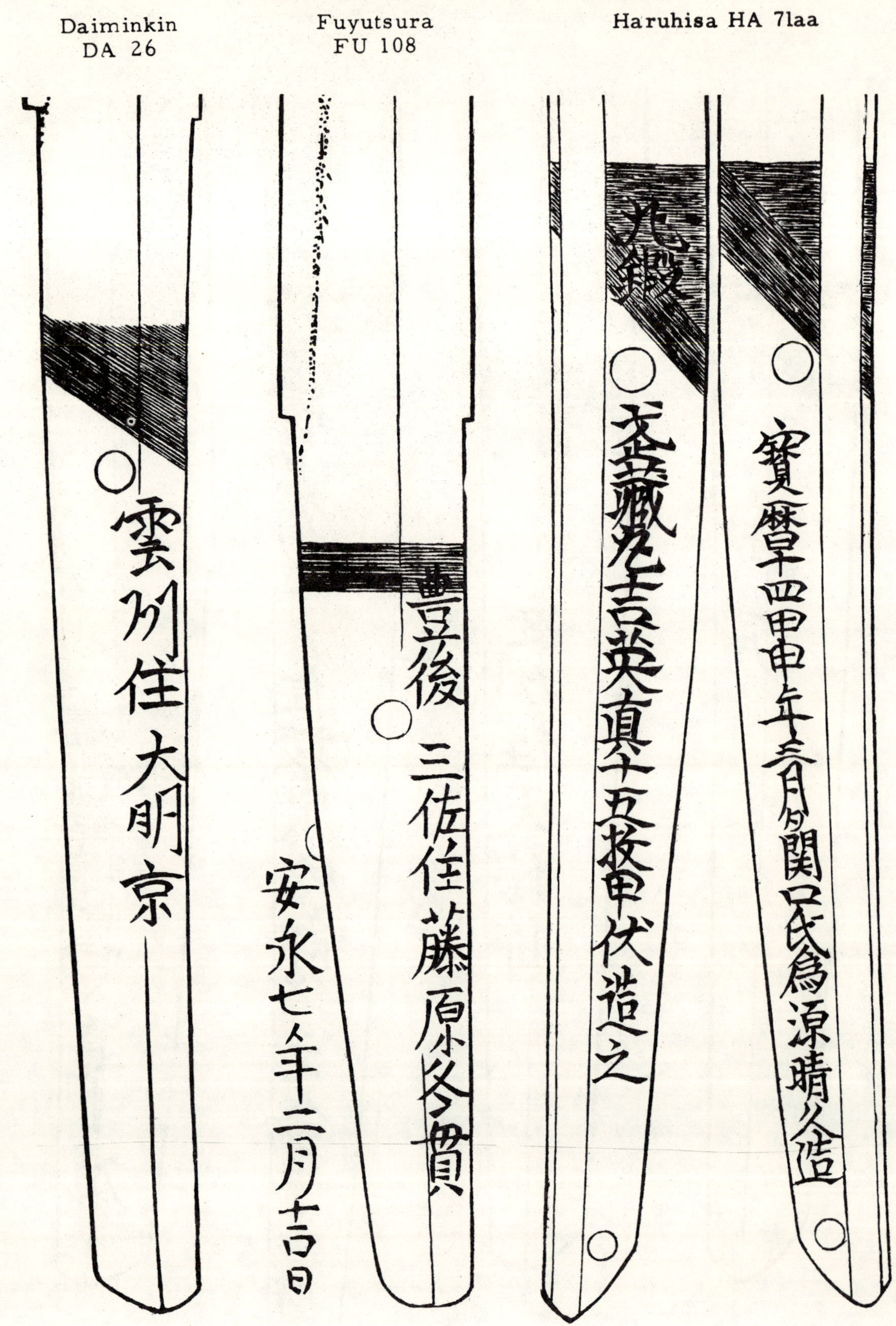

SHINTO BENGI OSHIGATA

Hankei HA 8   Hidekuni HI 31

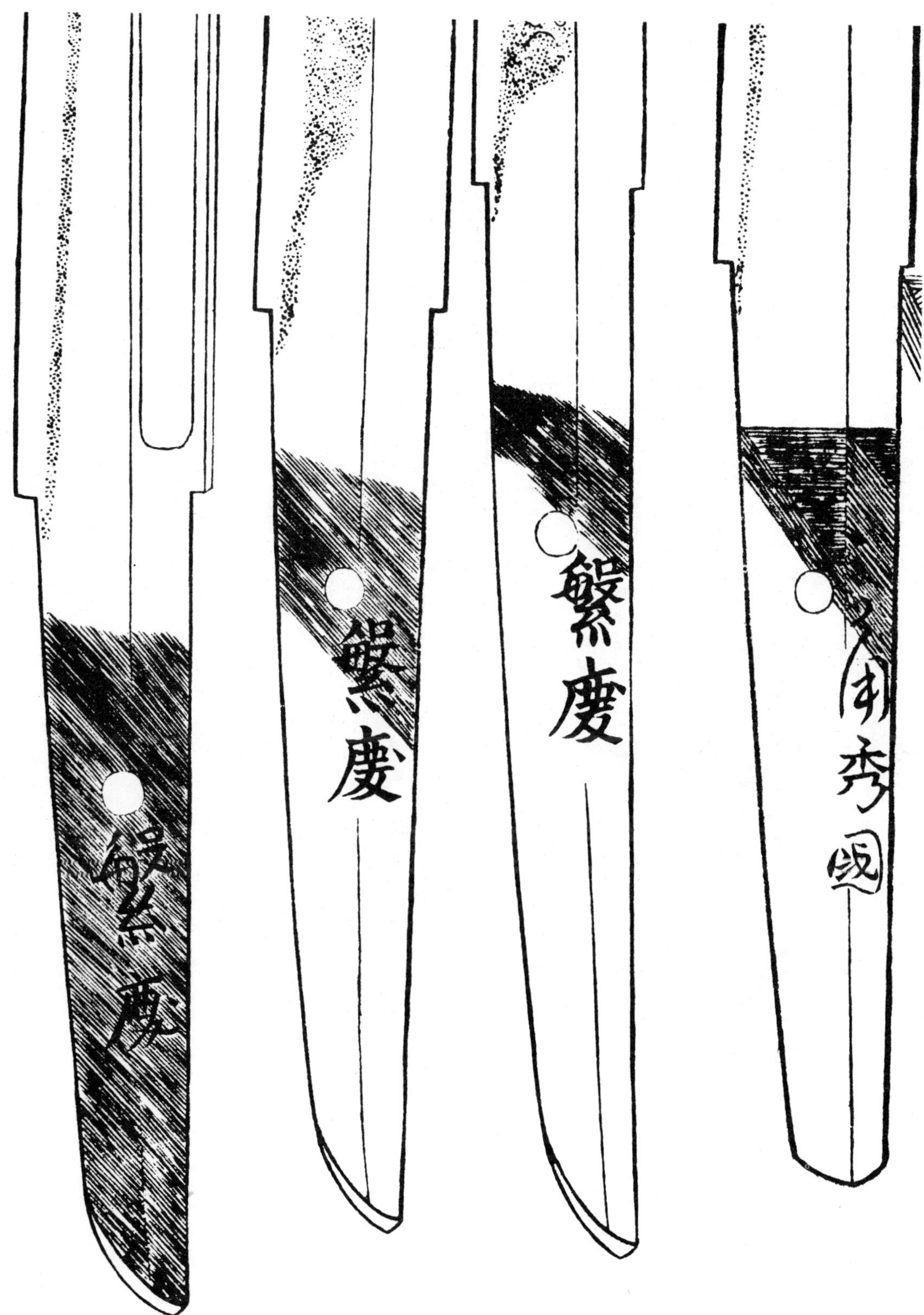

3

Harukuni HA 14
HA 14

Hirokane
HI 162

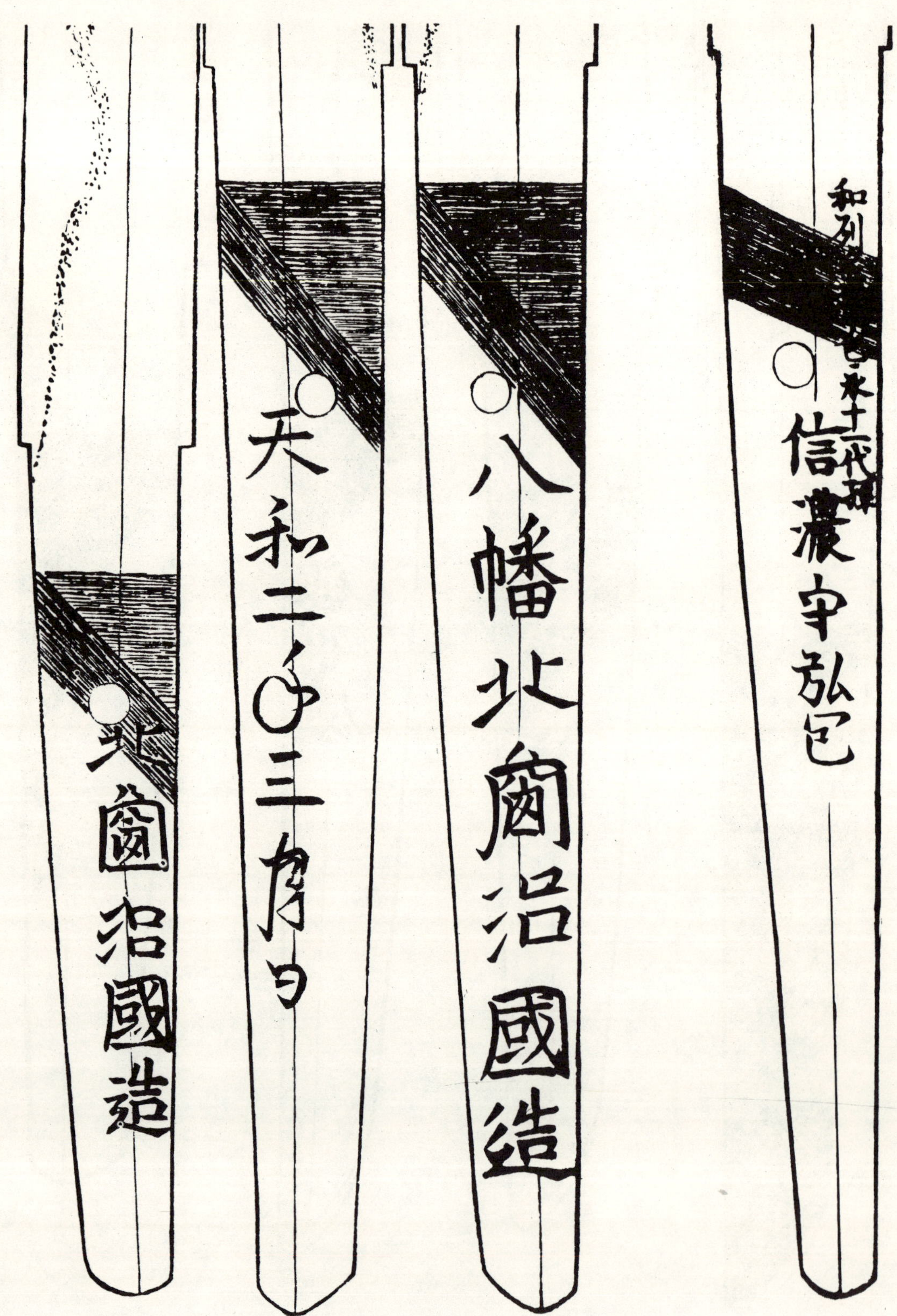

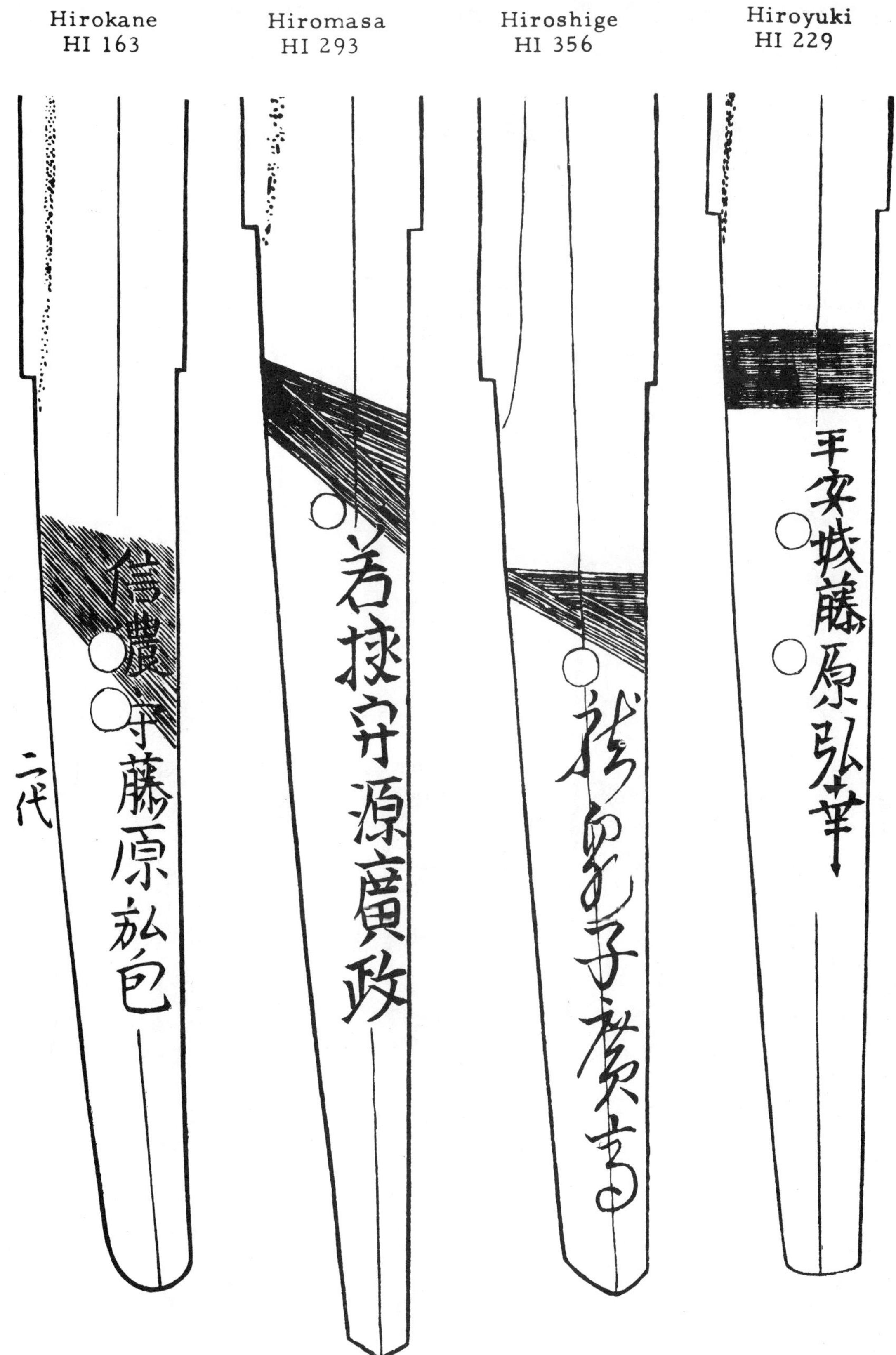
Hirokane
HI 163
Hiromasa
HI 293
Hiroshige
HI 356
Hiroyuki
HI 229

| Hiroyuki | Hirochika | Hiromasa | Hironobu | **Hironobu** |
| HI 229 | HI 255 | HI 293 | HI 321 | HI 327 |

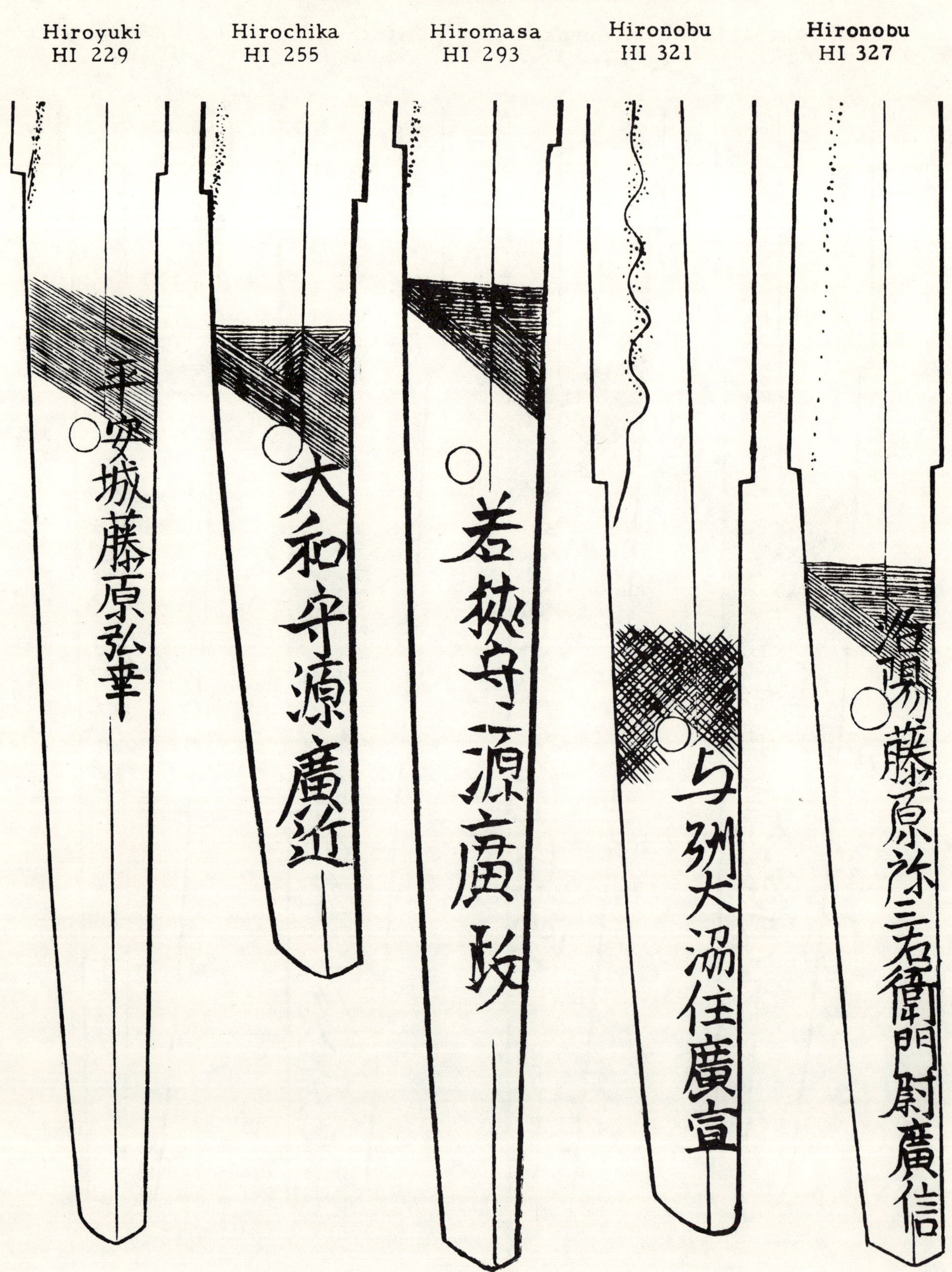

SHINTO BENGI OSHIGATA

Hironori HI 331	Hirosada HI 336	Hirosuke HI 360	Hirotaka HI 370	Hirotoki HI 379

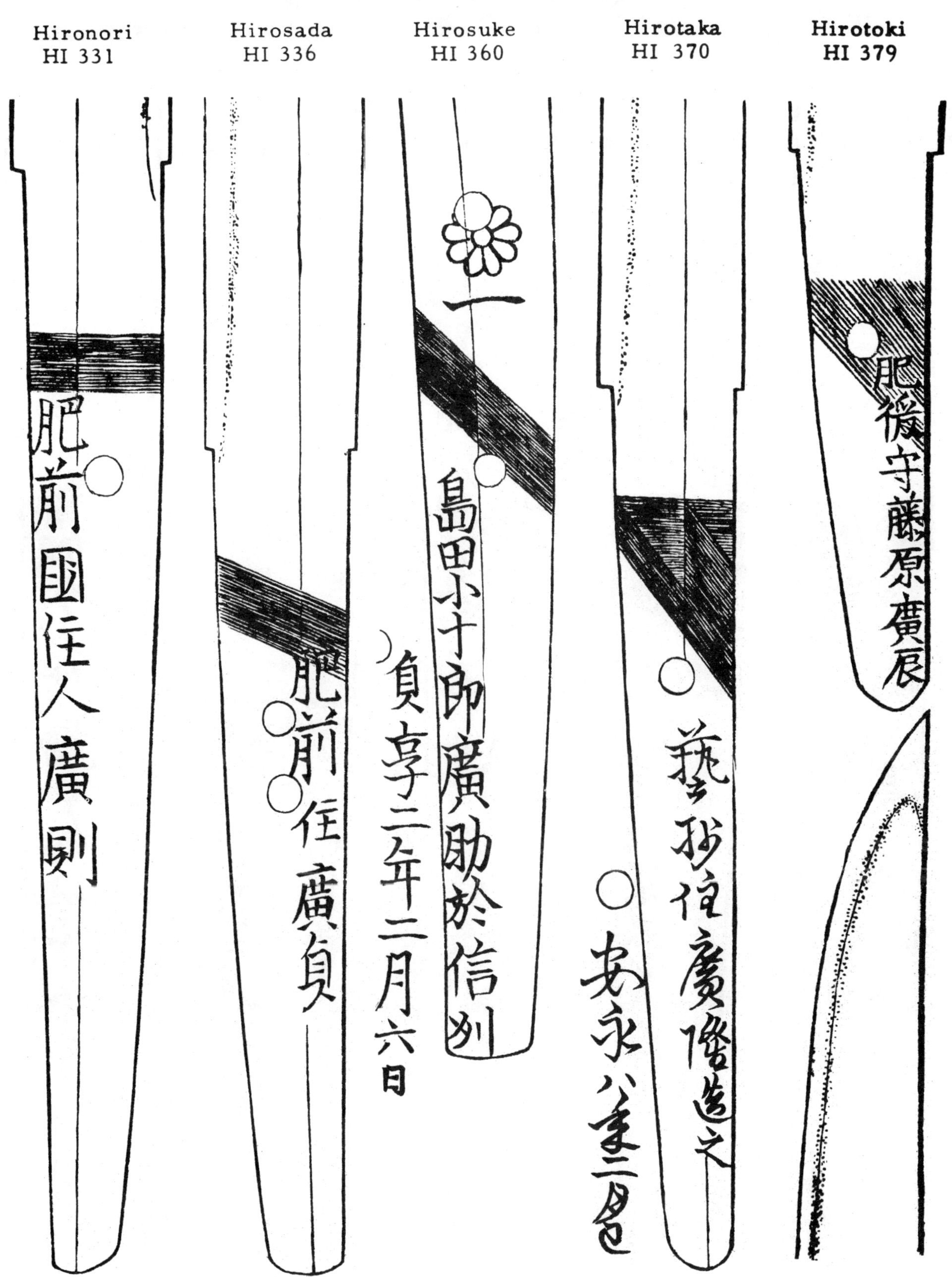

Hiroshige HI 356   Hiroyoshi HI 448   Hirotaro HI 373   Hiroyoshi HI 447

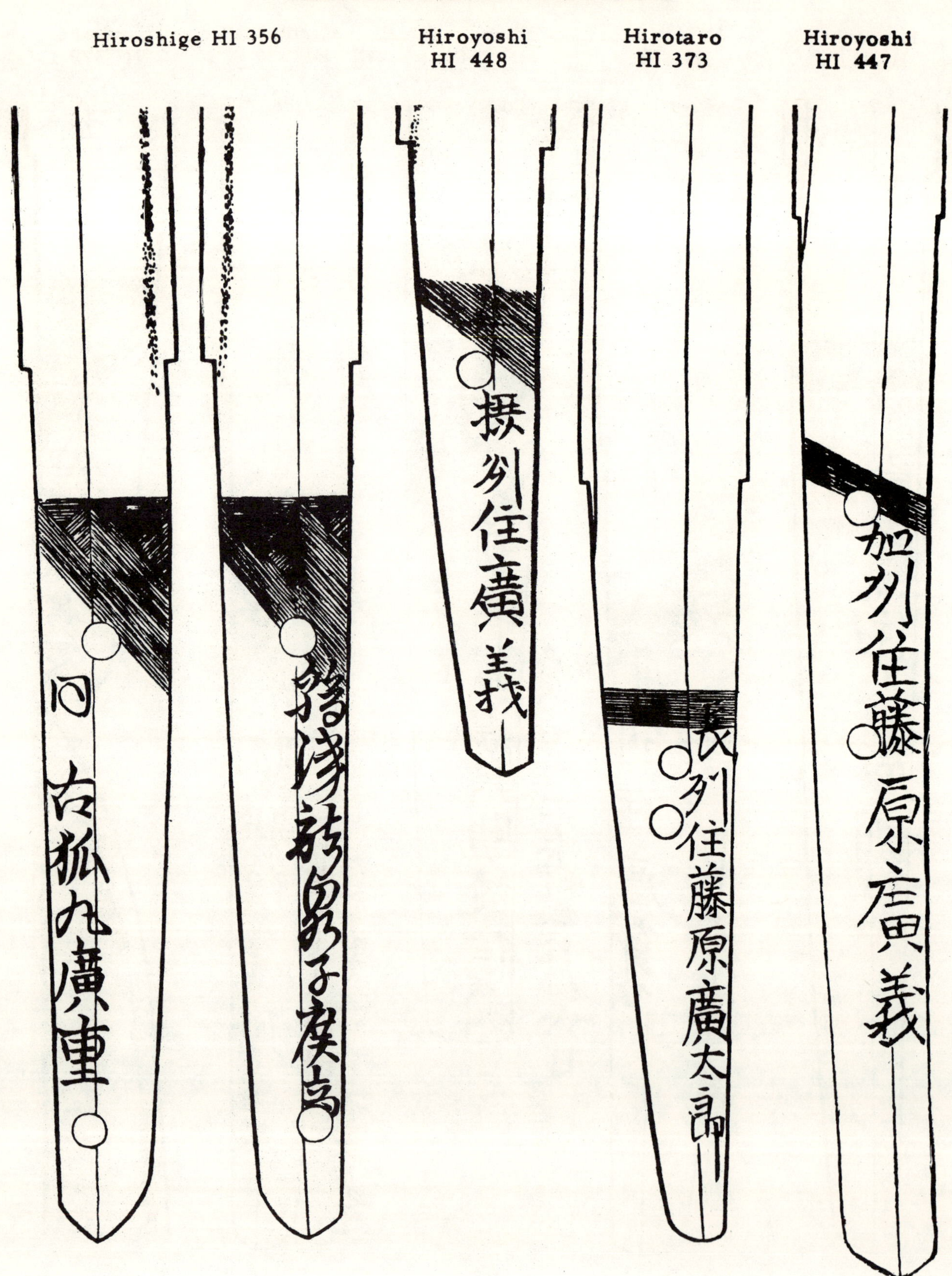

Hisakuni HI 472   Hisamichi HI 481

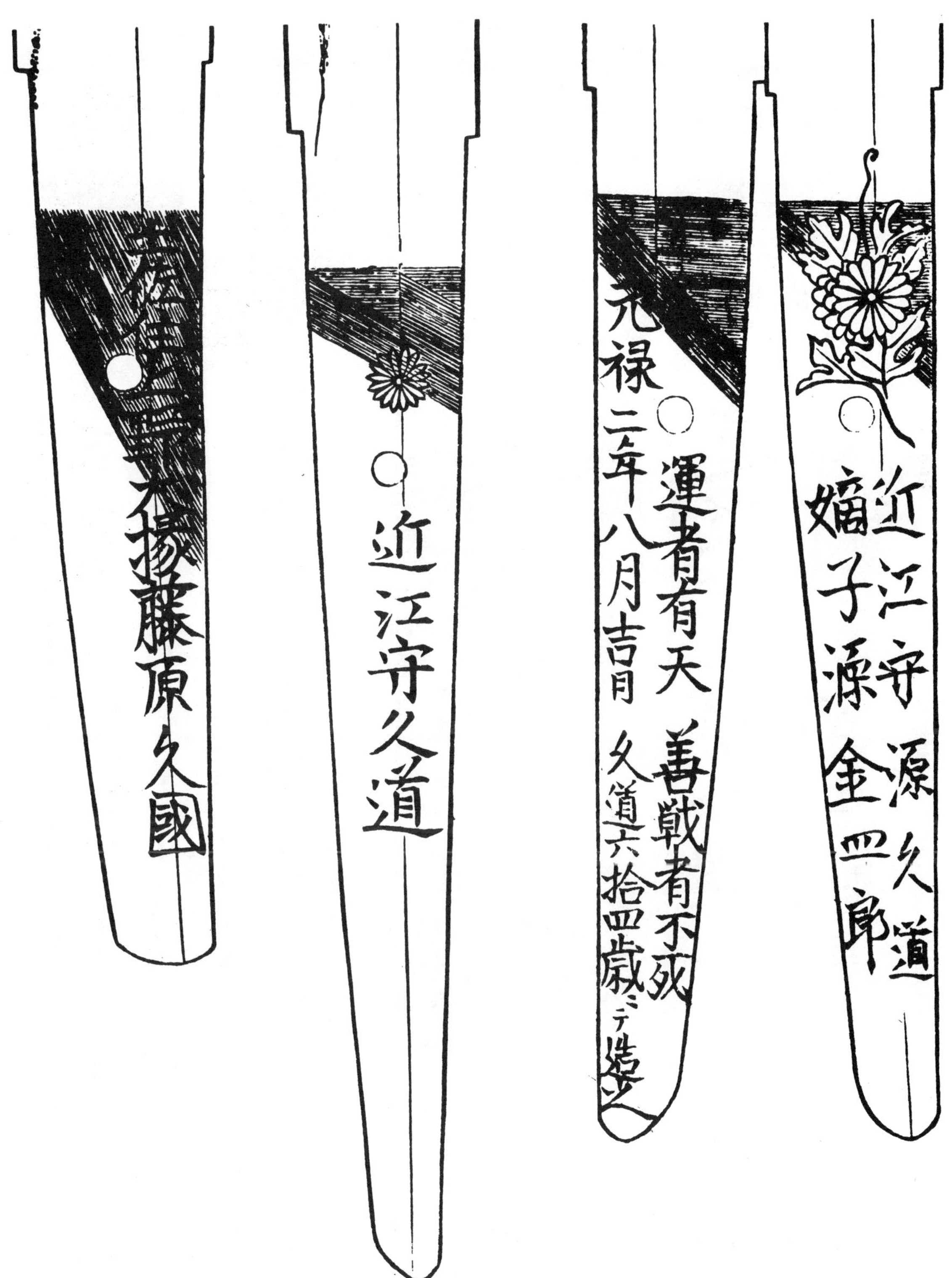

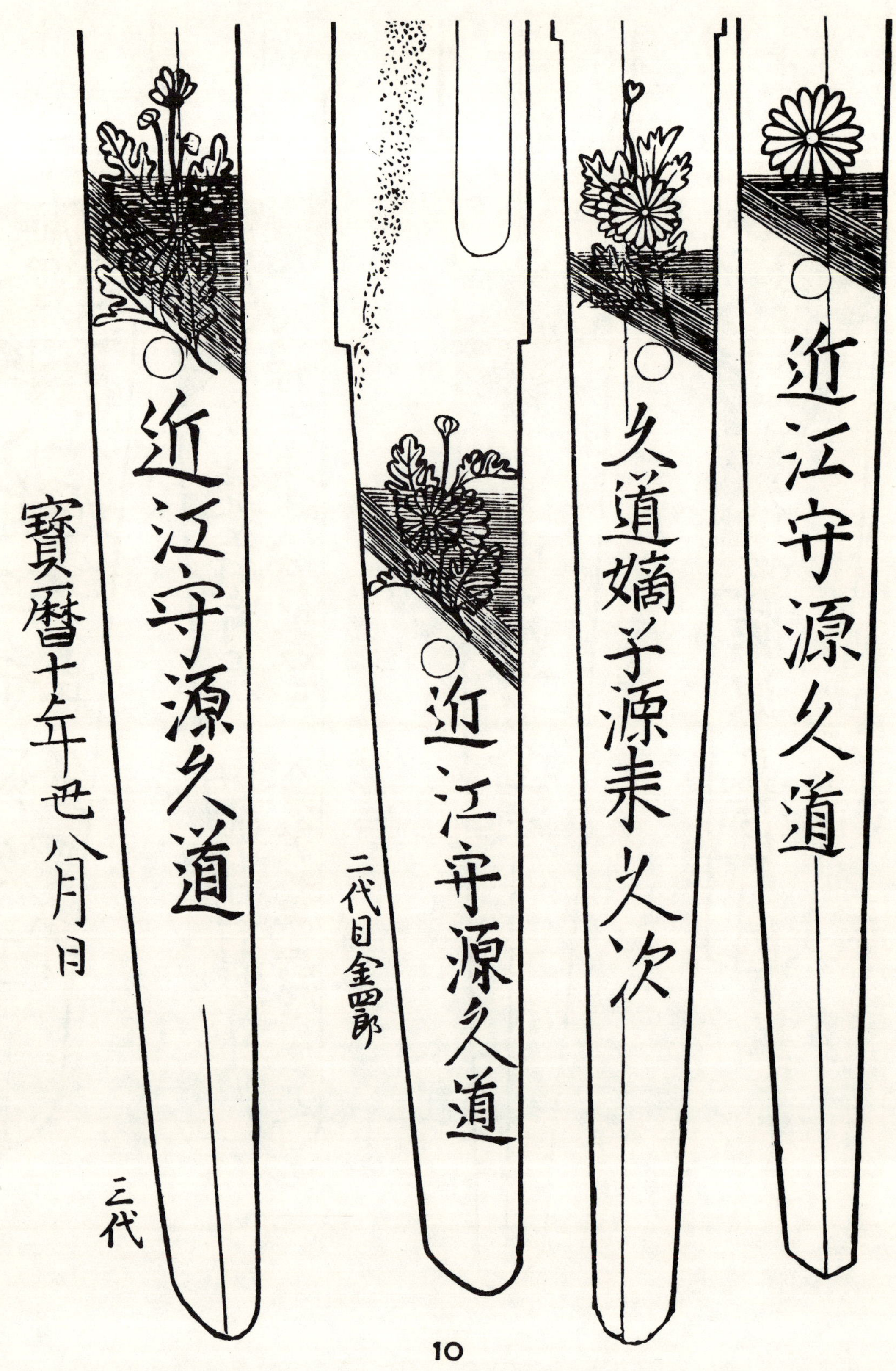
寶曆十五年廿八月日
近江守源久道
二代
二代目金四郎
近江守源久道
久道嫡子源未久次
近江守源久道

Ichiko IC 22   Ichiko IC 22   Ichiteru IC 37

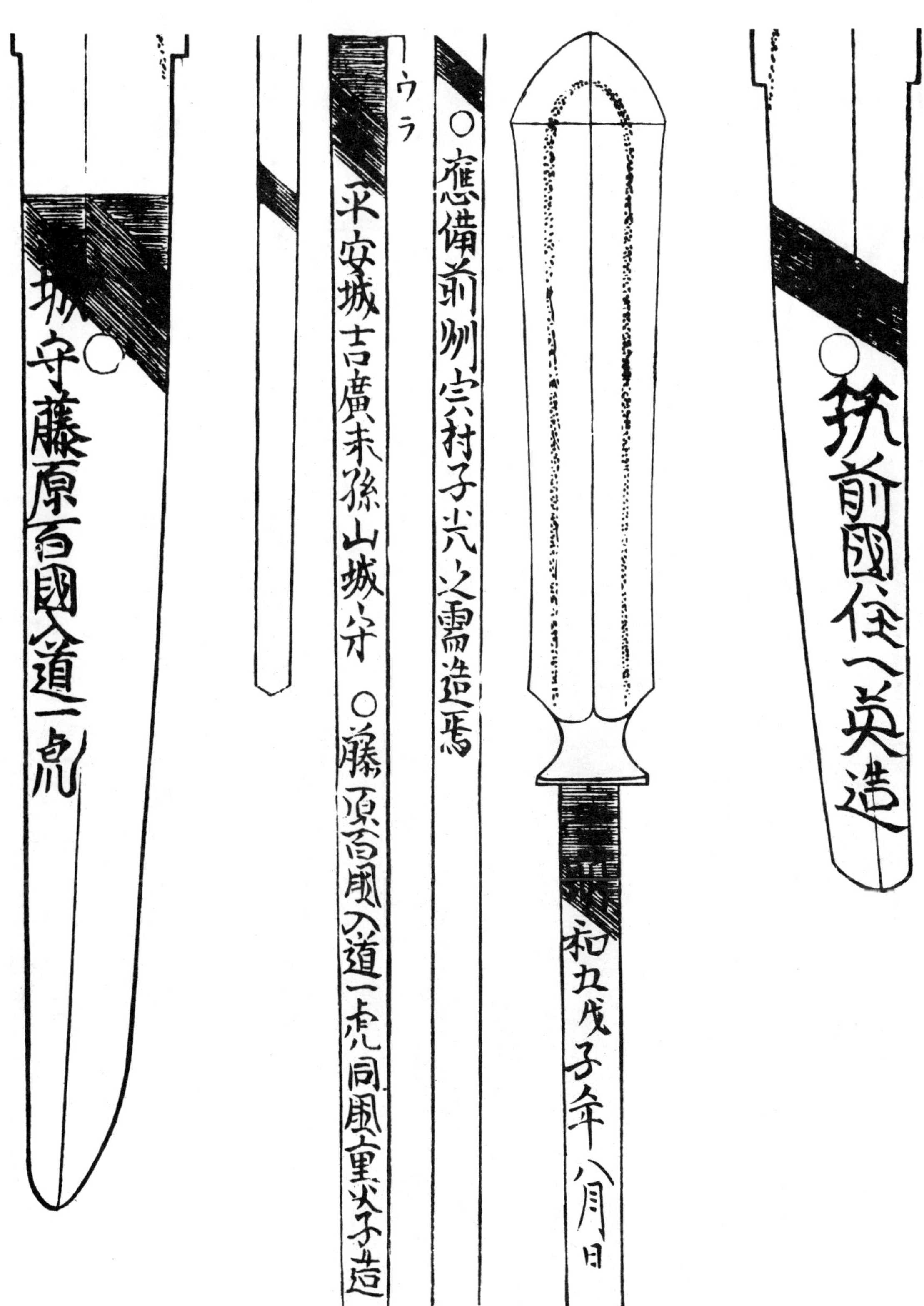

Hisasane
HI 509b

Hisatsugu
HI 523

Hōei HO 4

Inarimaru IN 1a

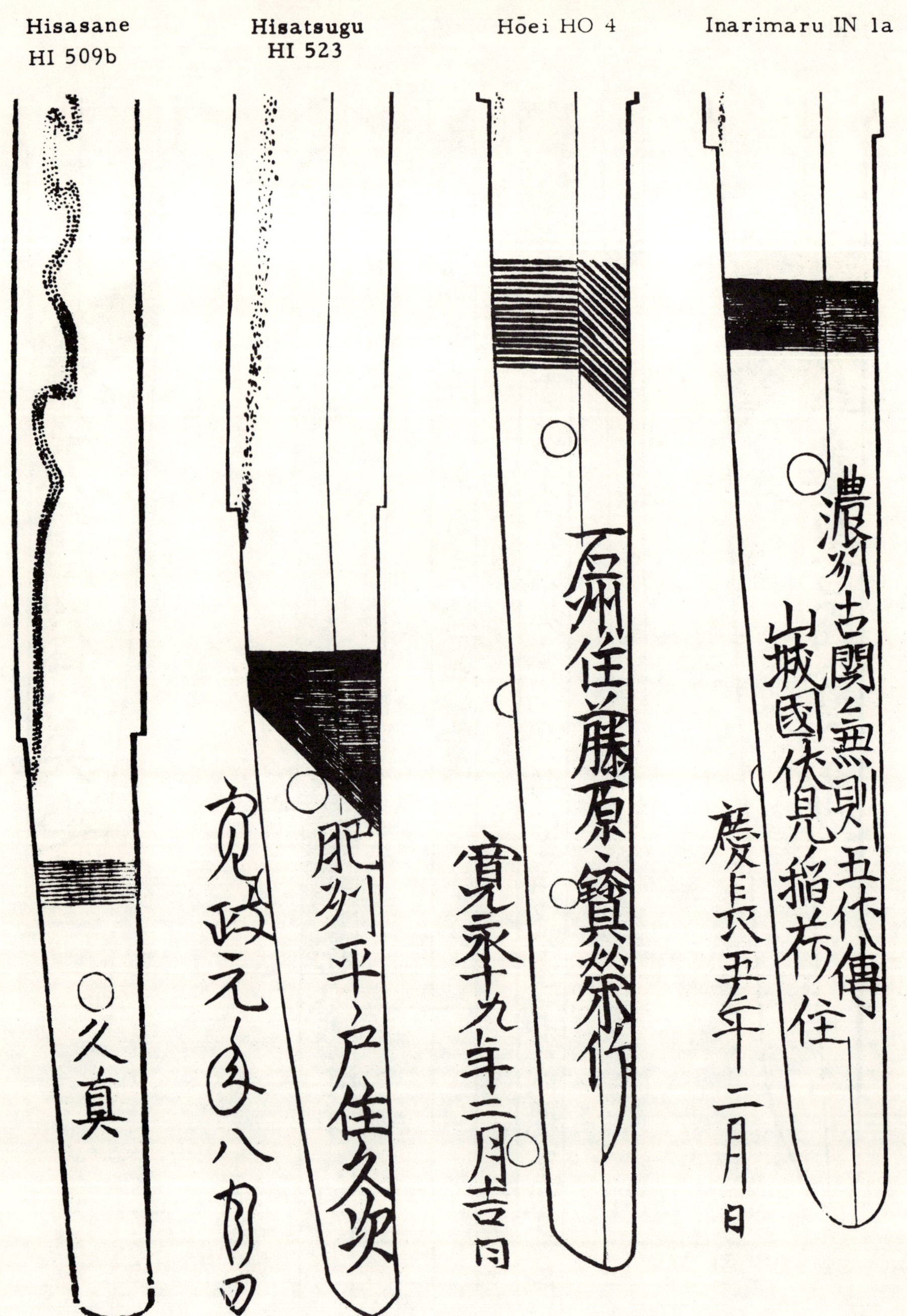

SHINTO BENGI OSHIGATA

Ippō IP 1   Iyehira IY 14   Iyetsugu
IY 209   Jumyo
JU 19-29 ?   JU 24

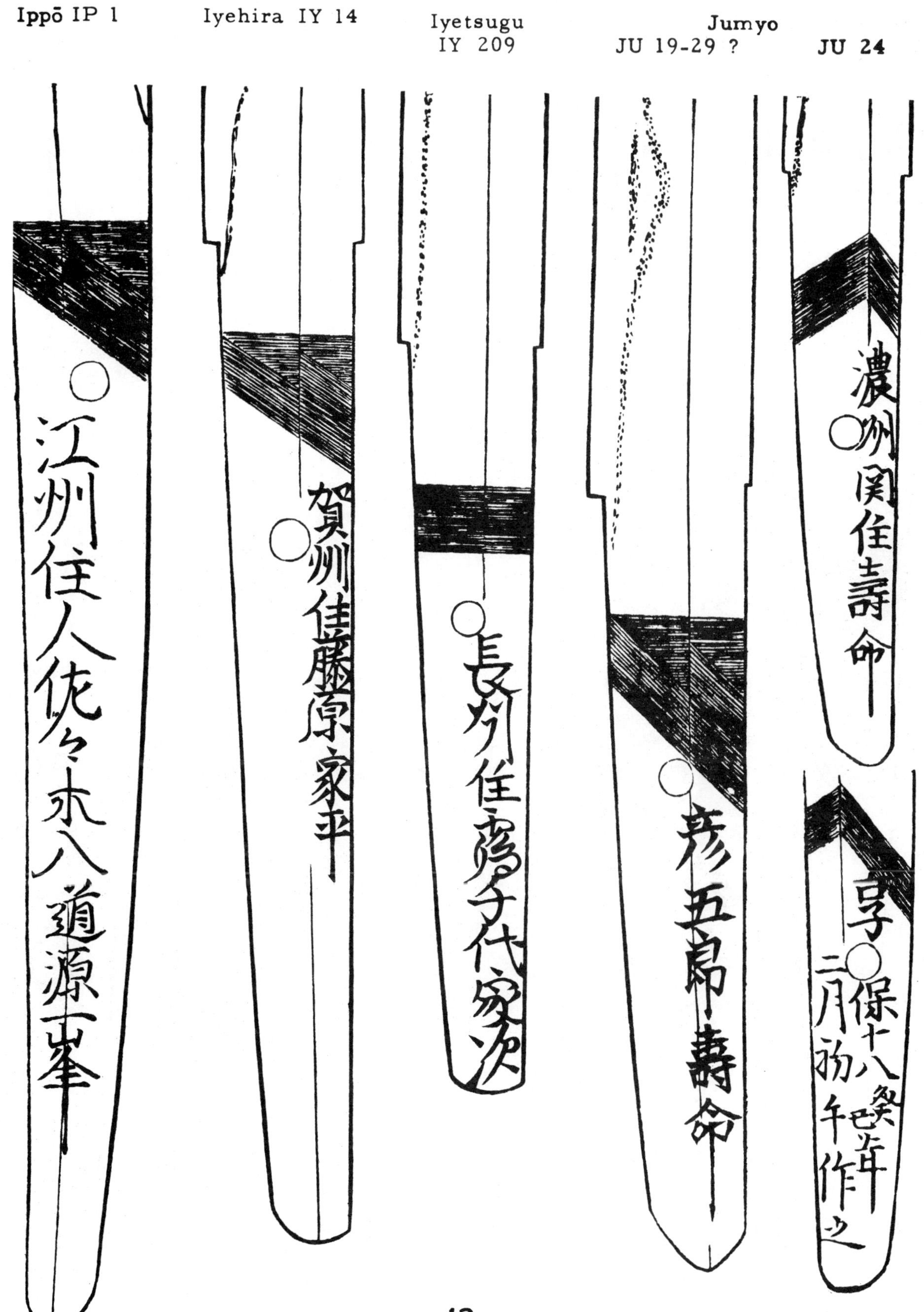

Kaboku KA 1   Kanekuni
KA 181

Kanesada
KA 278

Kanesada KA 278

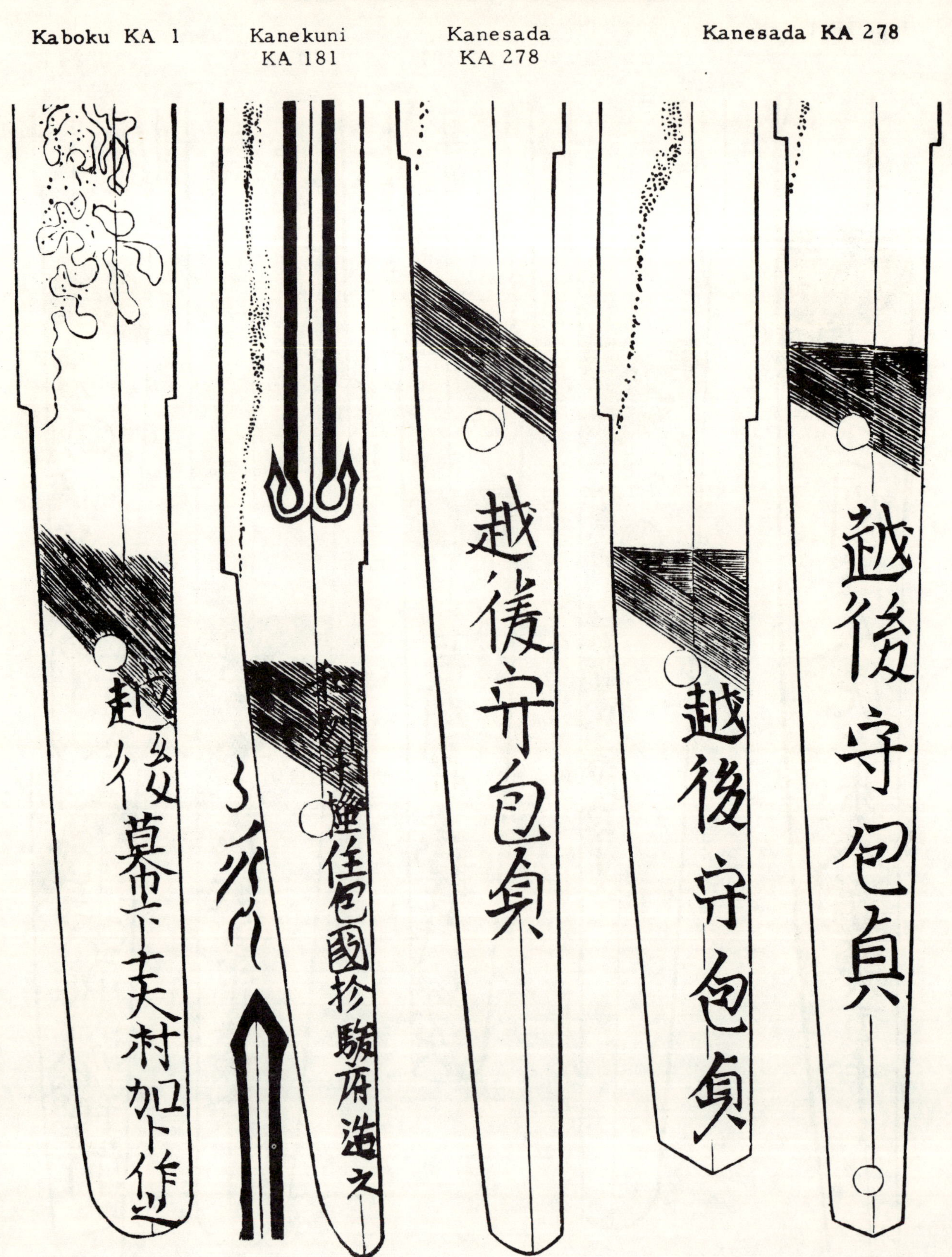

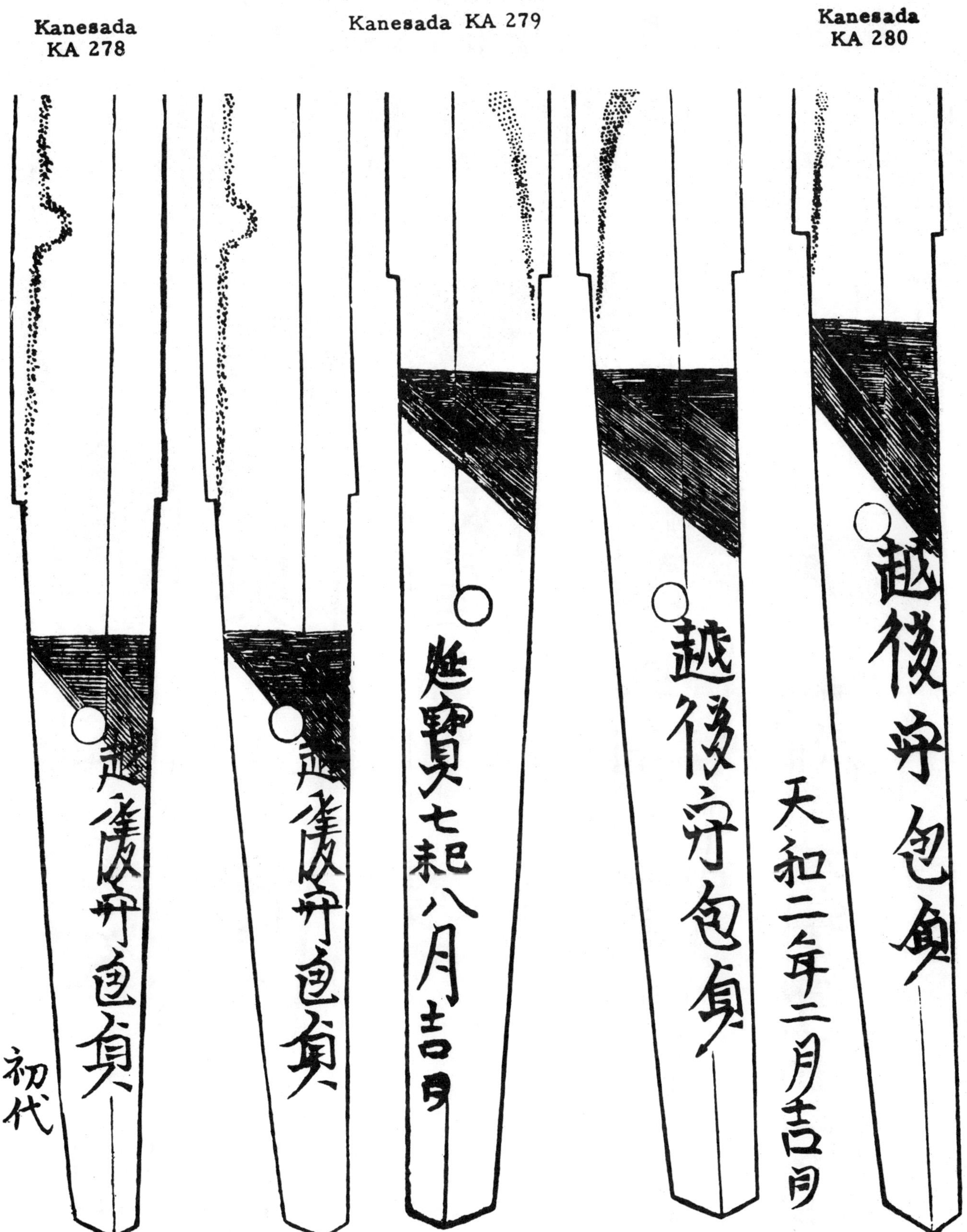

Kanesada
KA 278

Kanesada KA 279

Kanesada
KA 280

初代
越後守包貞
越後守包貞
延寶七秊八月吉日
越後守包貞
越後守包貞
天和二年二月吉日

Kaneshige KA 296   Kaneyasu
KA 349   Kaneyasu KA 351

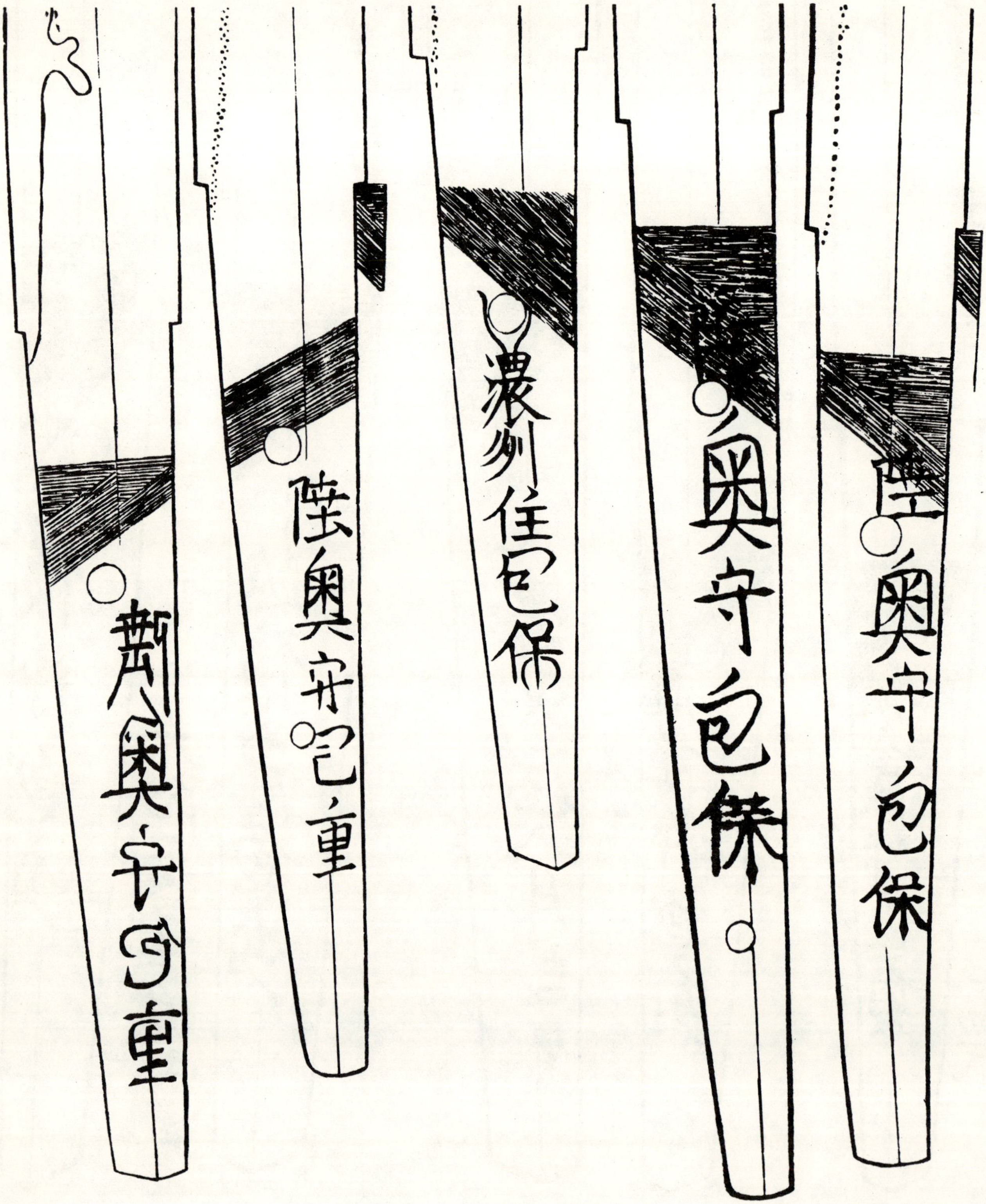

SHINTO BENGI OSHIGATA

Kaneyasu KA 350

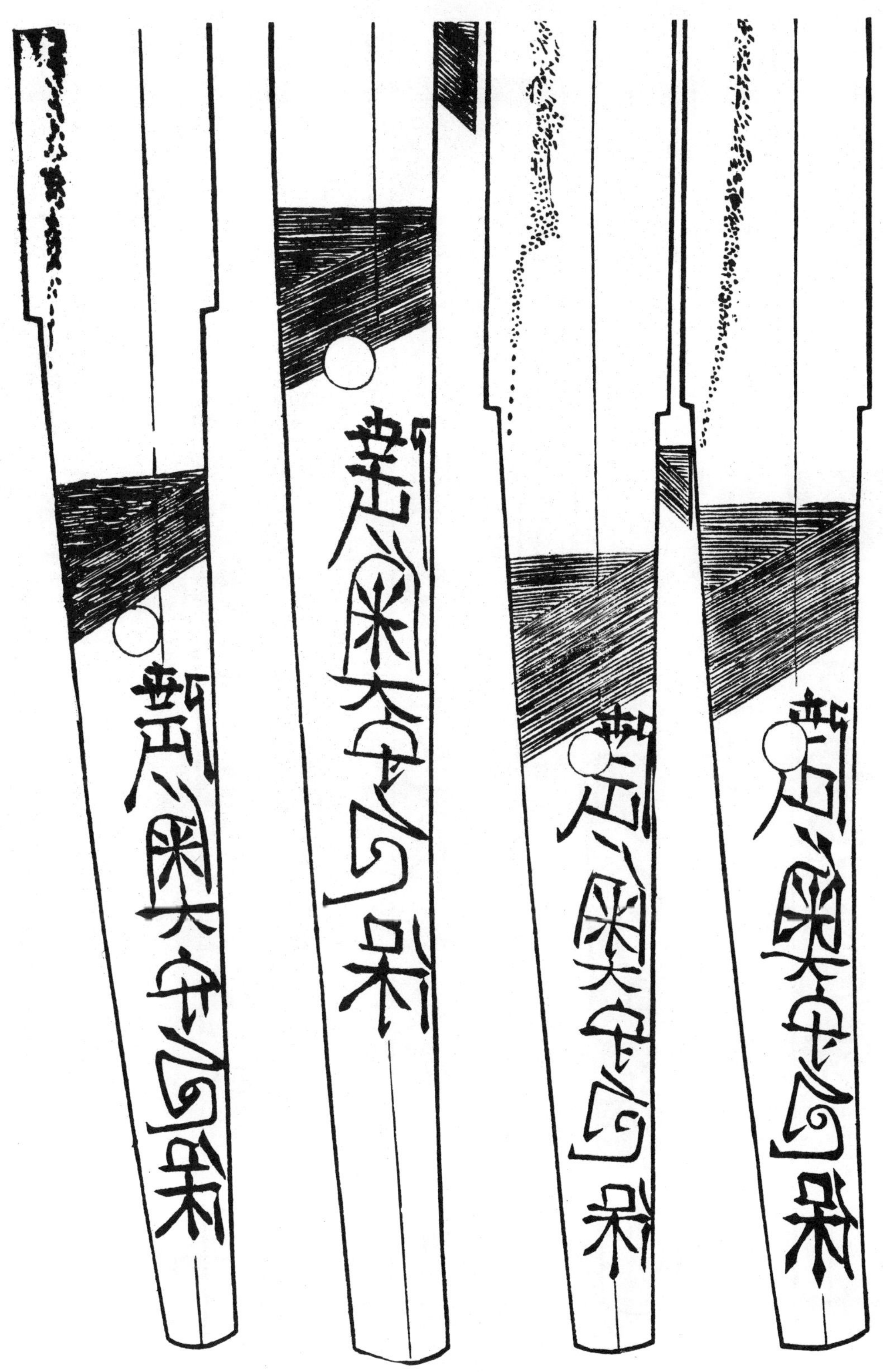

Kaneyasu KA 351

Kanefusa
KA 499

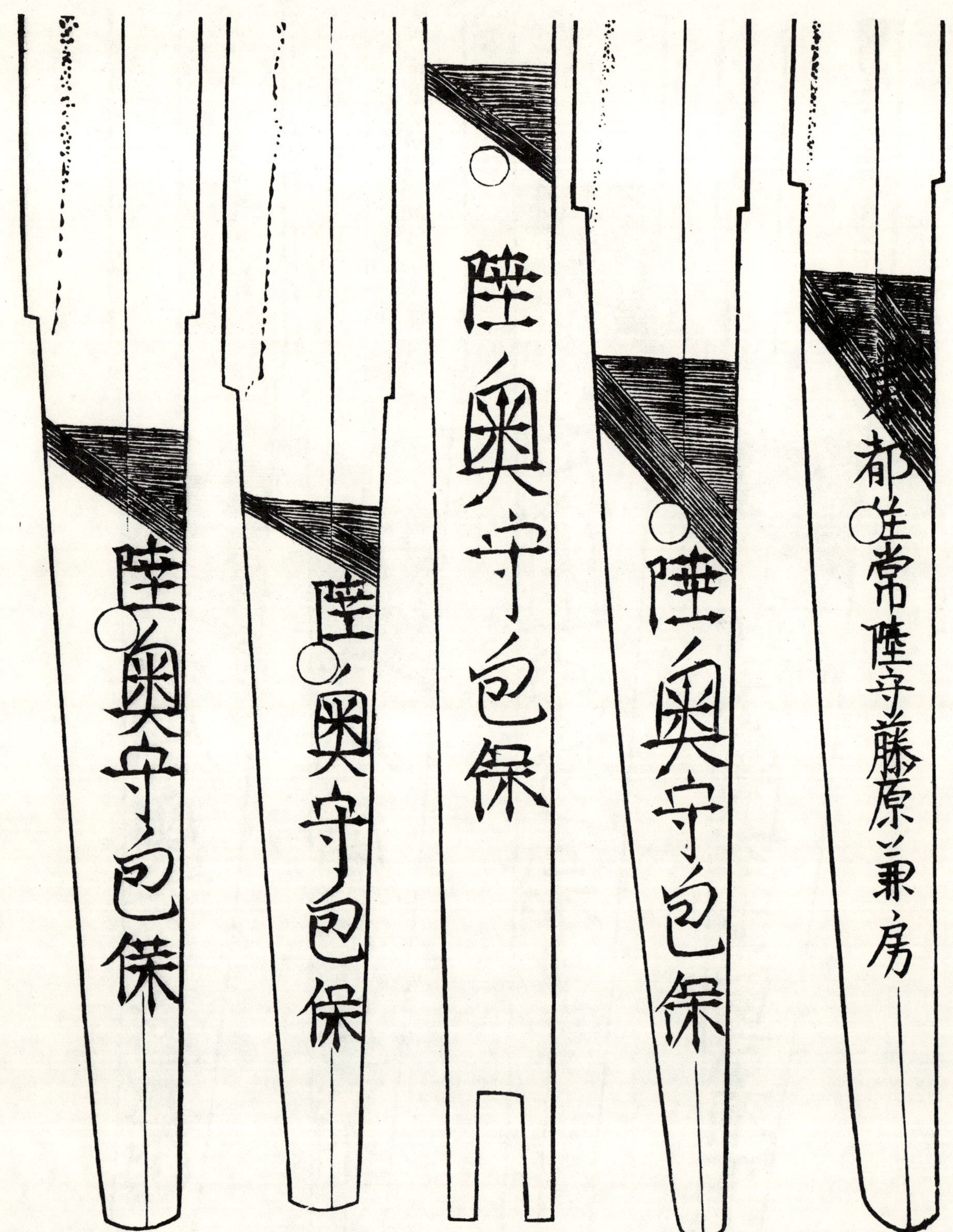

SHINTO BENGI OSHIGATA

Kanehiro
KA 531

Kanehiro
KA 544

Kanehiro KA 544
Made for Naganaka

Kaneiye
KA 576

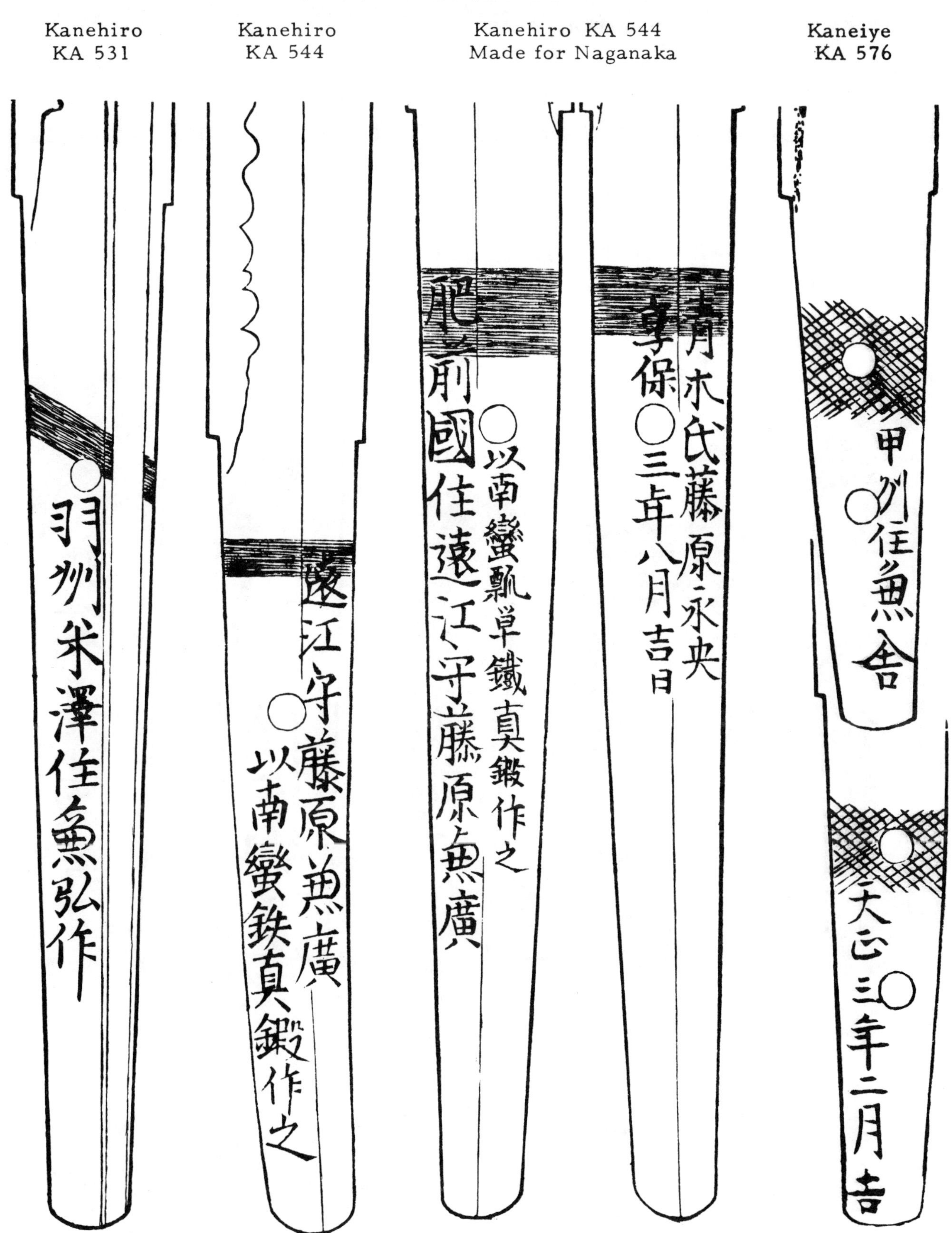

Kanekage
KA 605   Kanemichi KA 712   Kanemichi KA 713

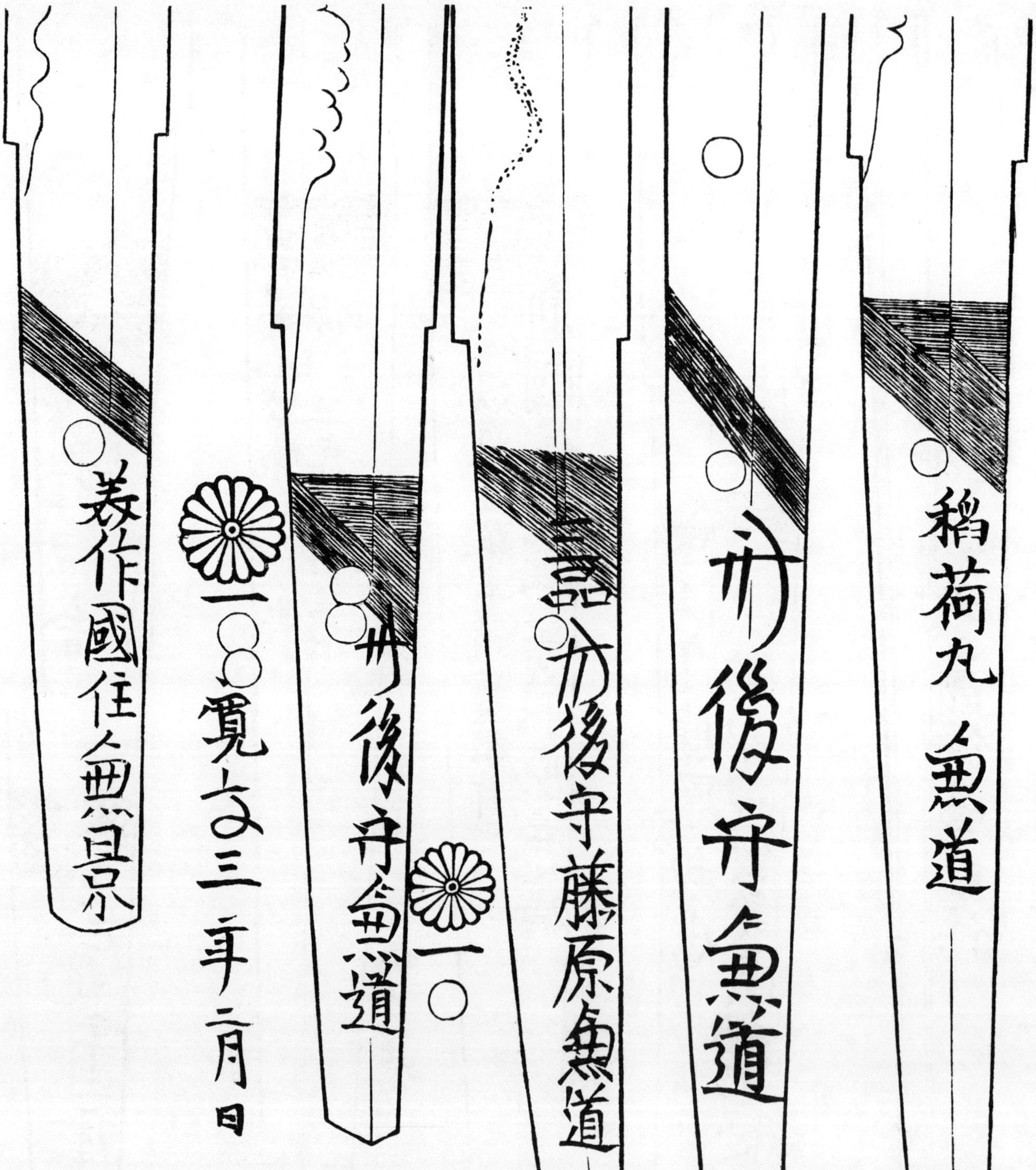

○義作國住人兼景

一○○寛文三年二月日

丹後守兼道　一○

嘉○丹後守藤原兼道

丹後守兼道

○稲荷丸　兼道

SHINTO BENGI OSHIGATA

Kanemichi KA 713   Kanenao
                                    KA 852

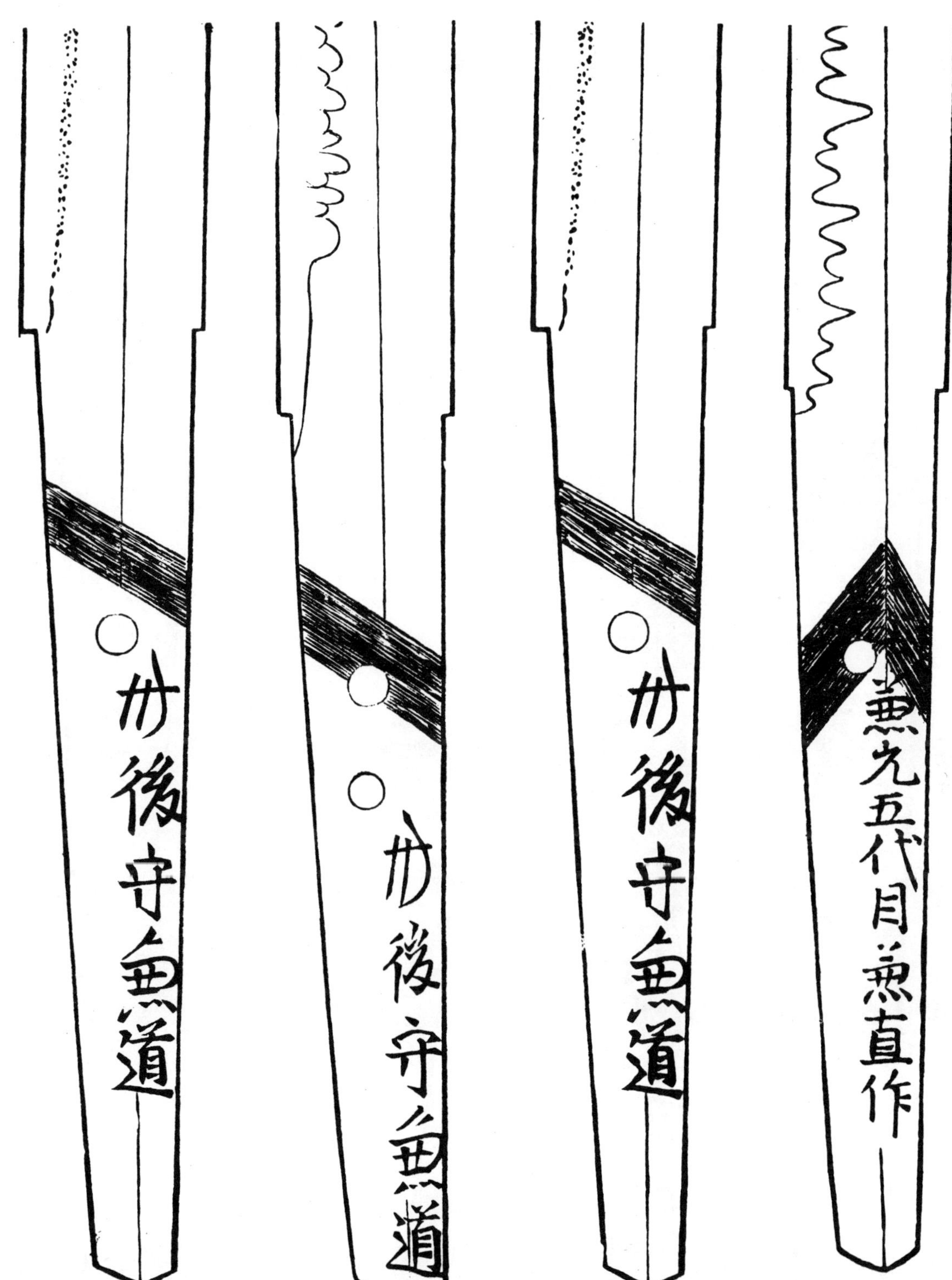

SHINTO BENGI OSHIGATA

Kanesada KA 961 ?

Kanesada
KA 981

Kanesaki
KA 999

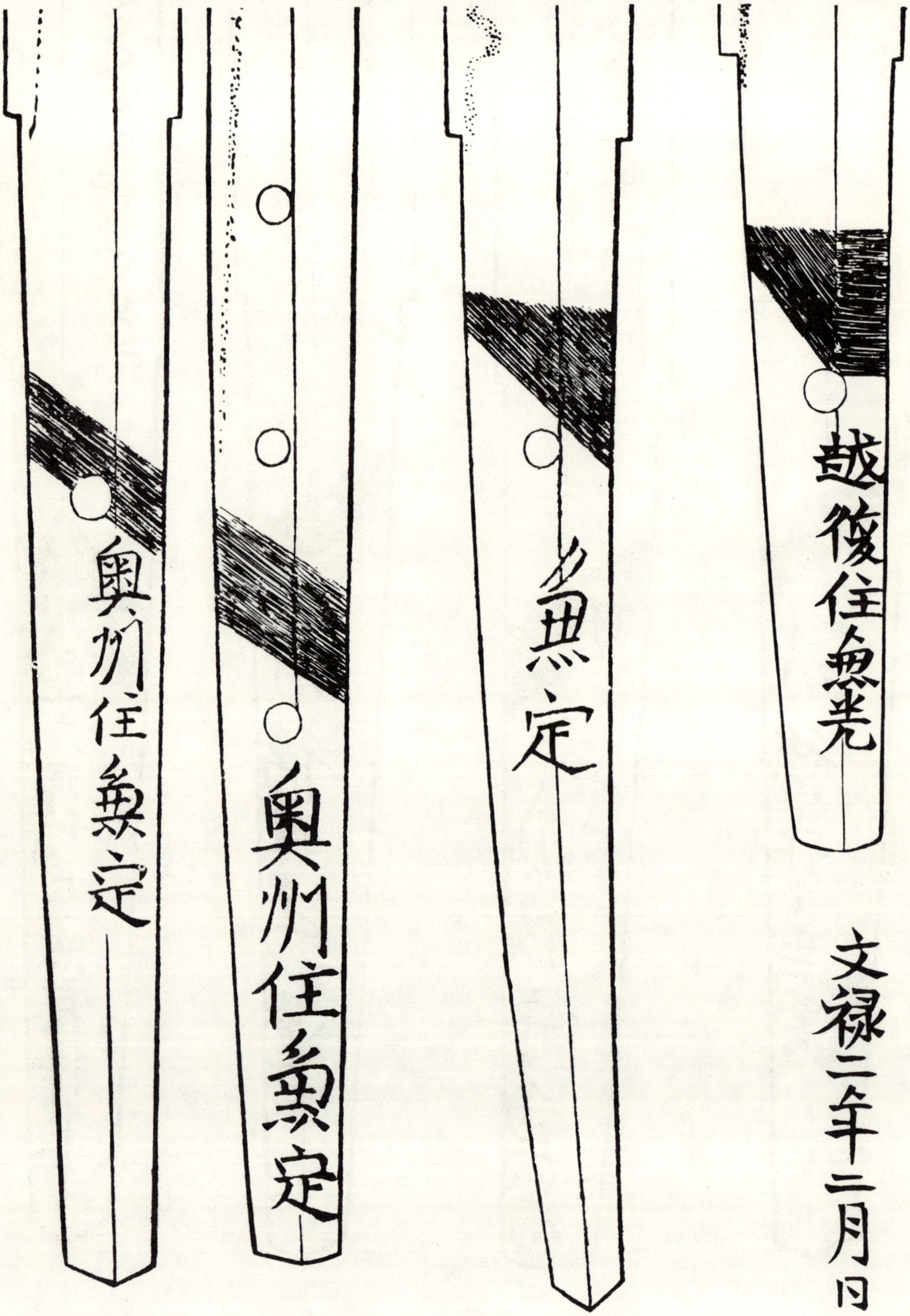

Kanesaki KA 1004   Kanesaki KA 1005

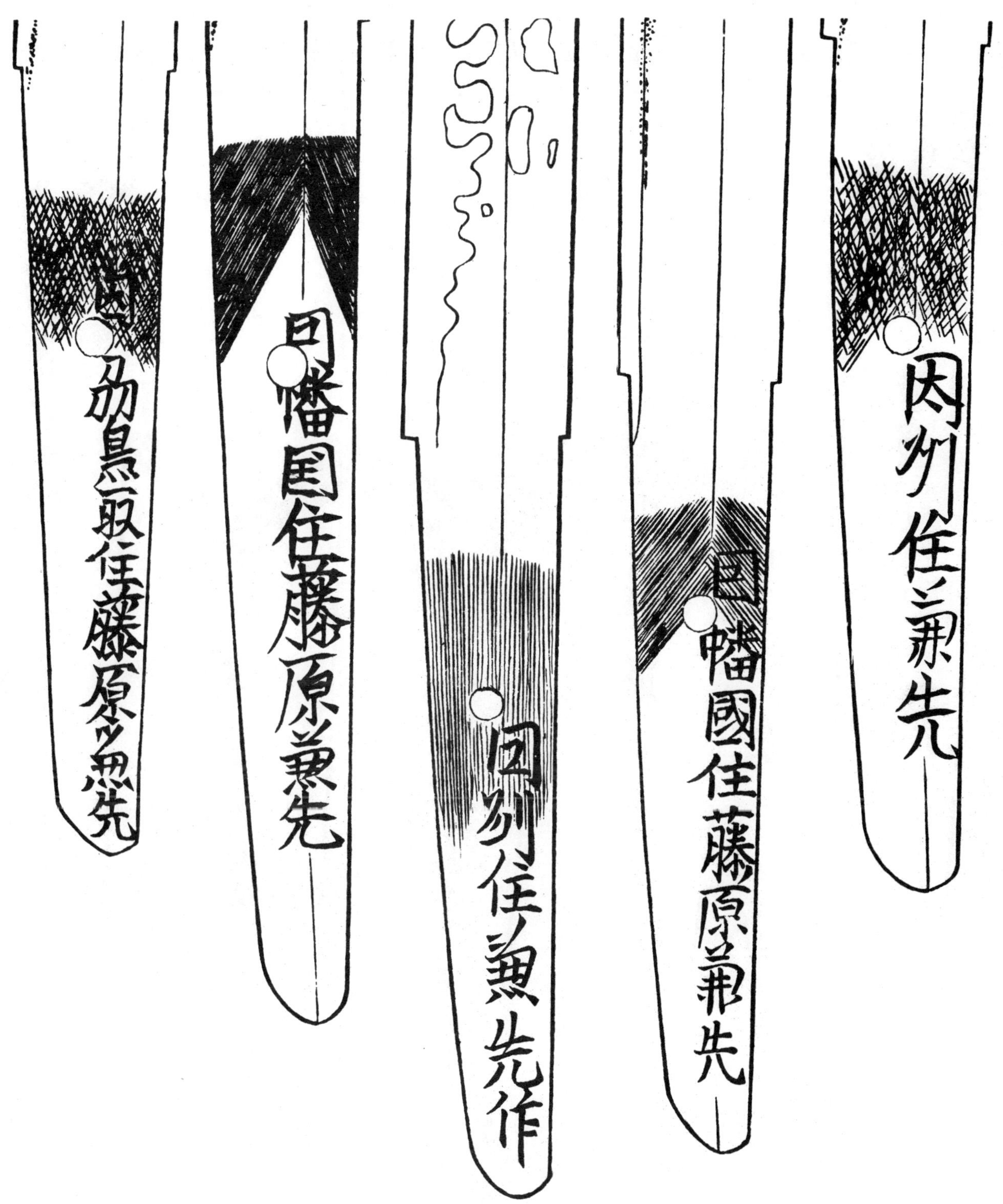

Kanesaki
KA 1010

Kanesaki
KA 1015

Kaneshige KA 1056

Kanesumi
KA 1078

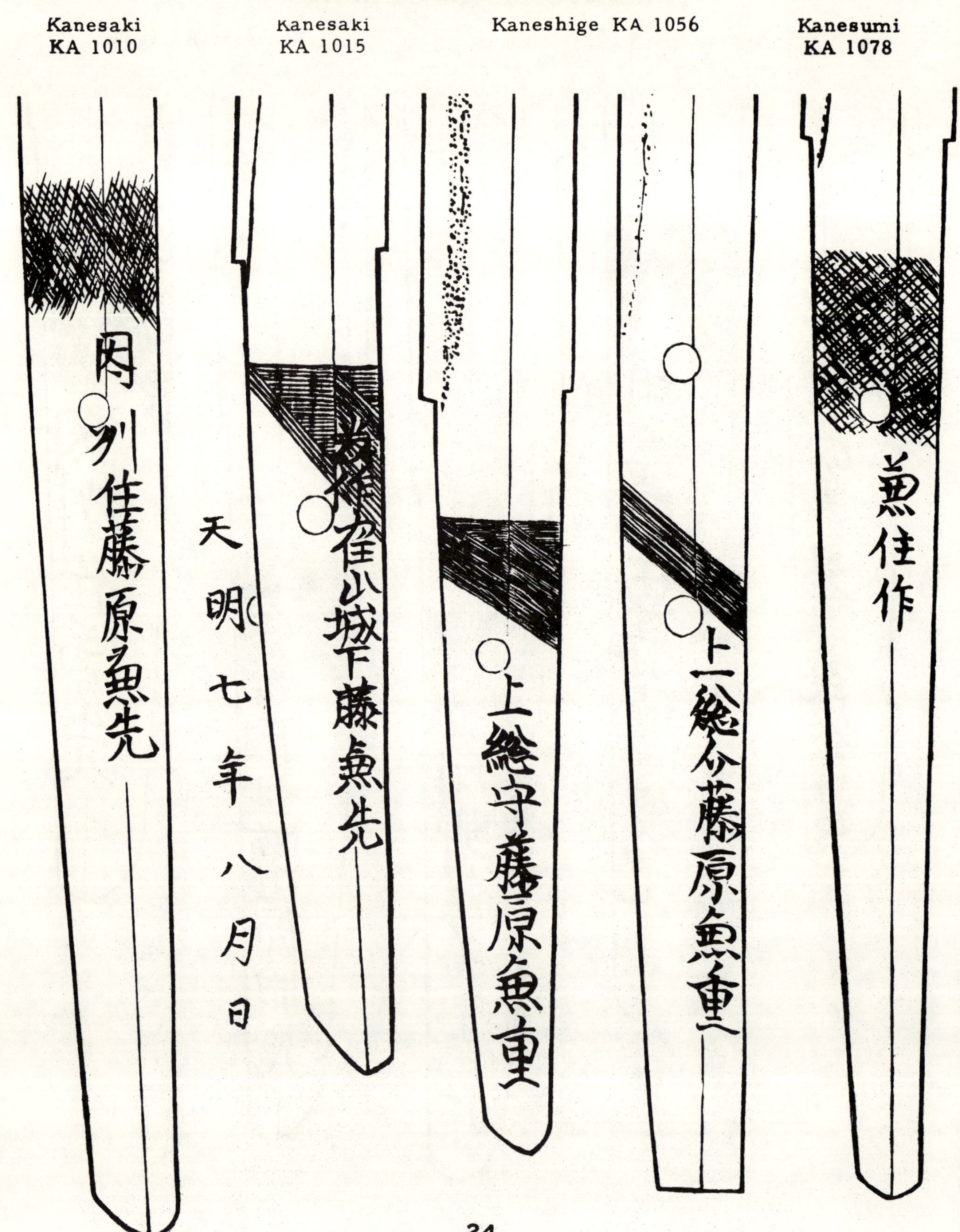

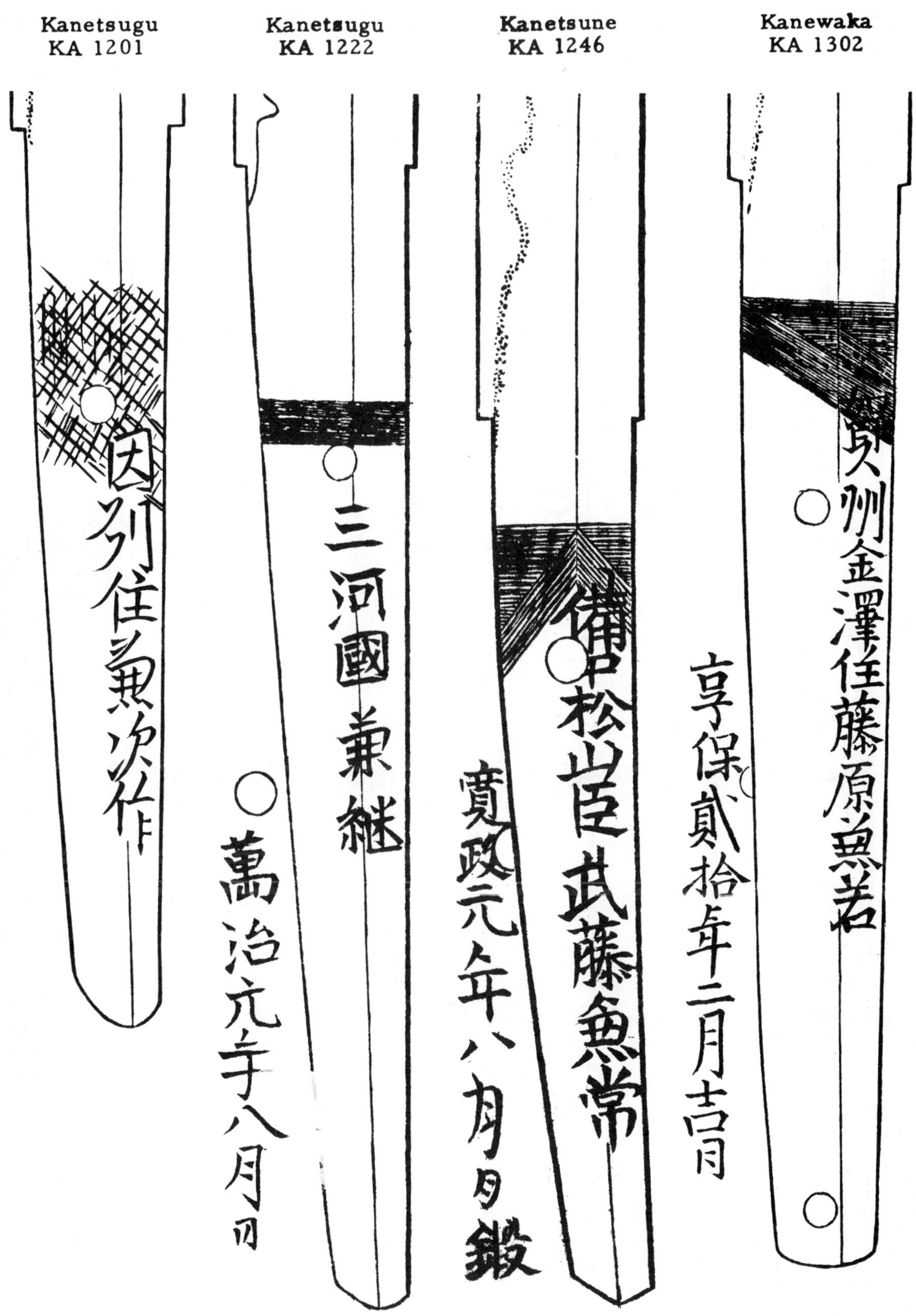

Kanetsugu
KA 1201

Kanetsugu
KA 1222

Kanetsune
KA 1246

Kanewaka
KA 1302

Kaneyasu	Kanetoki	Katsukuni	Katsuyoshi	**Kazumichi**
KA 1321a	KA 1365a	KA 1448	KA 1503	**KA 1516**

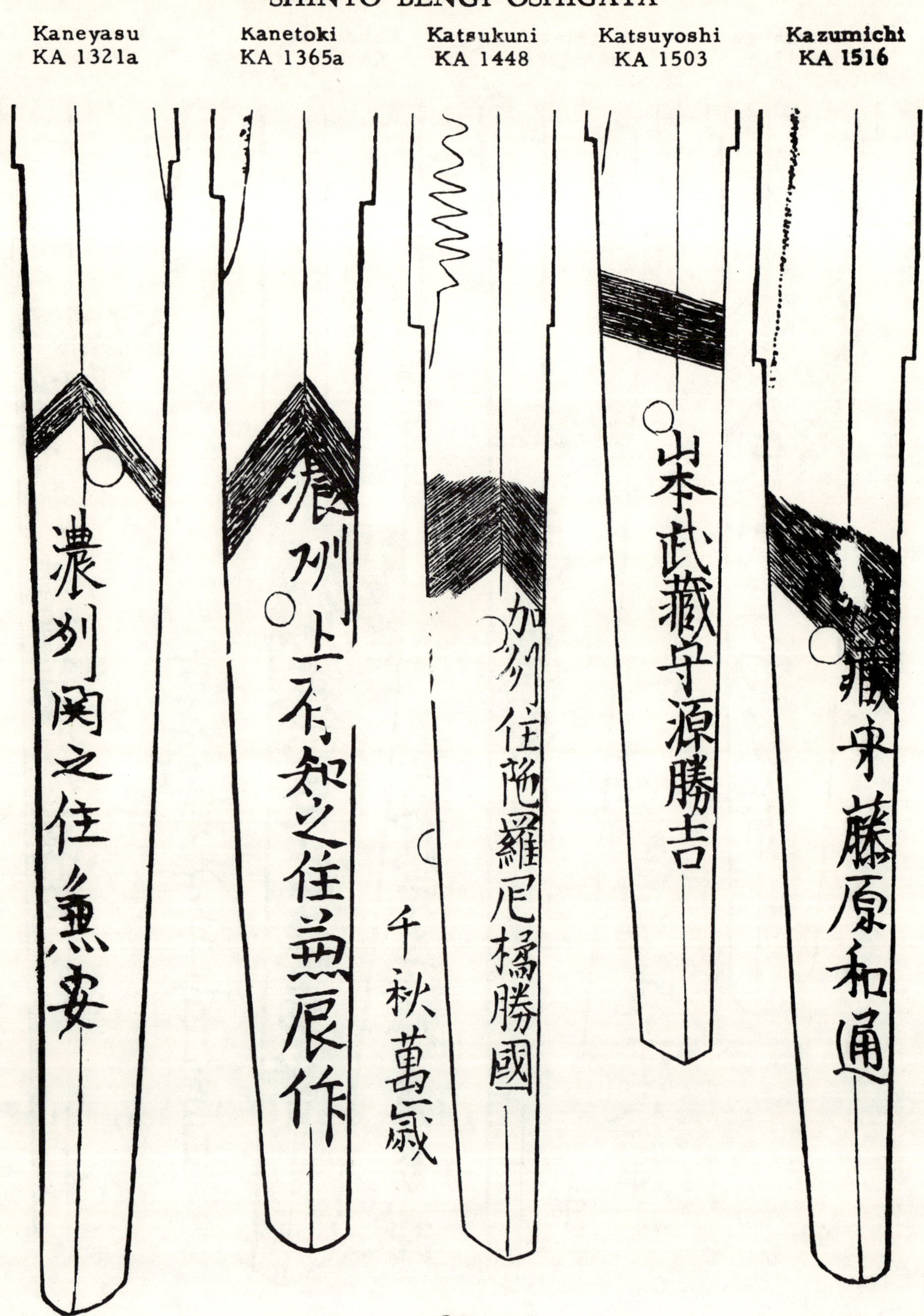

Kihō KI 5   Kunju KI 30   Kinmichi KI 43

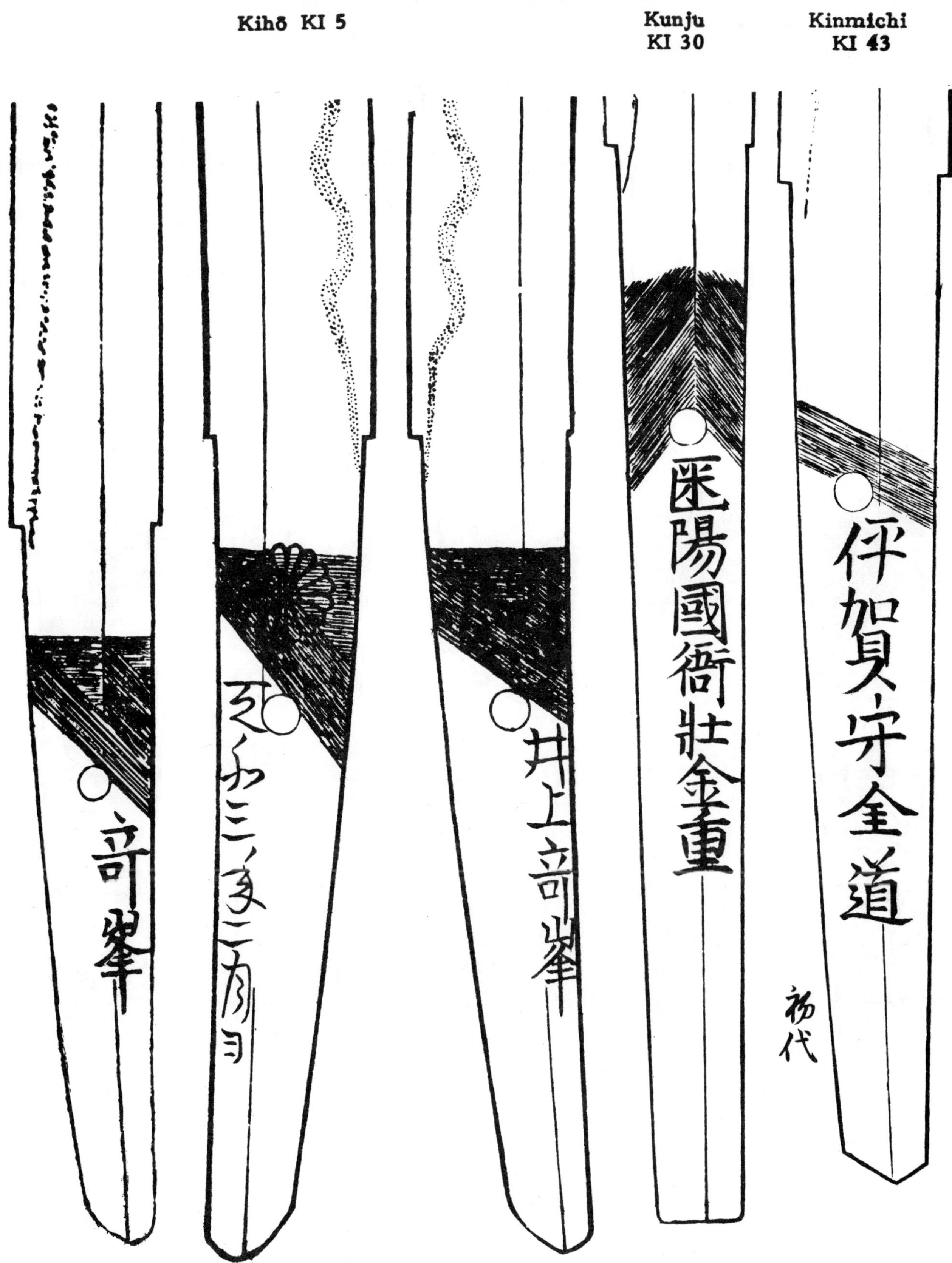

Kinmichi KI 43   Kinmichi KI 44

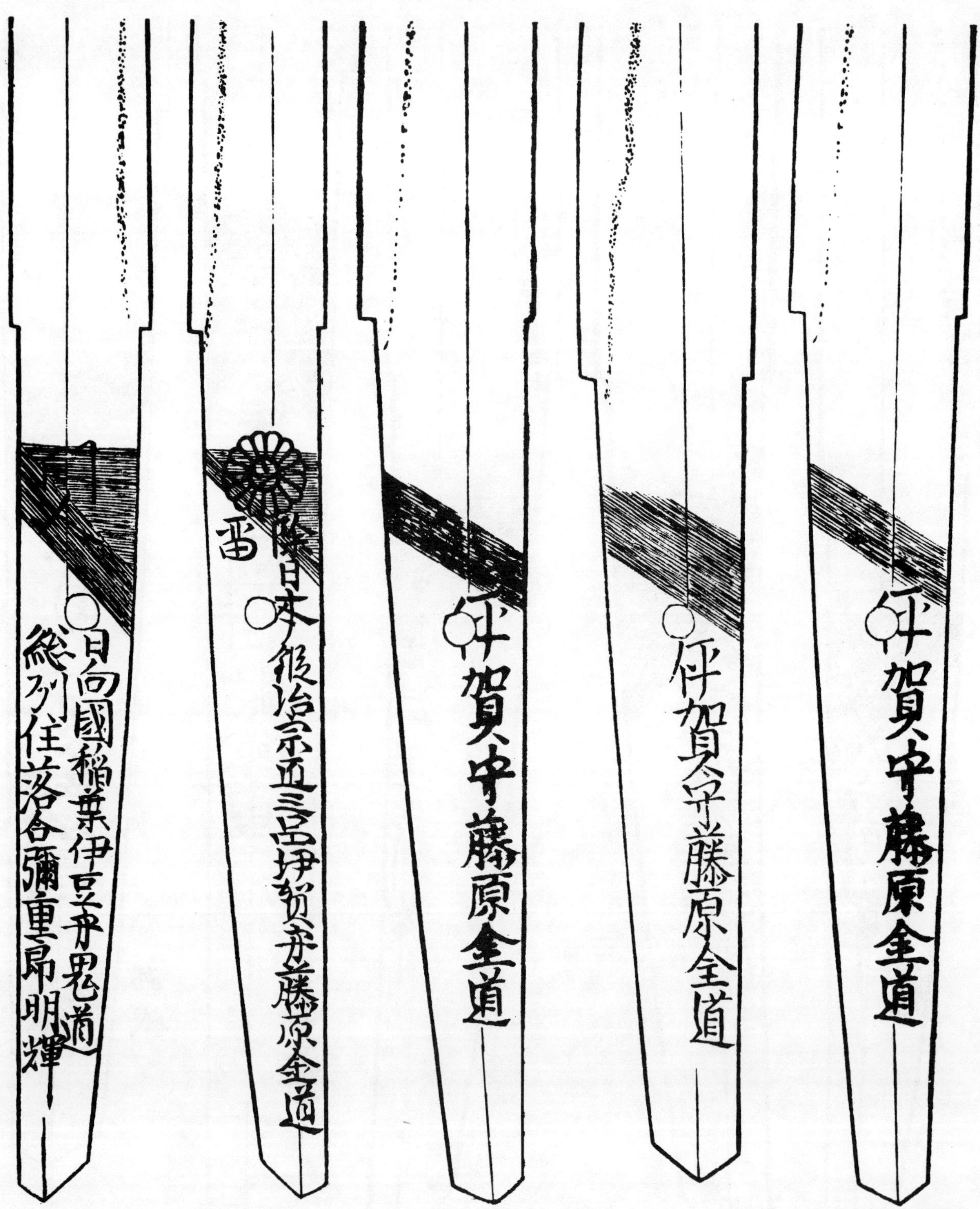

Kinmichi KI 45   Kinmichi KI 48

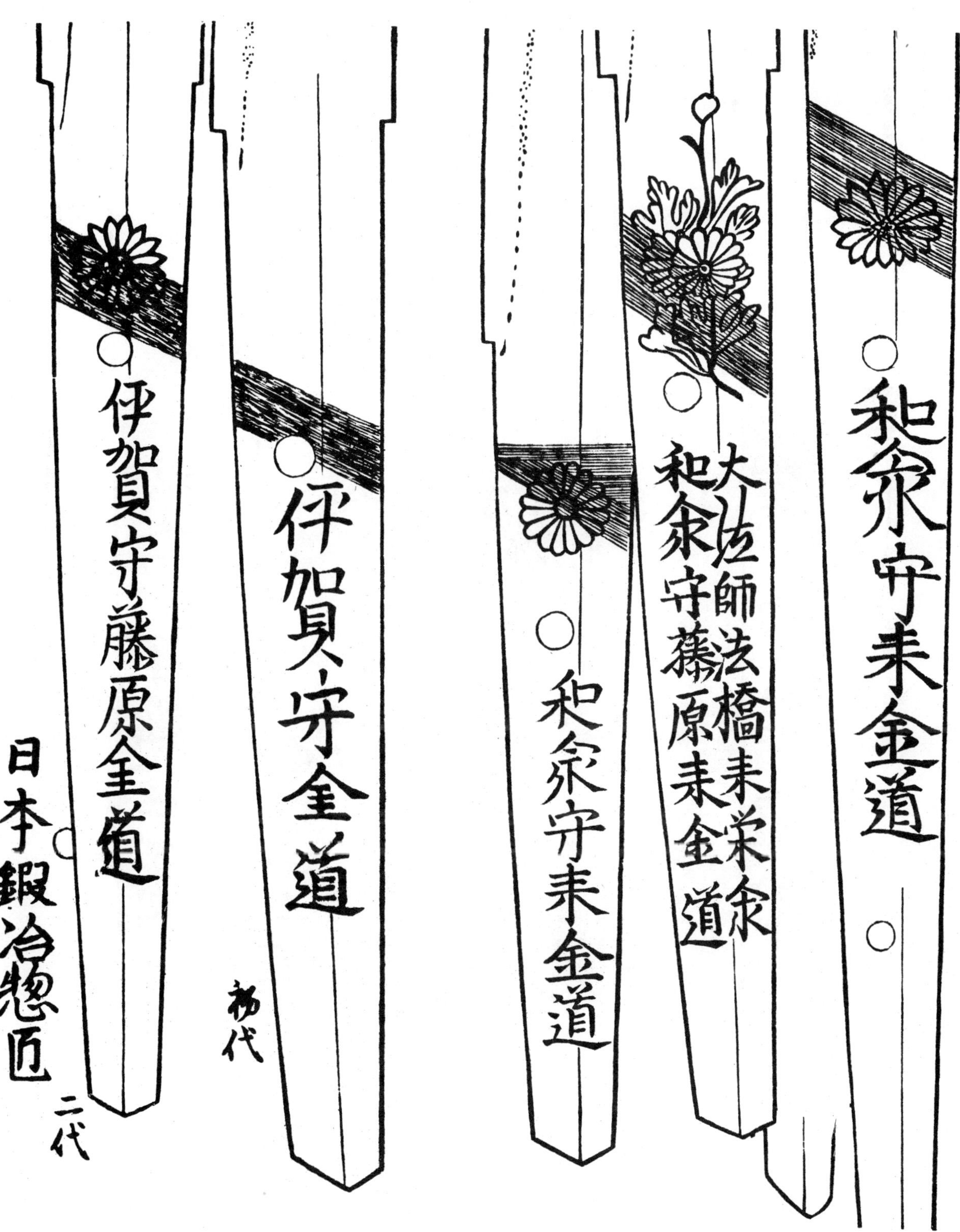

SHINTO BENGI OSHIGATA

Kiyokazu	Kiyomasa	Kiyonobu
KI 107	KI 116	KI 200

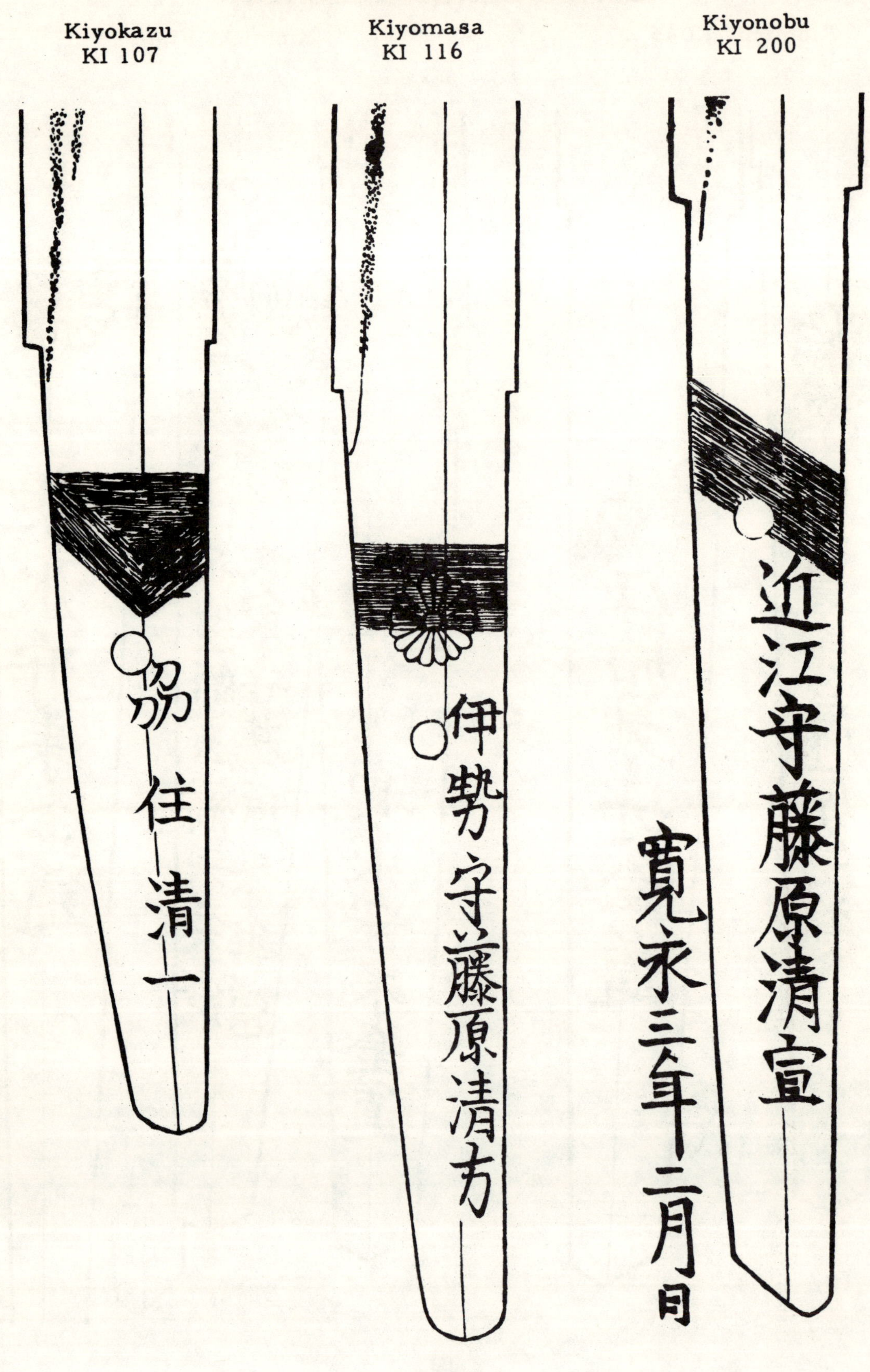

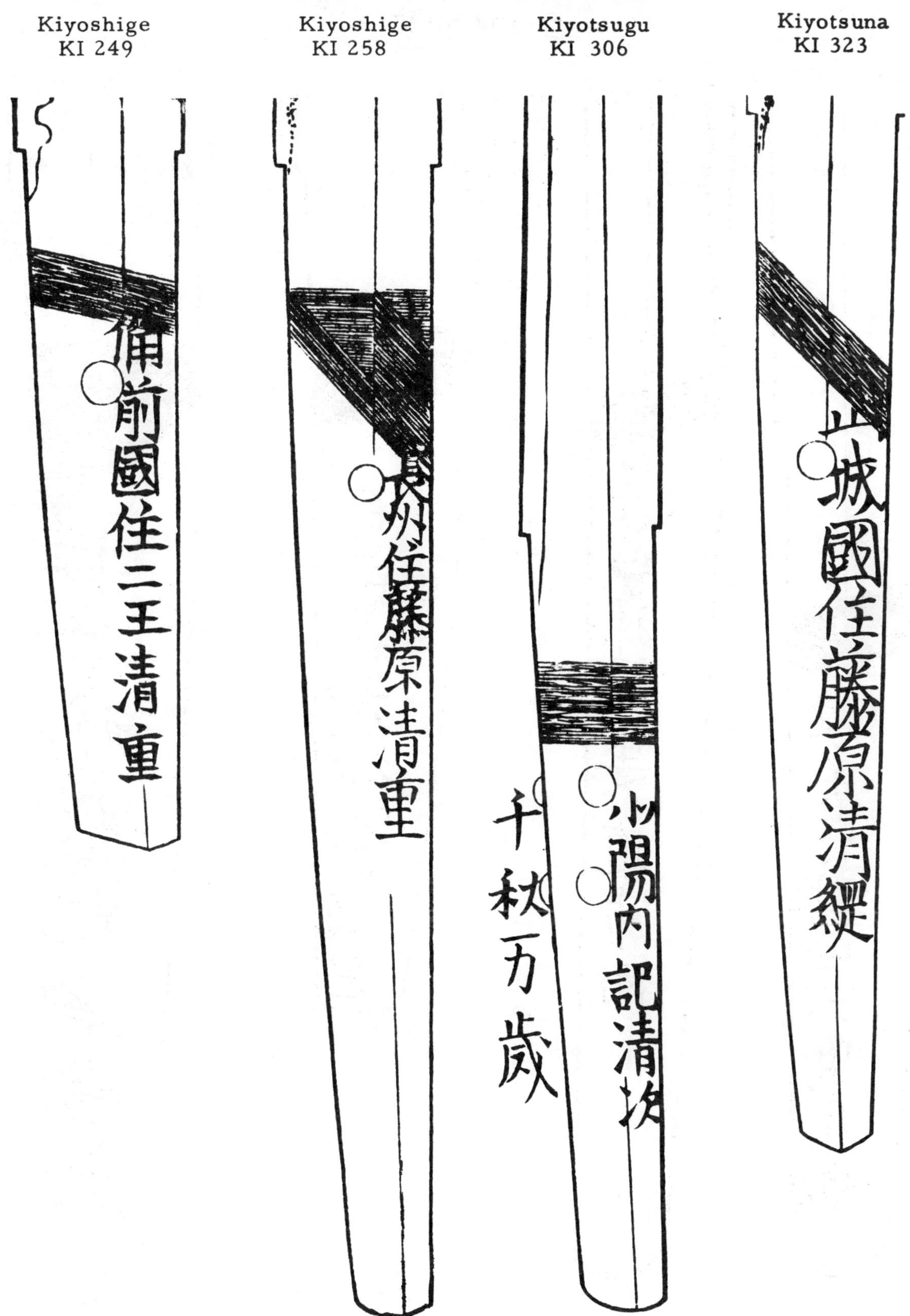
Kiyoshige
KI 249

Kiyoshige
KI 258

Kiyotsugu
KI 306

Kiyotsuna
KI 323

備前國住三王清重

長州住藤原清重

千秋万歳

山陽内記清次

山城國住藤原清綱

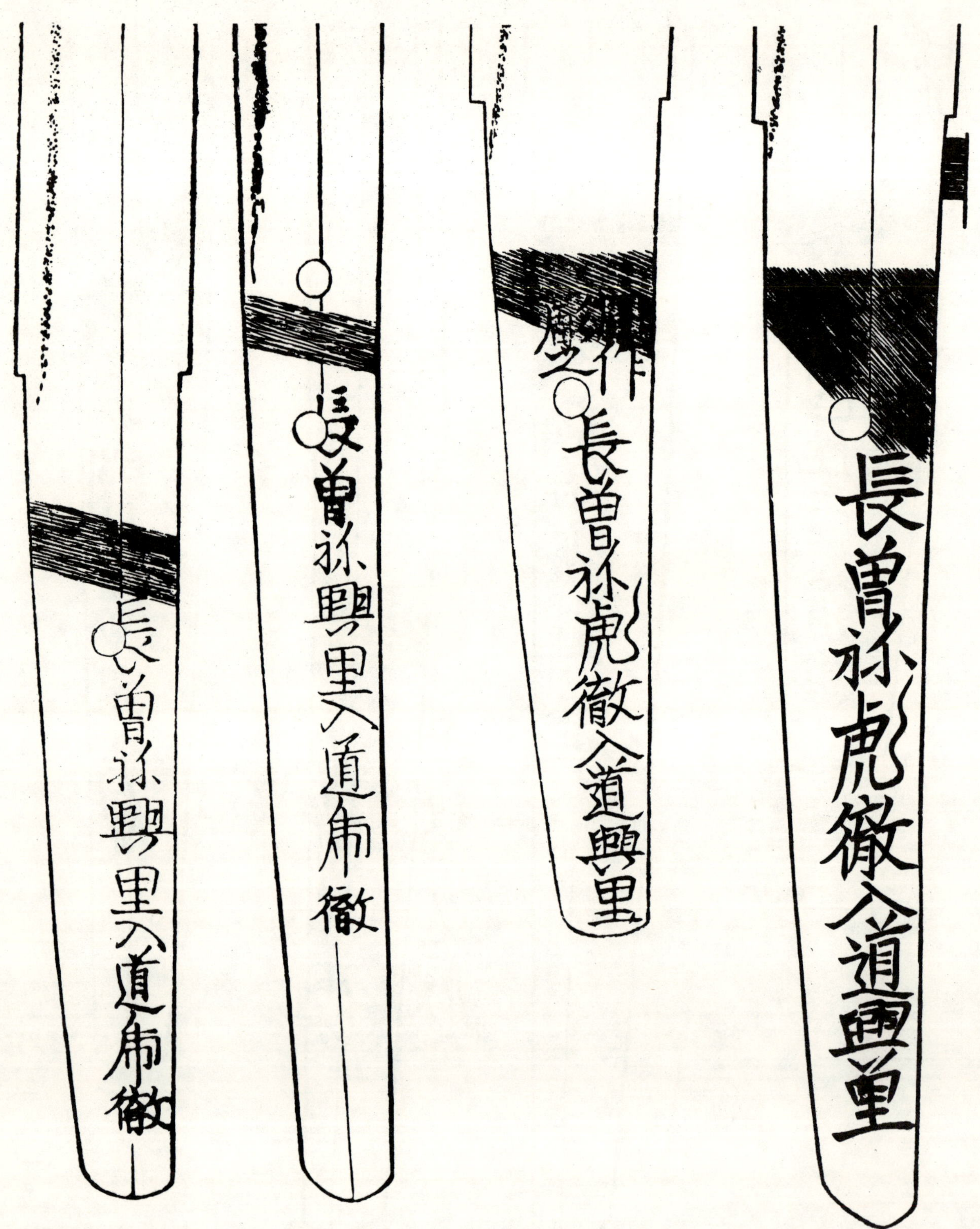

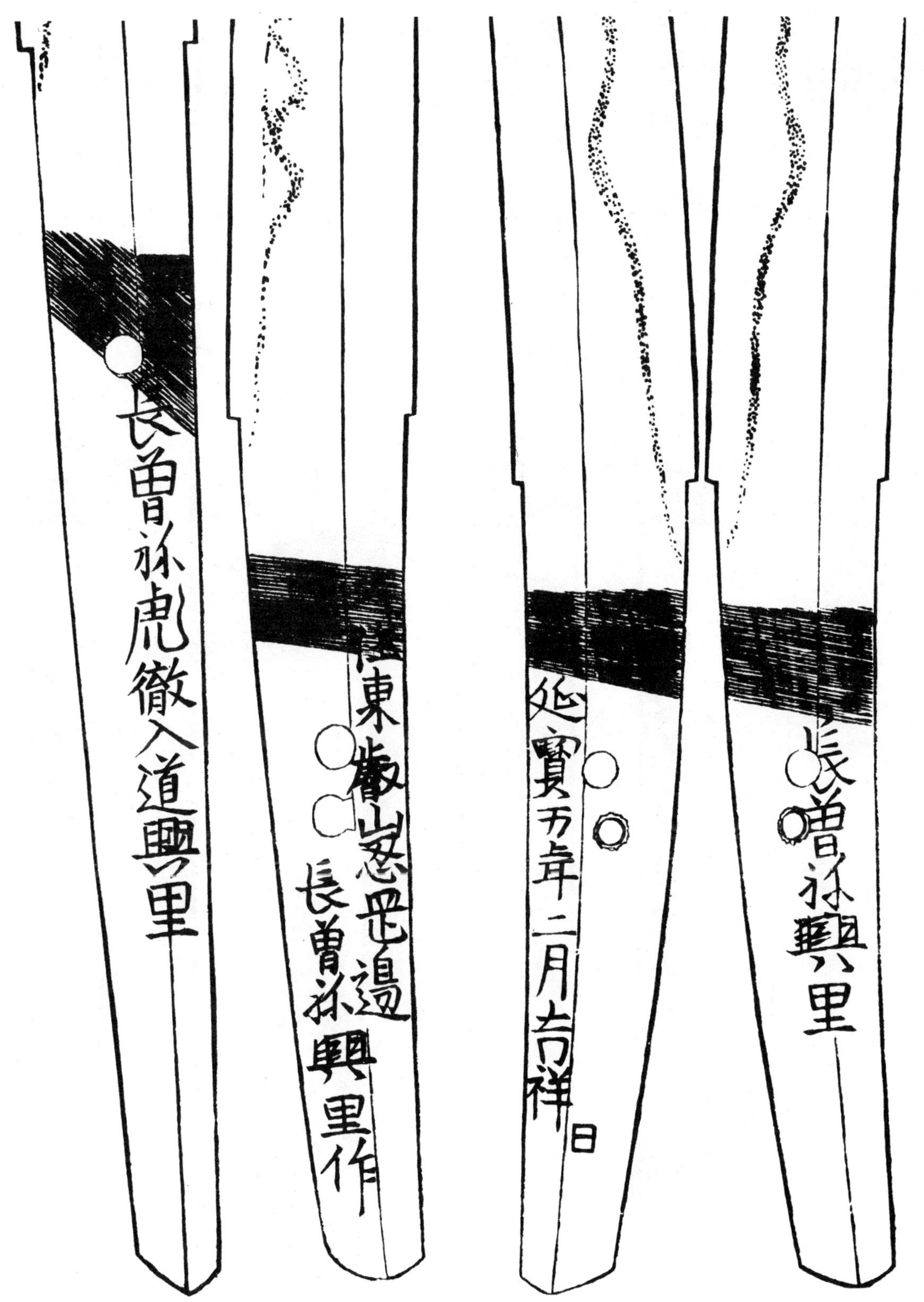

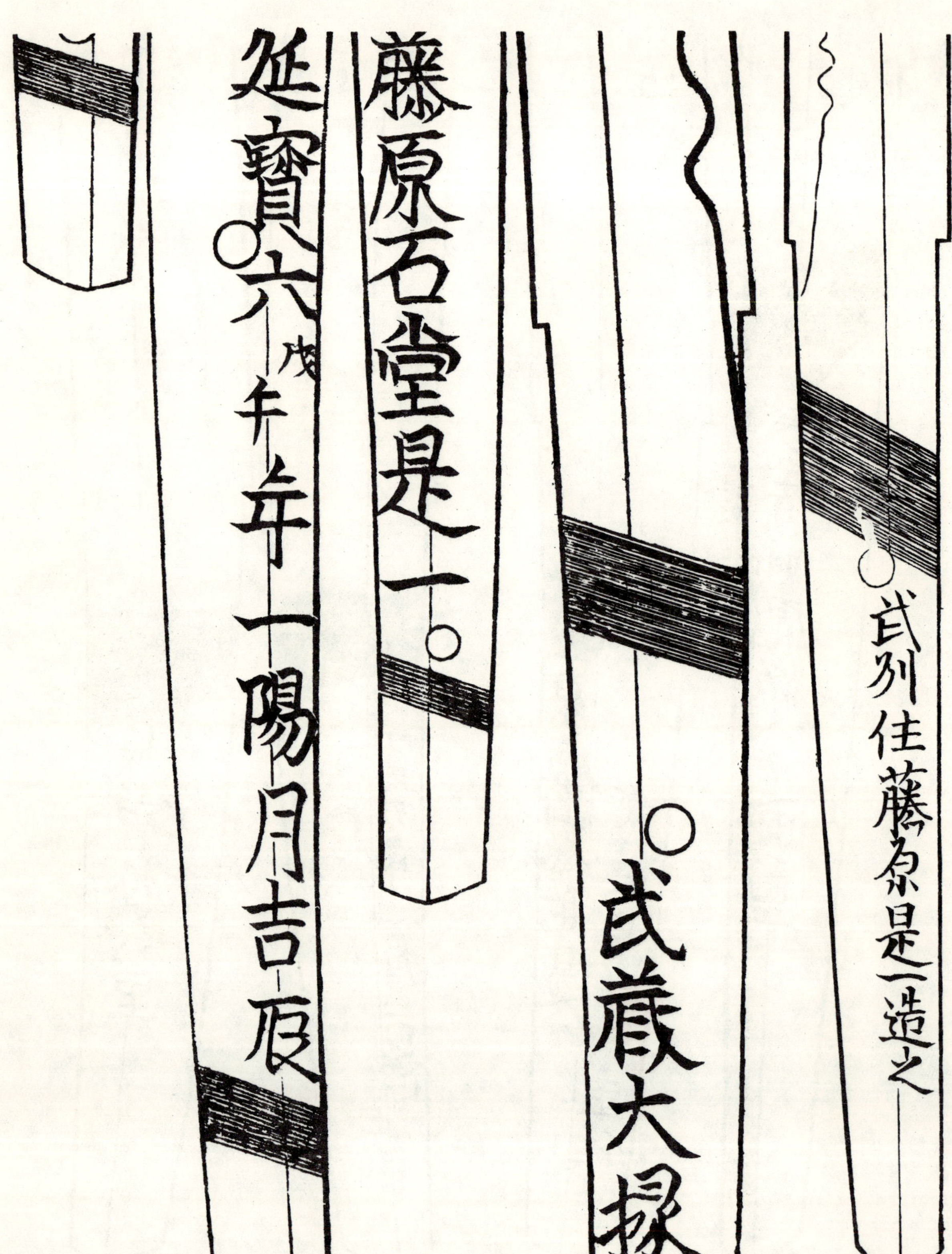

SHINTO BENGI OSHIGATA

Kikuhiro KI 19	Kunifusa KU 42	Kuniharu KU 47	Kunihide KU 58

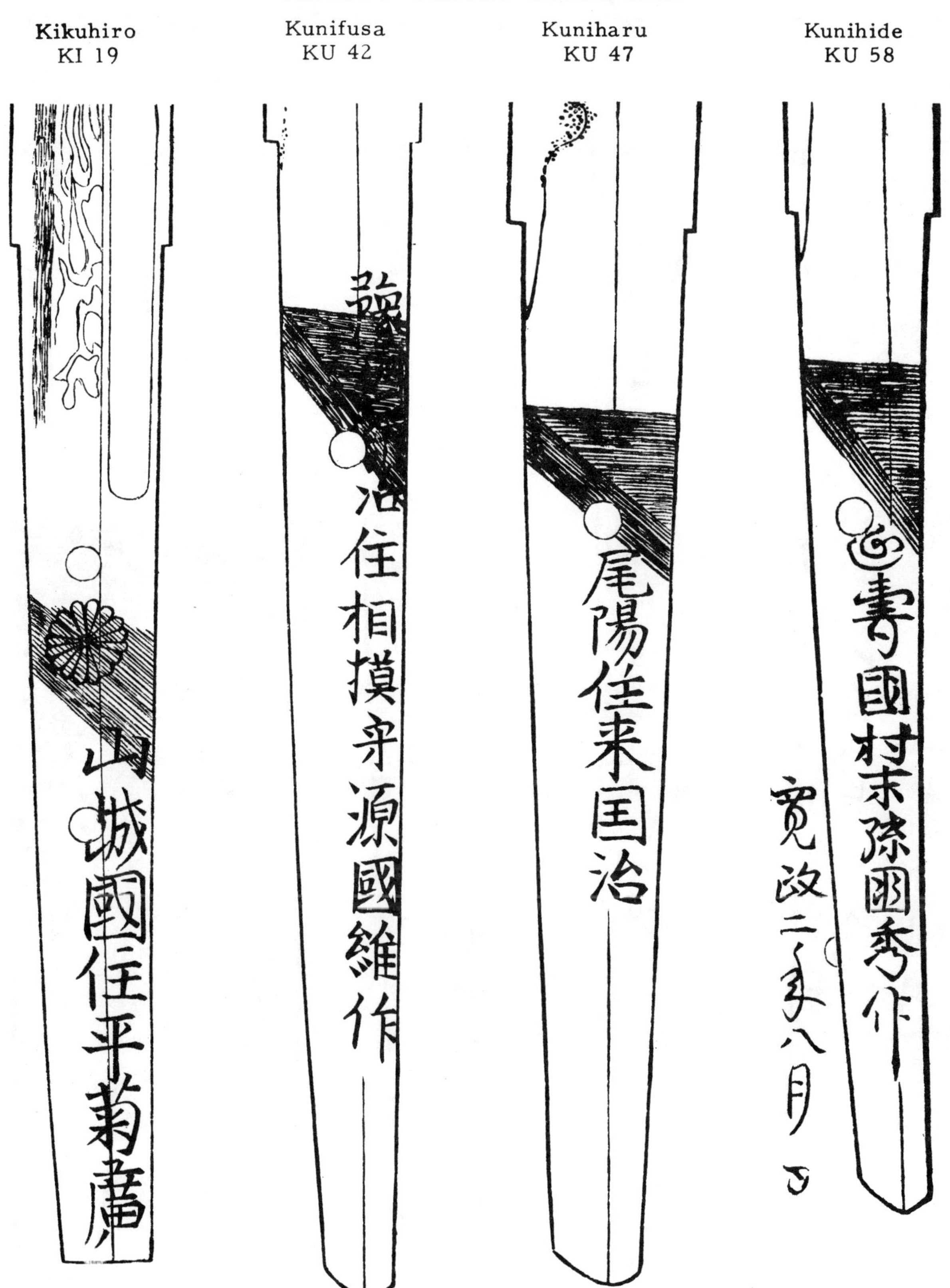

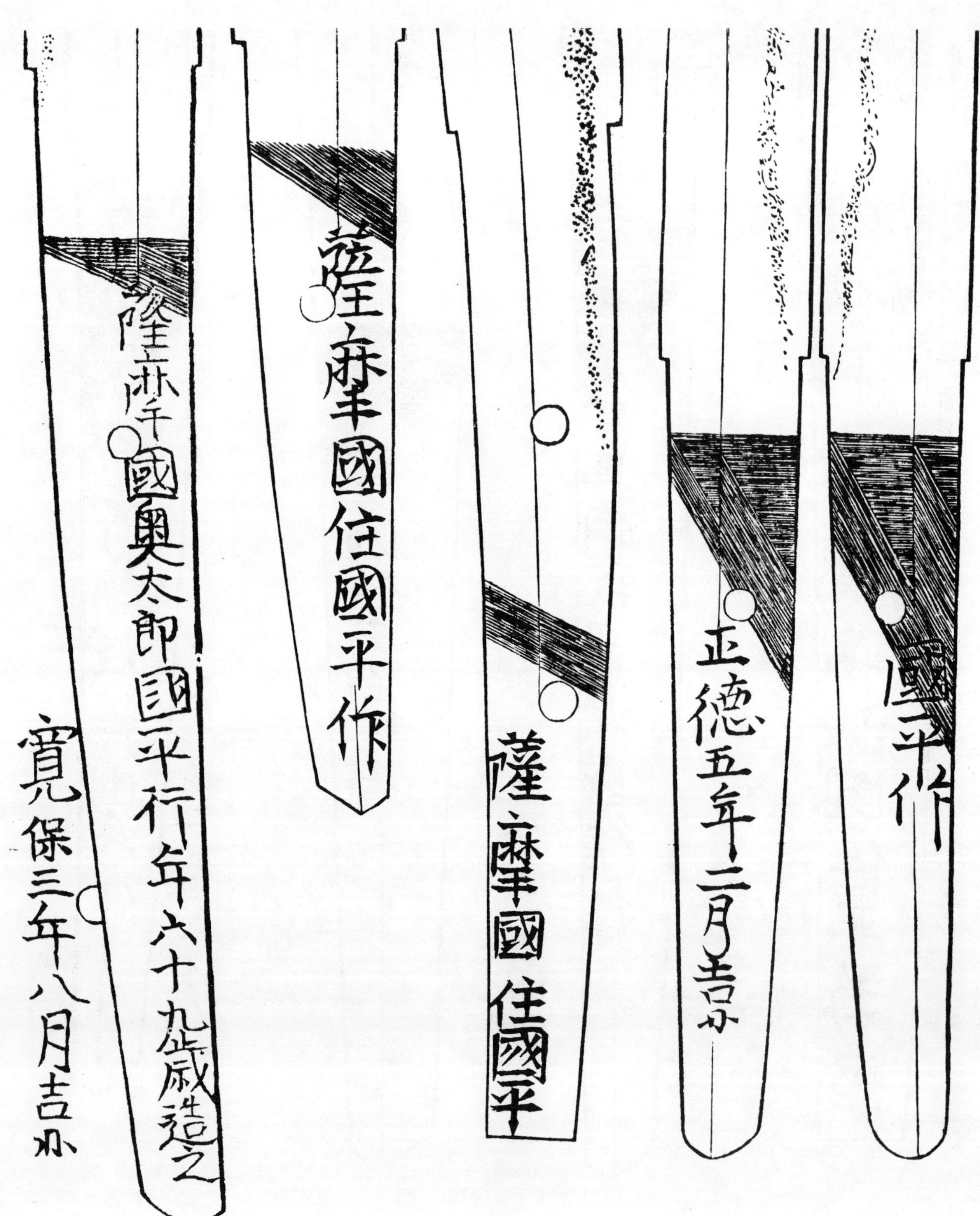
寛保三年八月吉
陸奥國奥太郎國平行年六十九歳造之
薩摩國住國平作
薩摩國住國平
正德五年二月吉
國平作

Kunihira
KU 80

Kunihiro
KU 99

Kunihiro KU 107

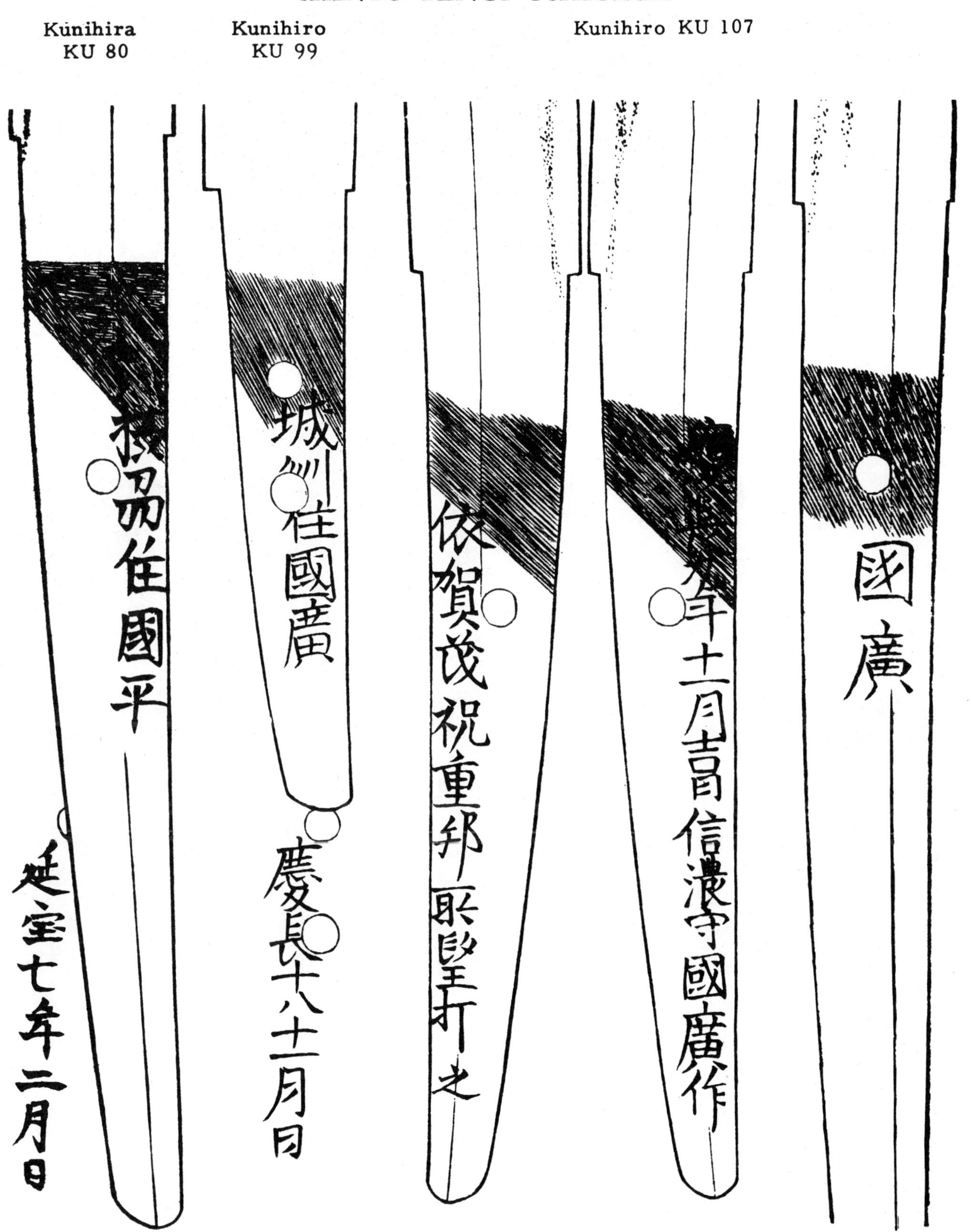

SHINTO BENGI OSHIGATA

Kunihiro. KU 107   Kunihiro KU ?   Kunihiro KU 109a   Kunihiro KU 123

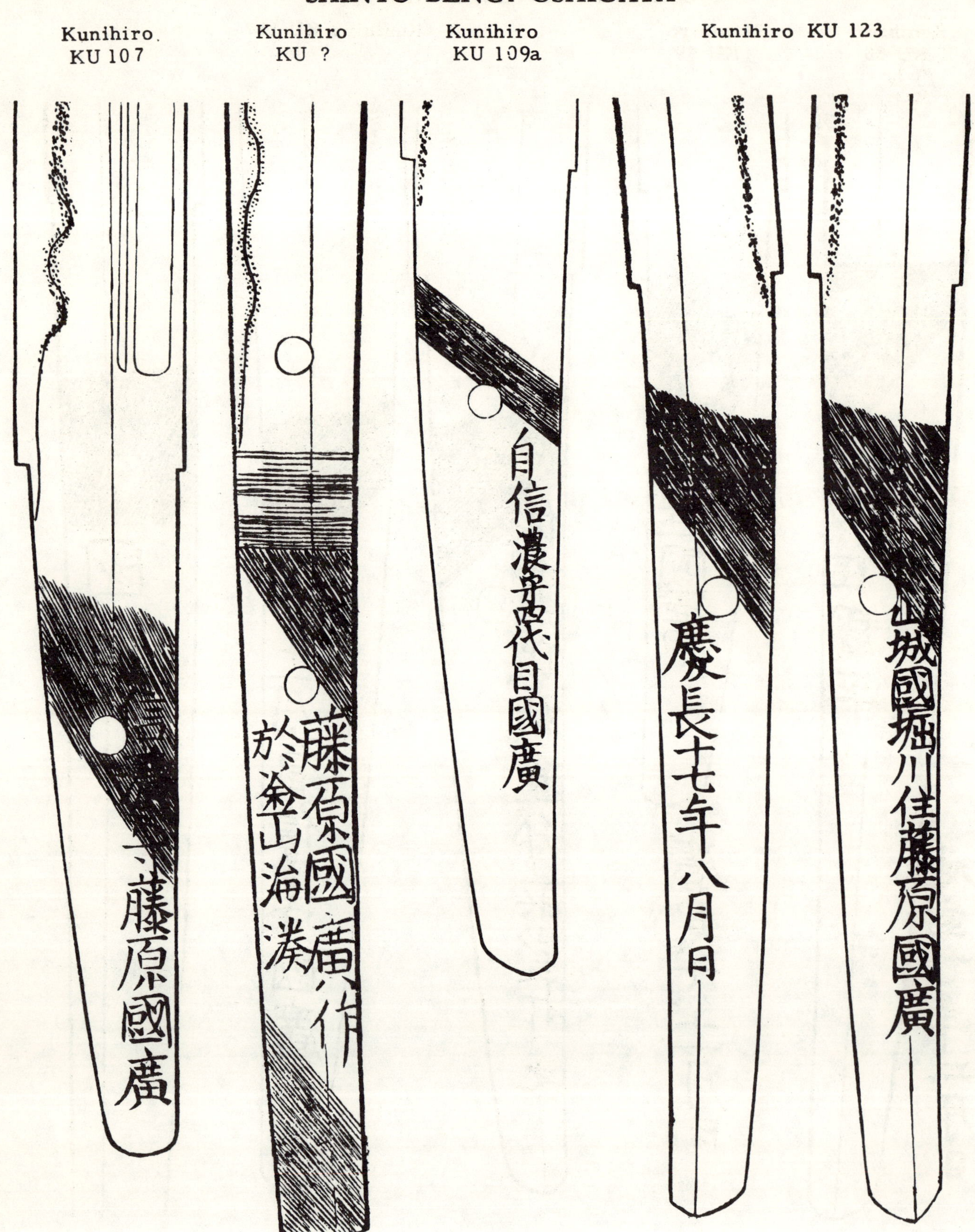

SHINTO BENGI OSHIGATA

Kunikane KU 159	Kunikane KU 162	Kunikane KU 163	Kunikane KU 168	Kunikiyo KU 196

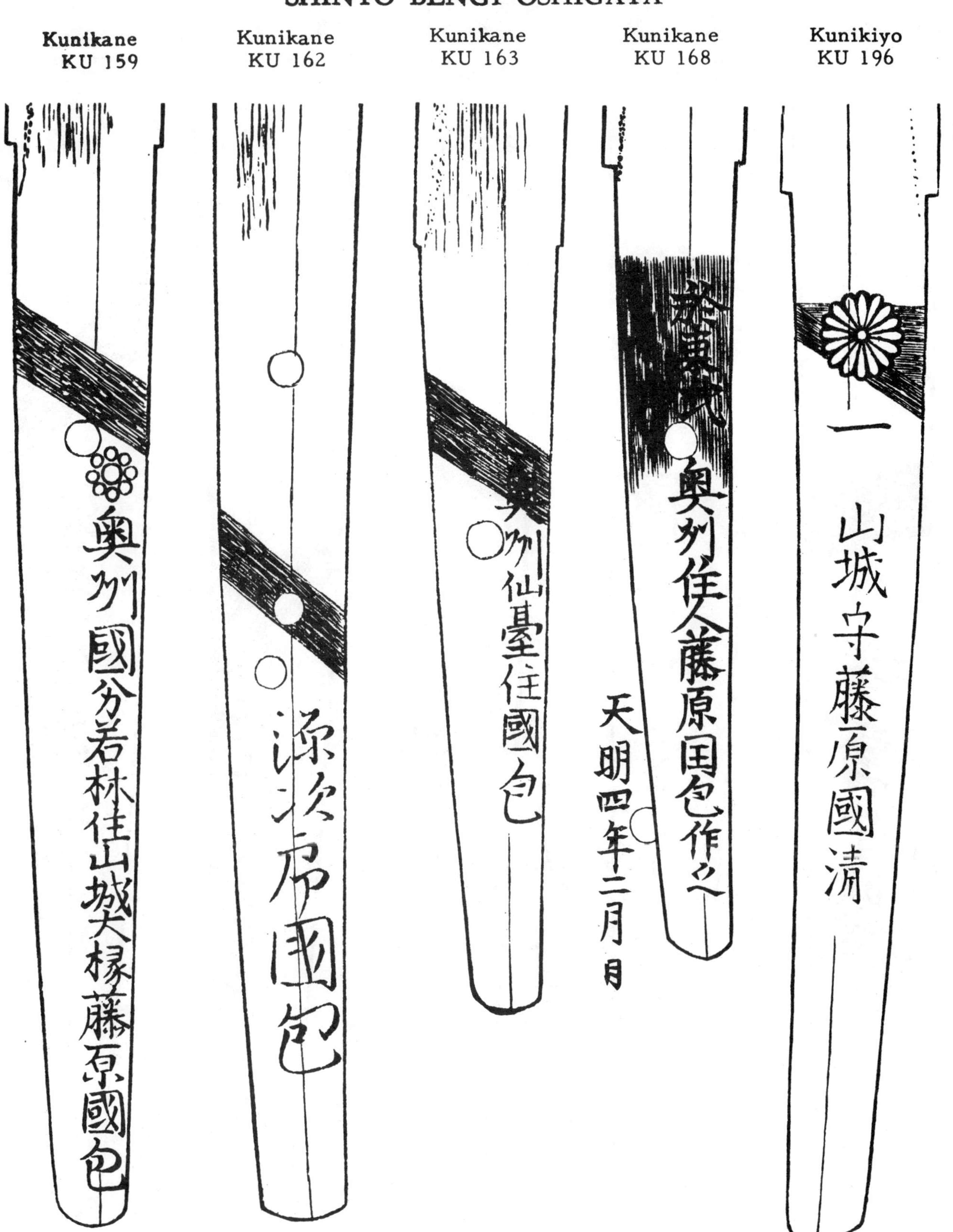

Kunikiyo KU 201	Kunimasa KU 235	Kunimasa KU 245	Kunimichi KU 257	Kunimitsu KU 288

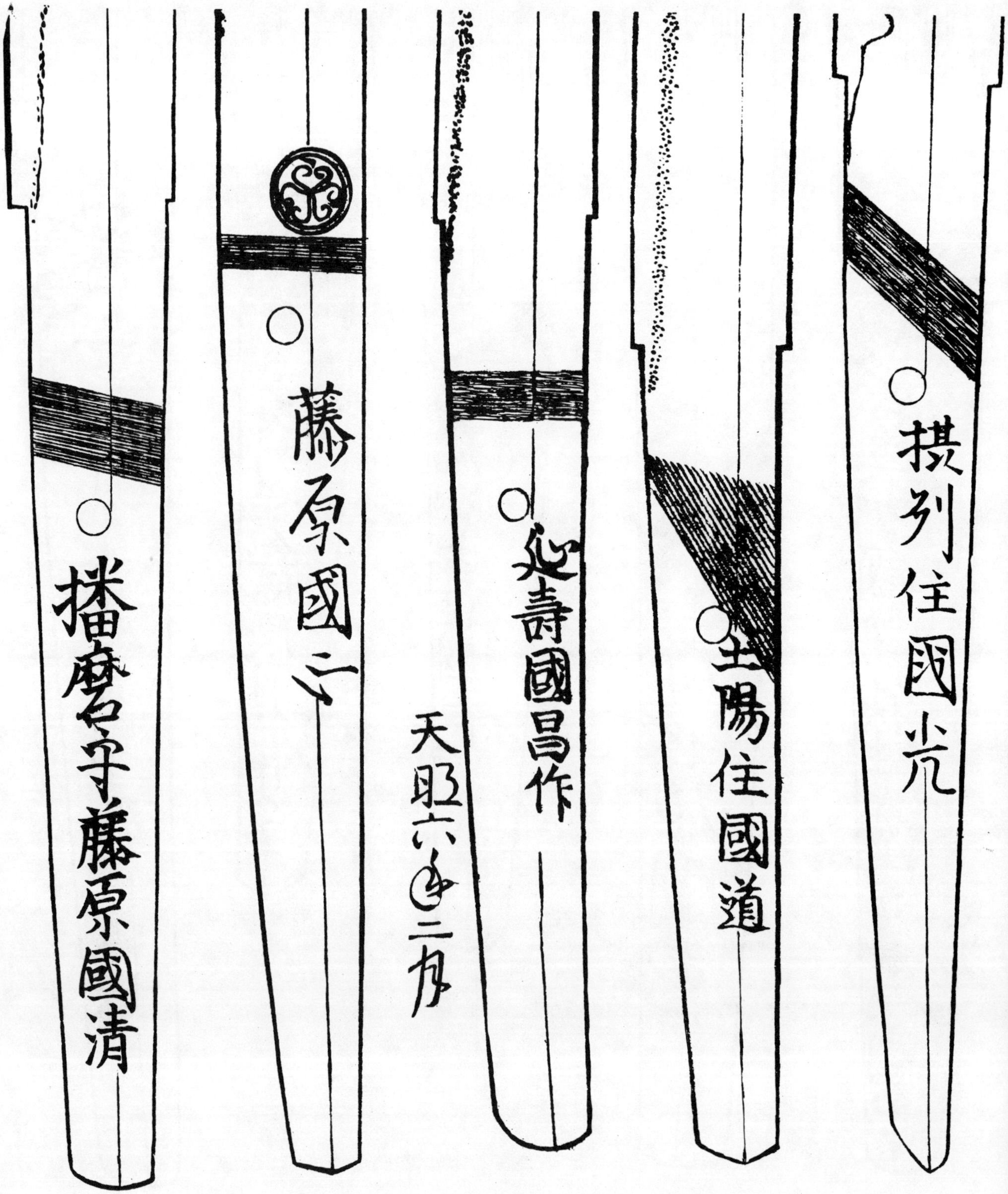

Kunimichi KU 259   Kunimichi KU 260   Kunimichi
                                                     KU 261

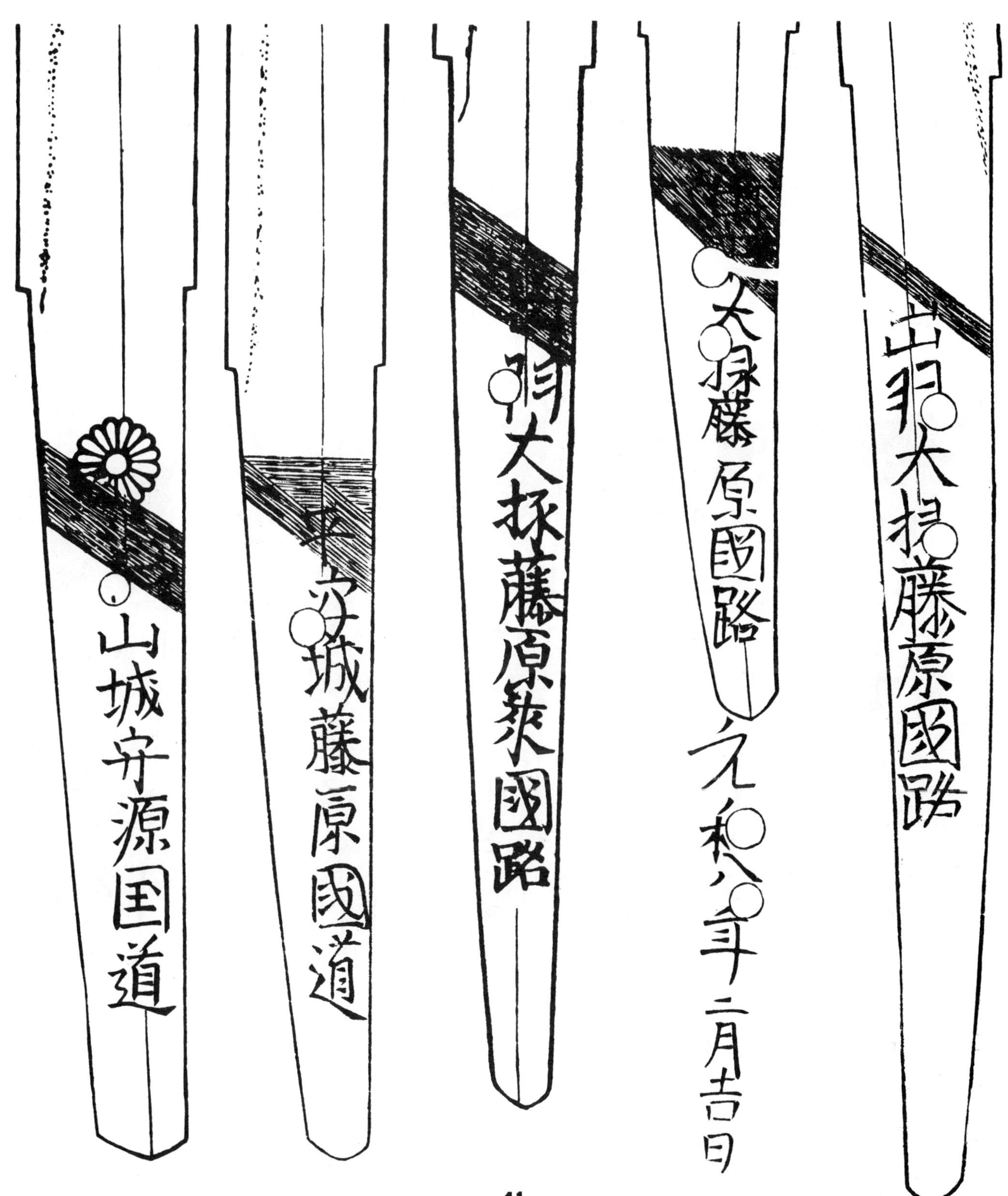

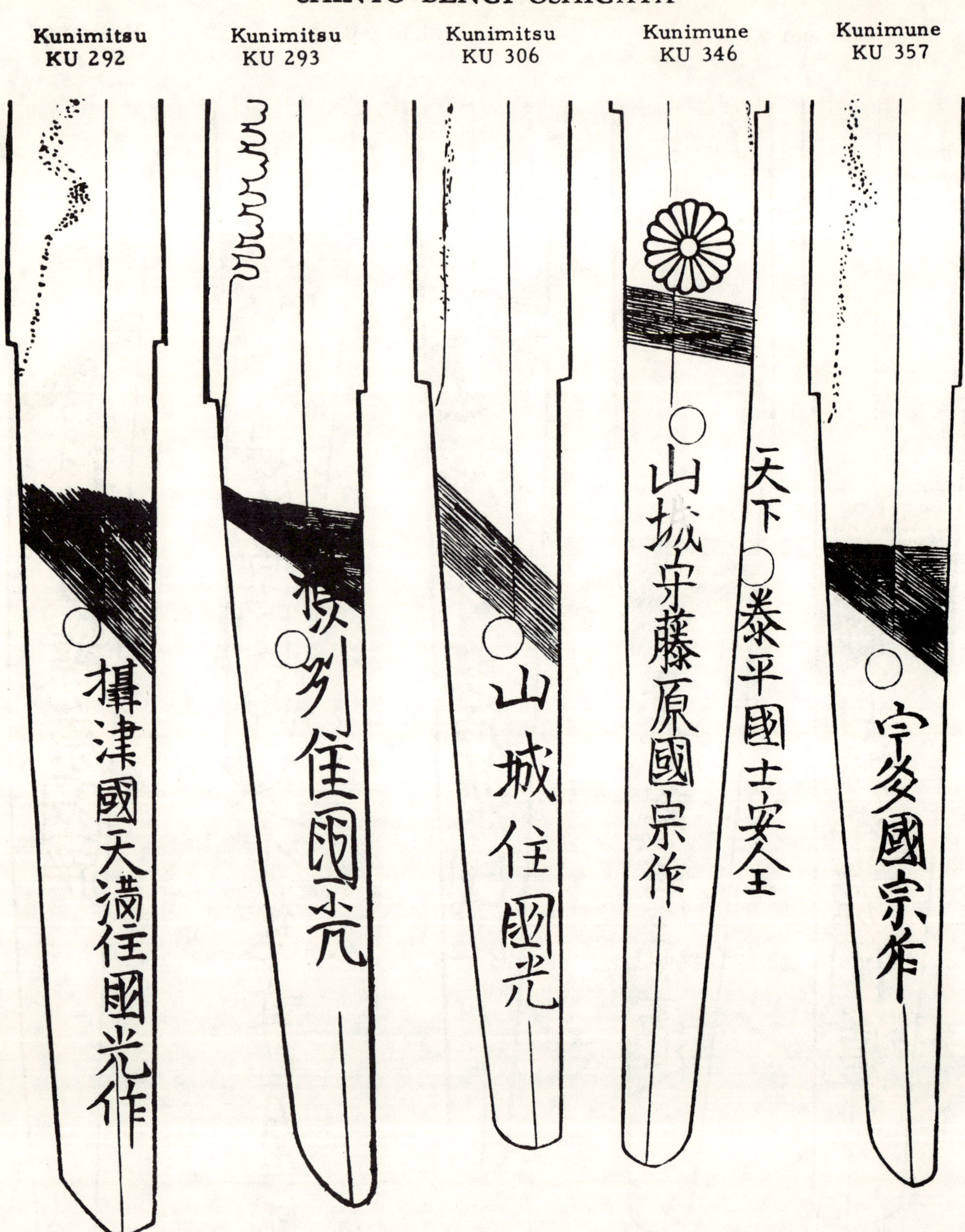
Kunimitsu
KU 292
Kunimitsu
KU 293
Kunimitsu
KU 306
Kunimune
KU 346
Kunimune
KU 357
攝津國天満住國光作
攝州住國光
山城住國光
山城守藤原國宗作
天下泰平國土安全
宇多國宗作

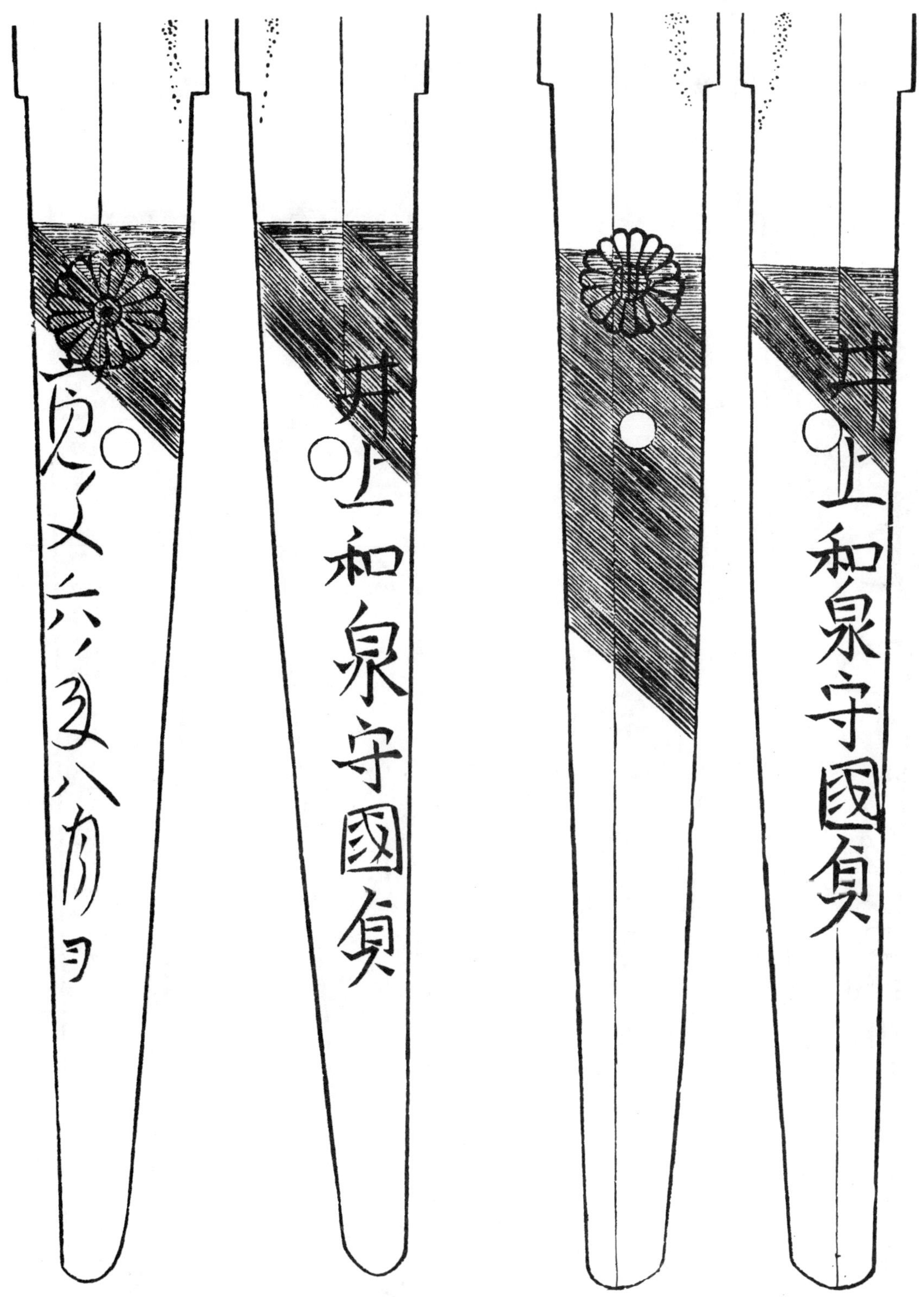

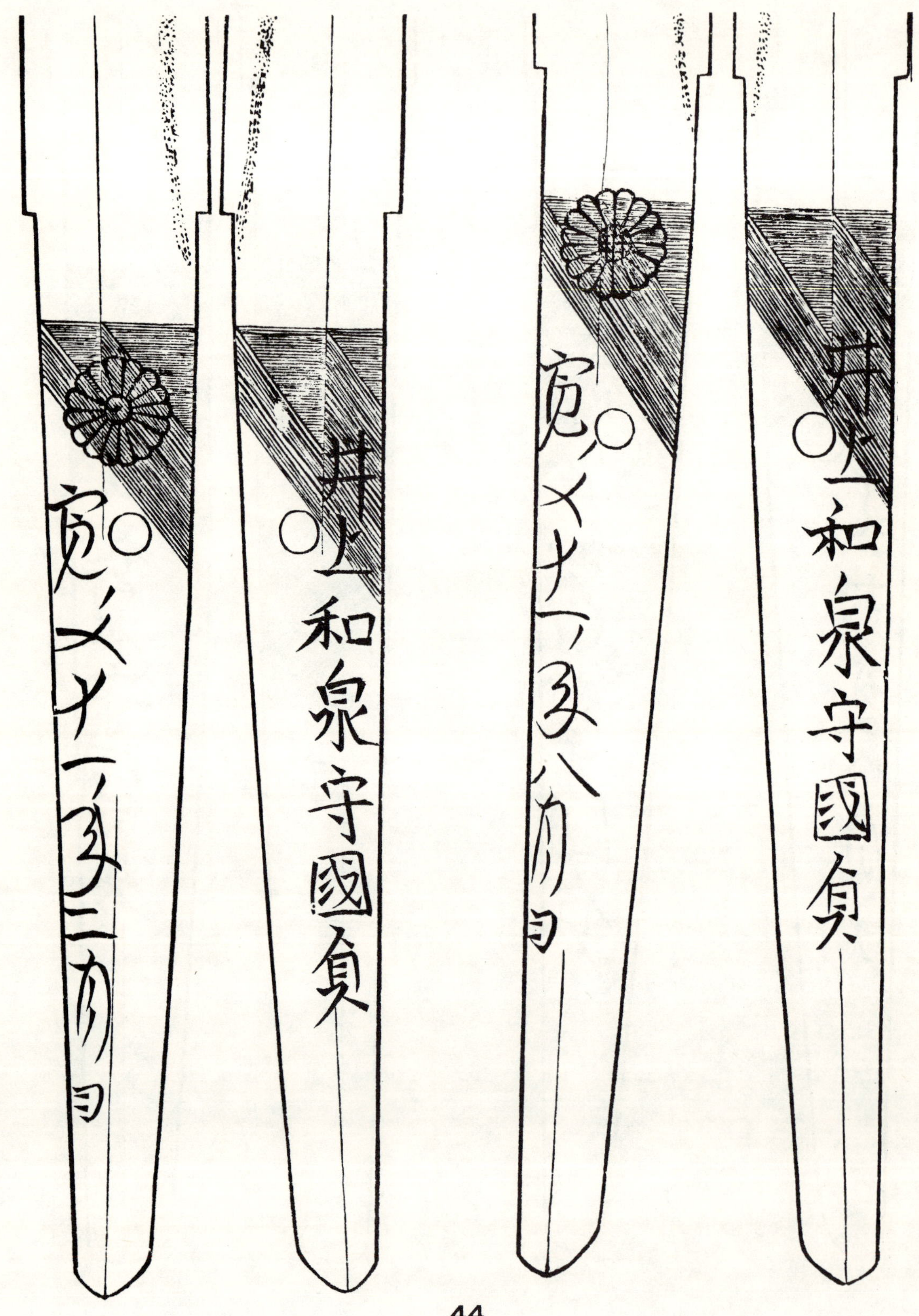

Kunisada
KU 498

Kunisada & Kunisuke
KU 498   KU 618

Kunisada KU 499

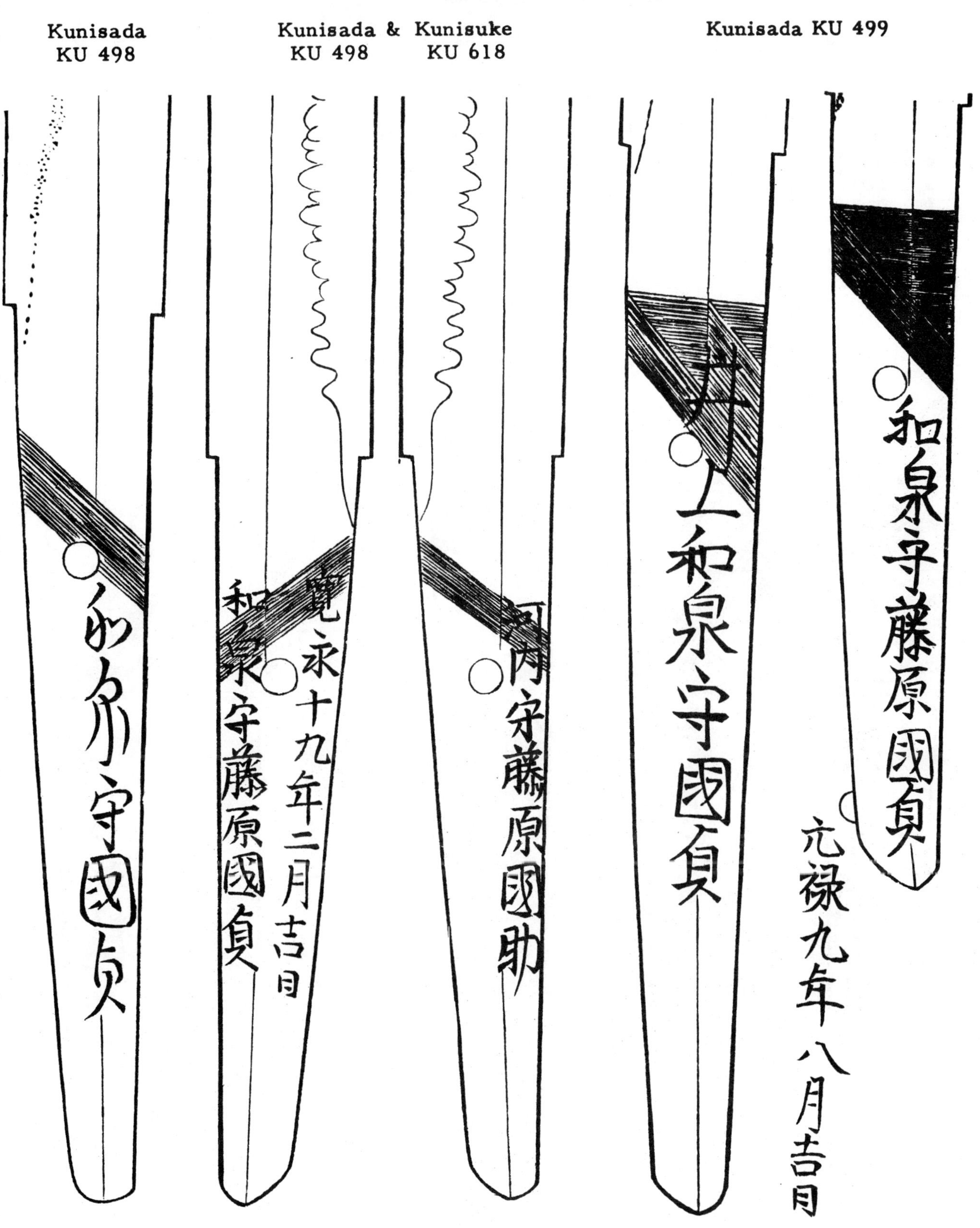

Kunisada KU 497   Kunisada KU 498

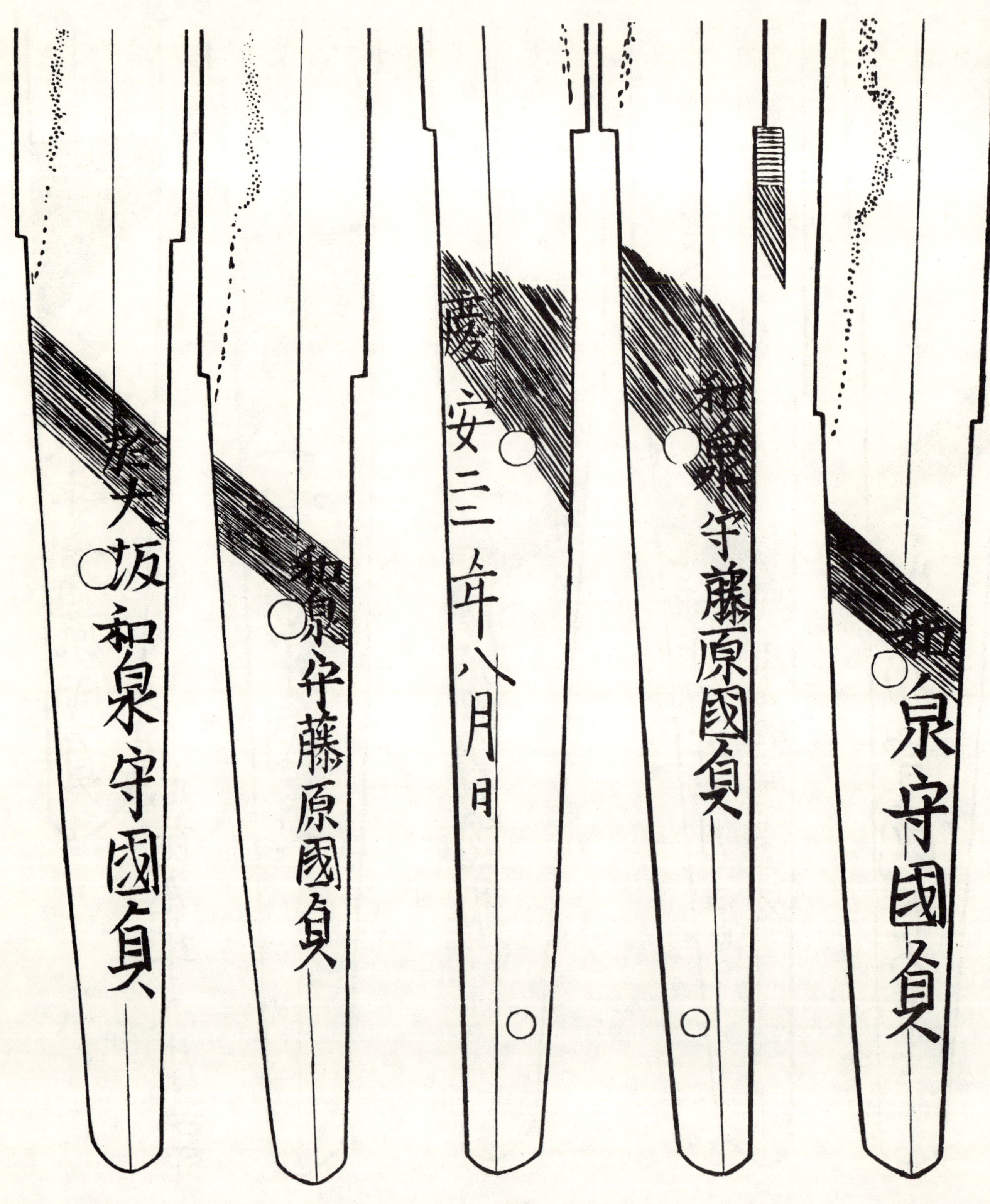

SHINTO BENGI OSHIGATA

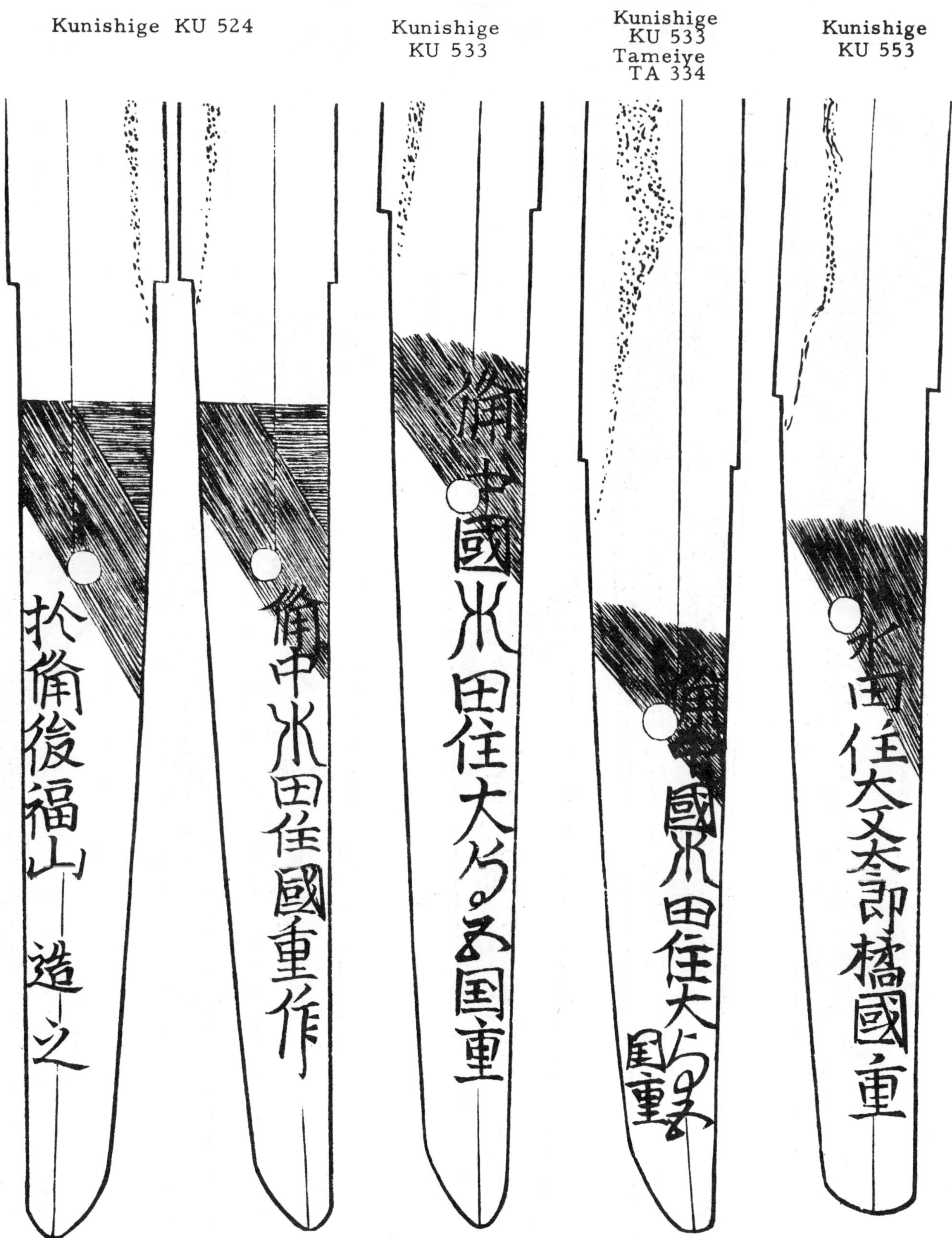

Kunishige KU 542	Kunishige KU 554	Kunishige KU 565	Kunishige KU 586	Kunishige KU 581

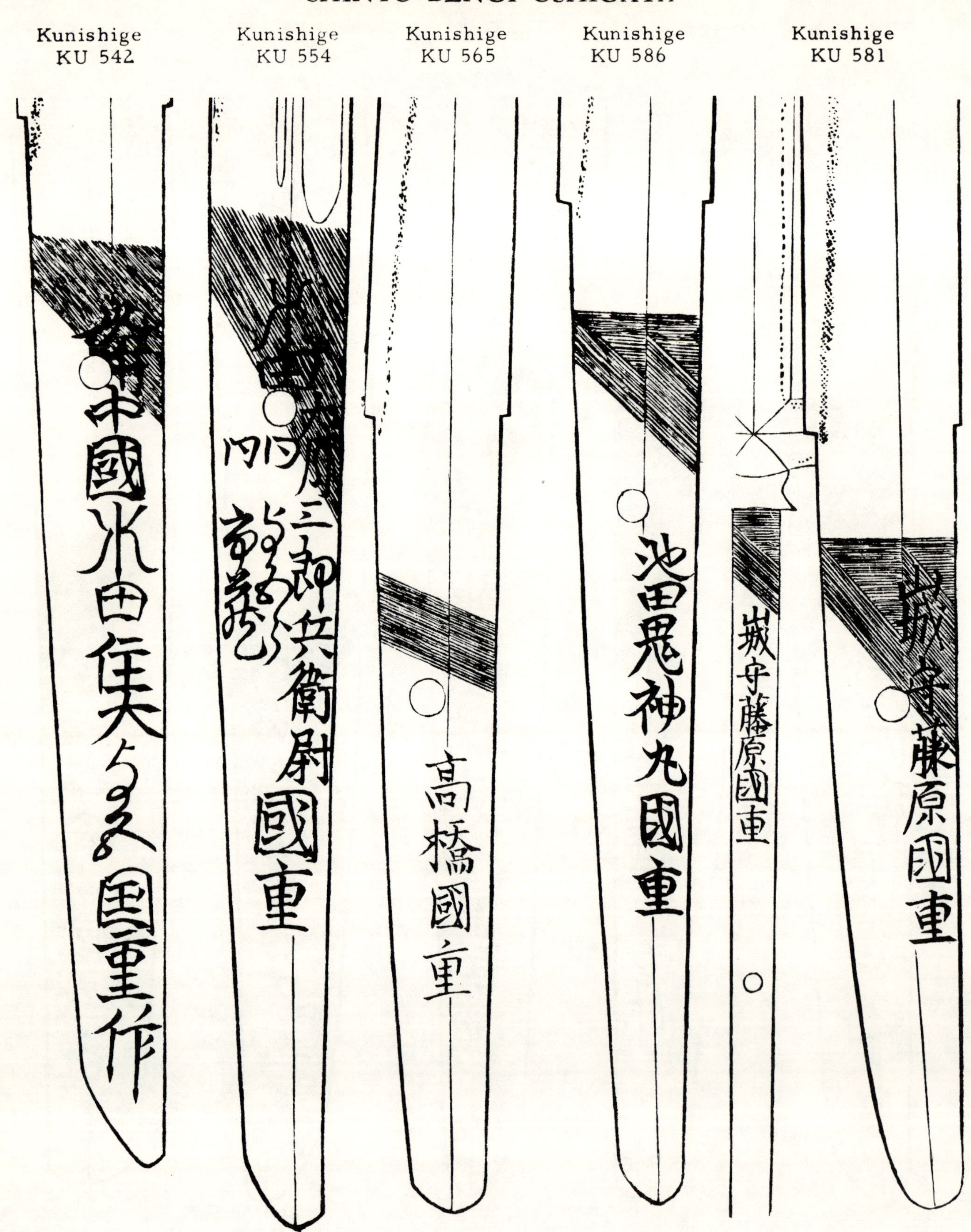

Kunisuke
KU 603

Kunisuke
KU 617

Kunisuke KU 619

Kunisuke
KU 620

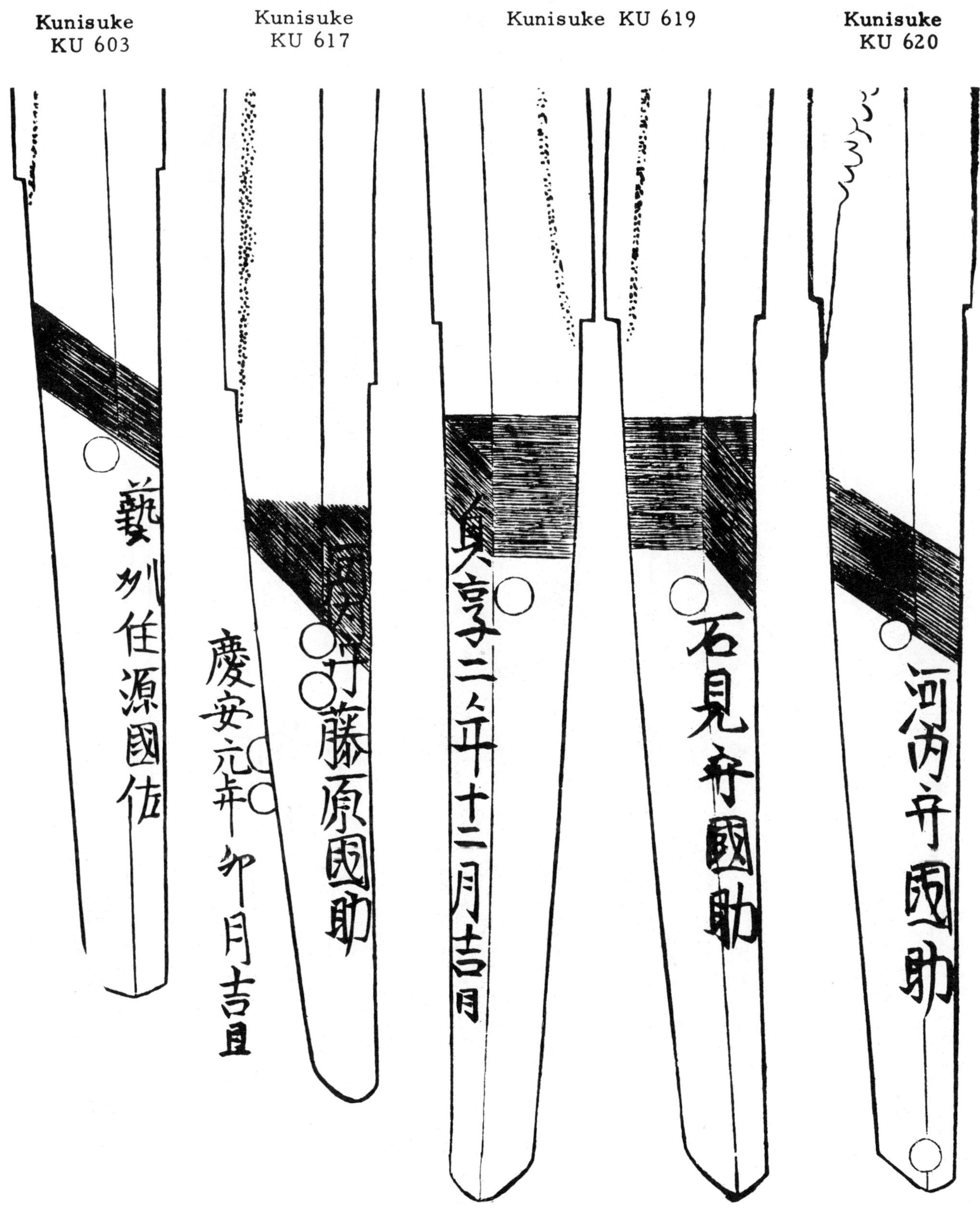

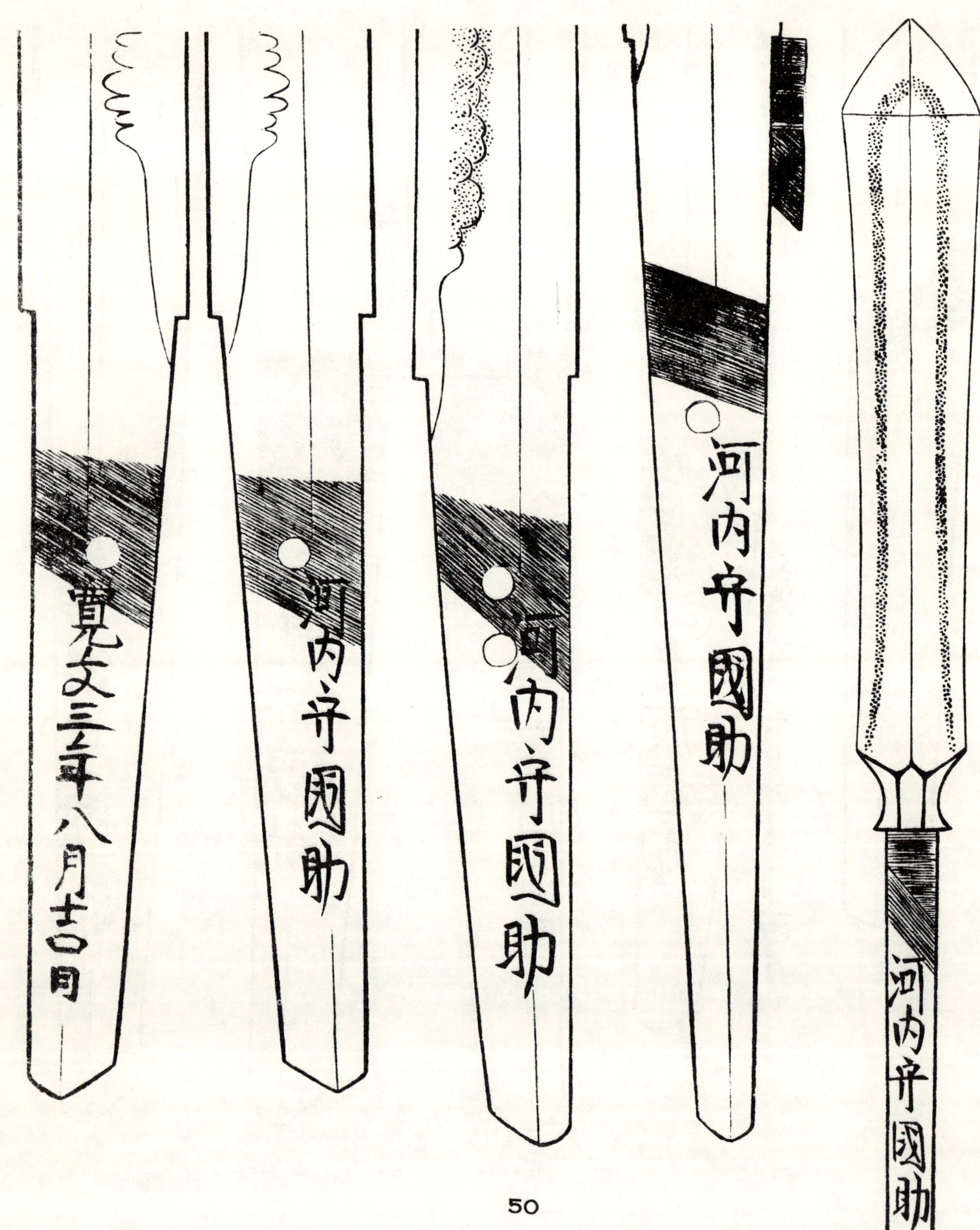

Kunisuke KU 618   Kunisuke KU 620   Kunisumi
                                                  KU 631

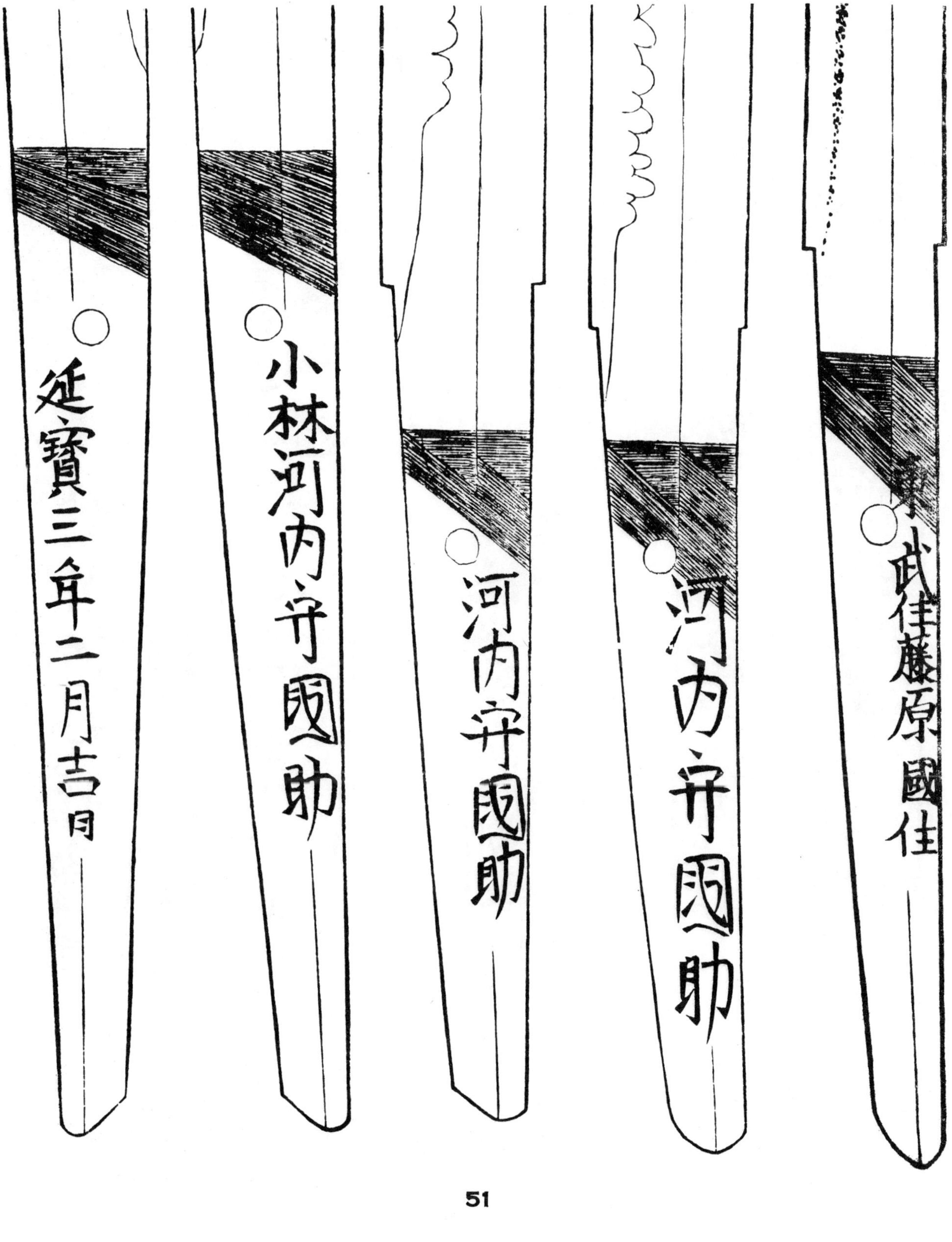

延寶三年二月吉日

小林河内守國助

河内守國助

河内守國助

武佳藤原國住

SHINTO BENGI OSHIGATA

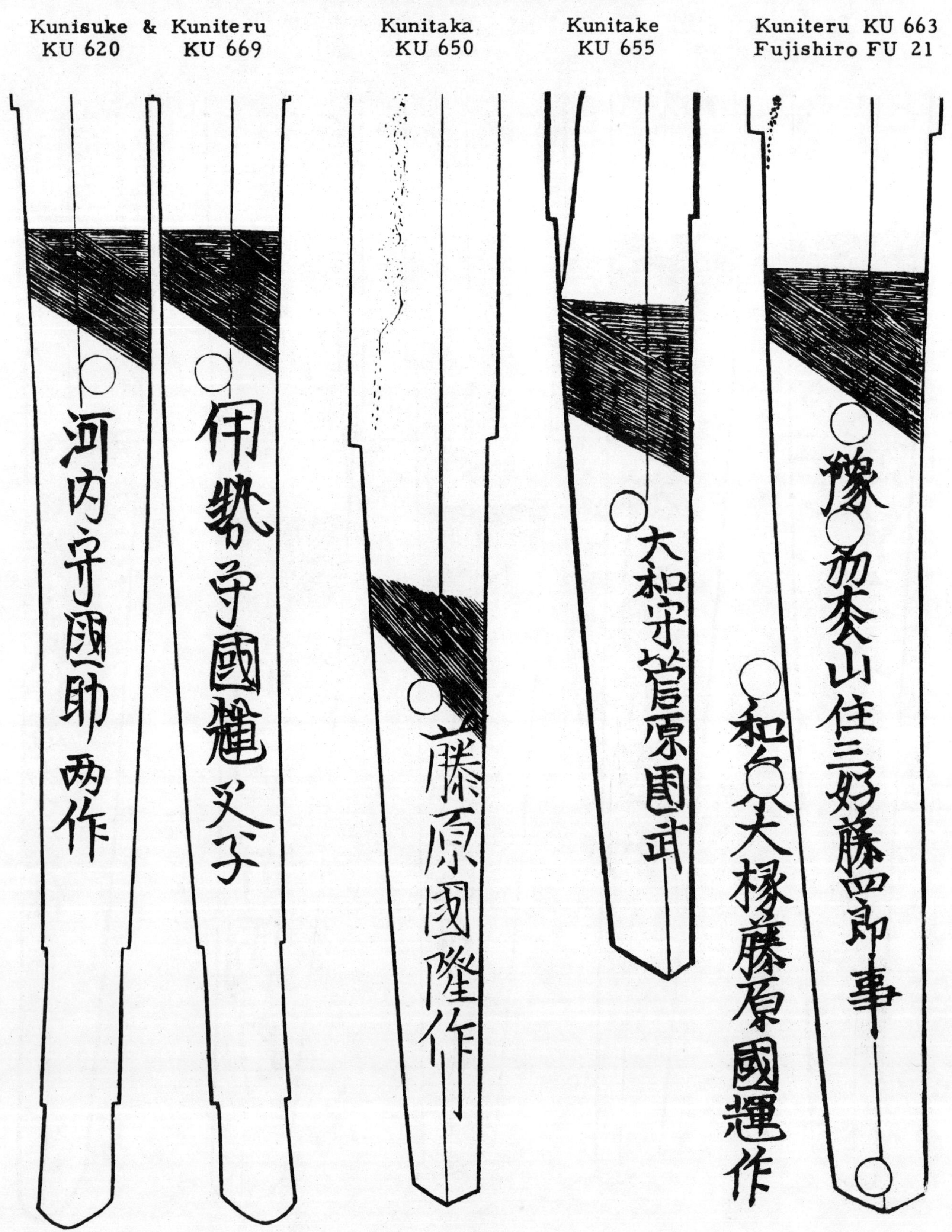

SHINTO BENGI OSHIGATA

Kuniteru
KU 667

Kuniteru KU 669

Horimono by
Kuniteru

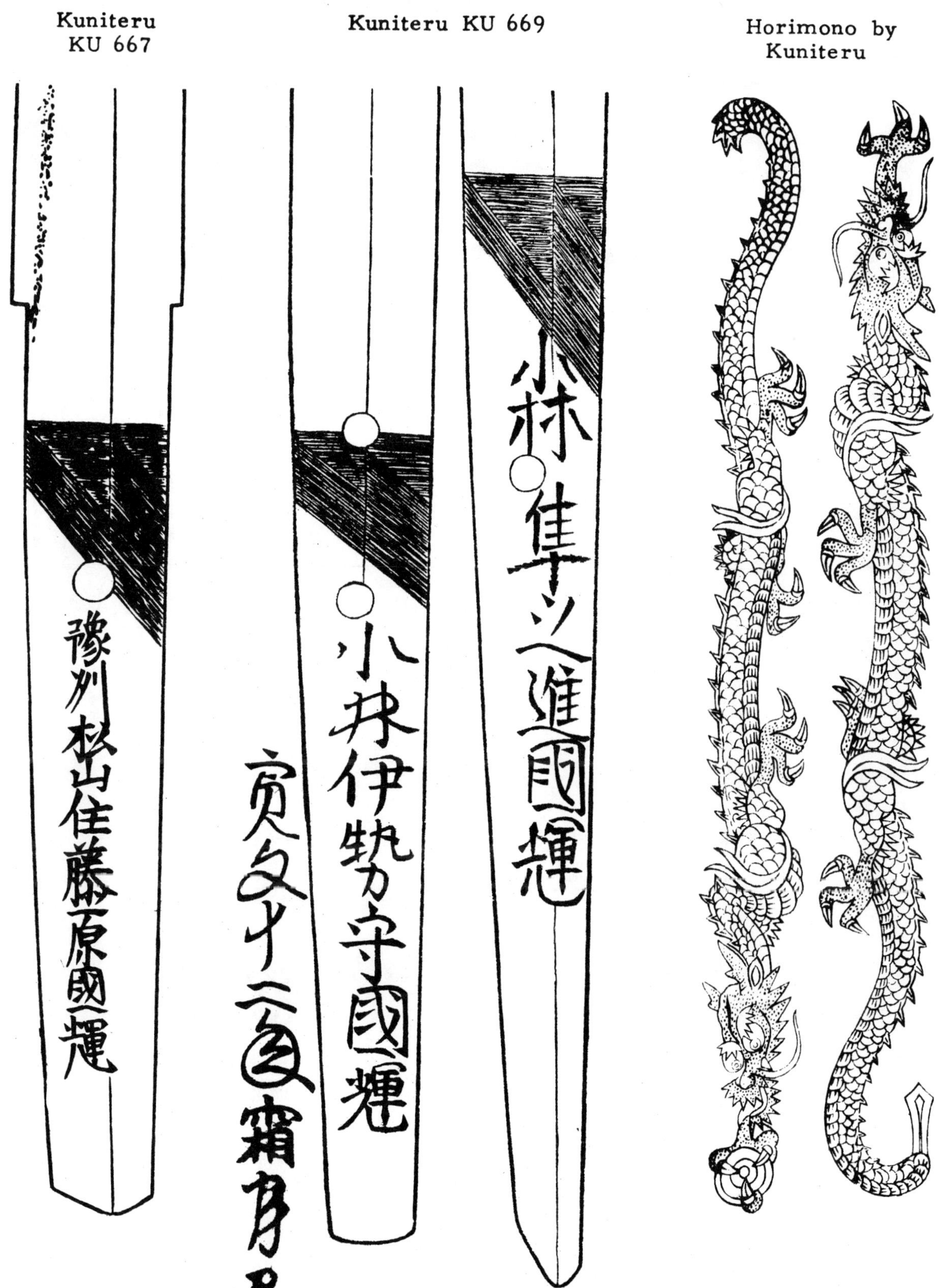

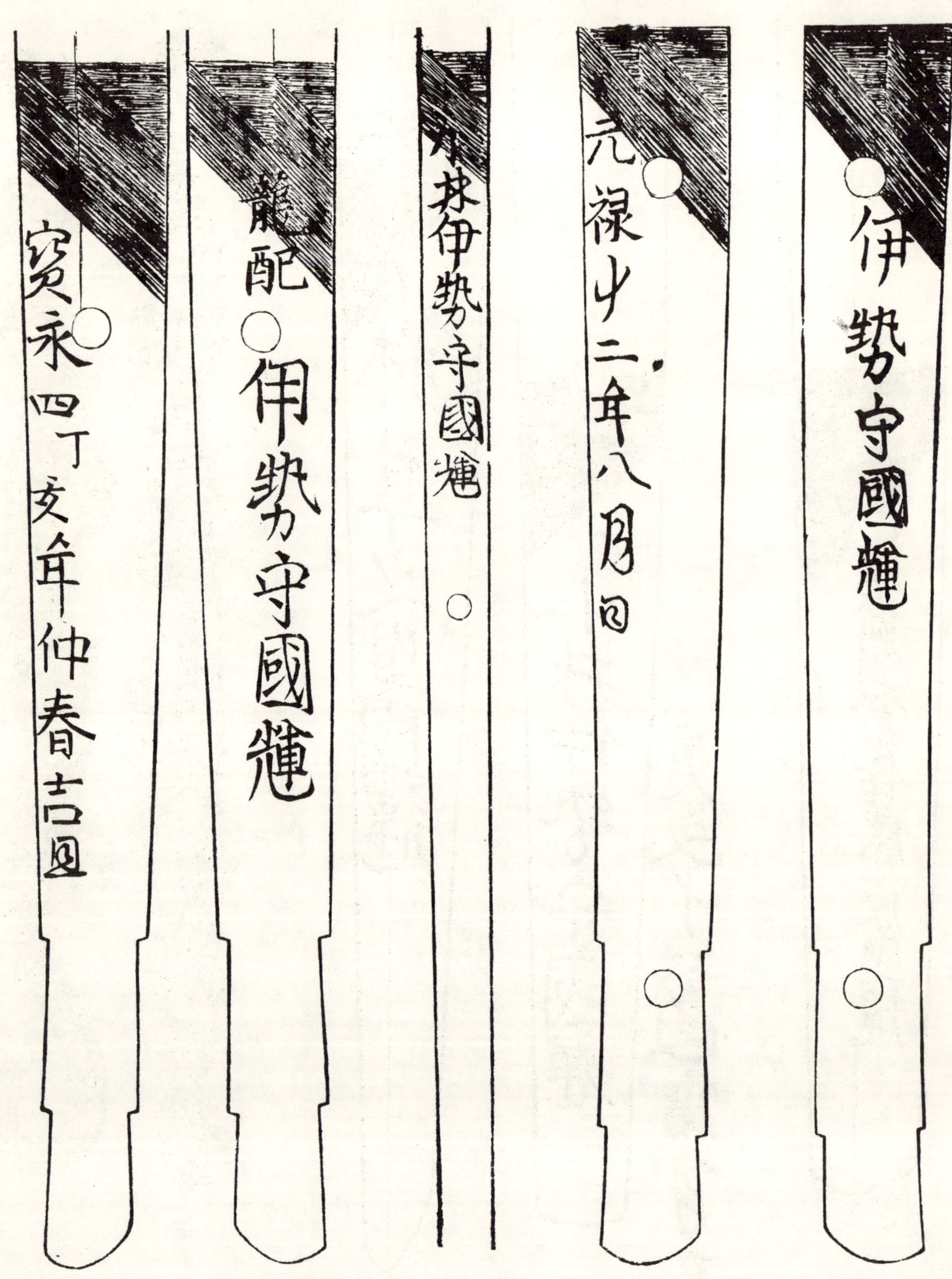

○小林伊勢守國輝

三月日

小林伊勢守國輝

小林伊勢守國輝

佐○渡守國富元喜作

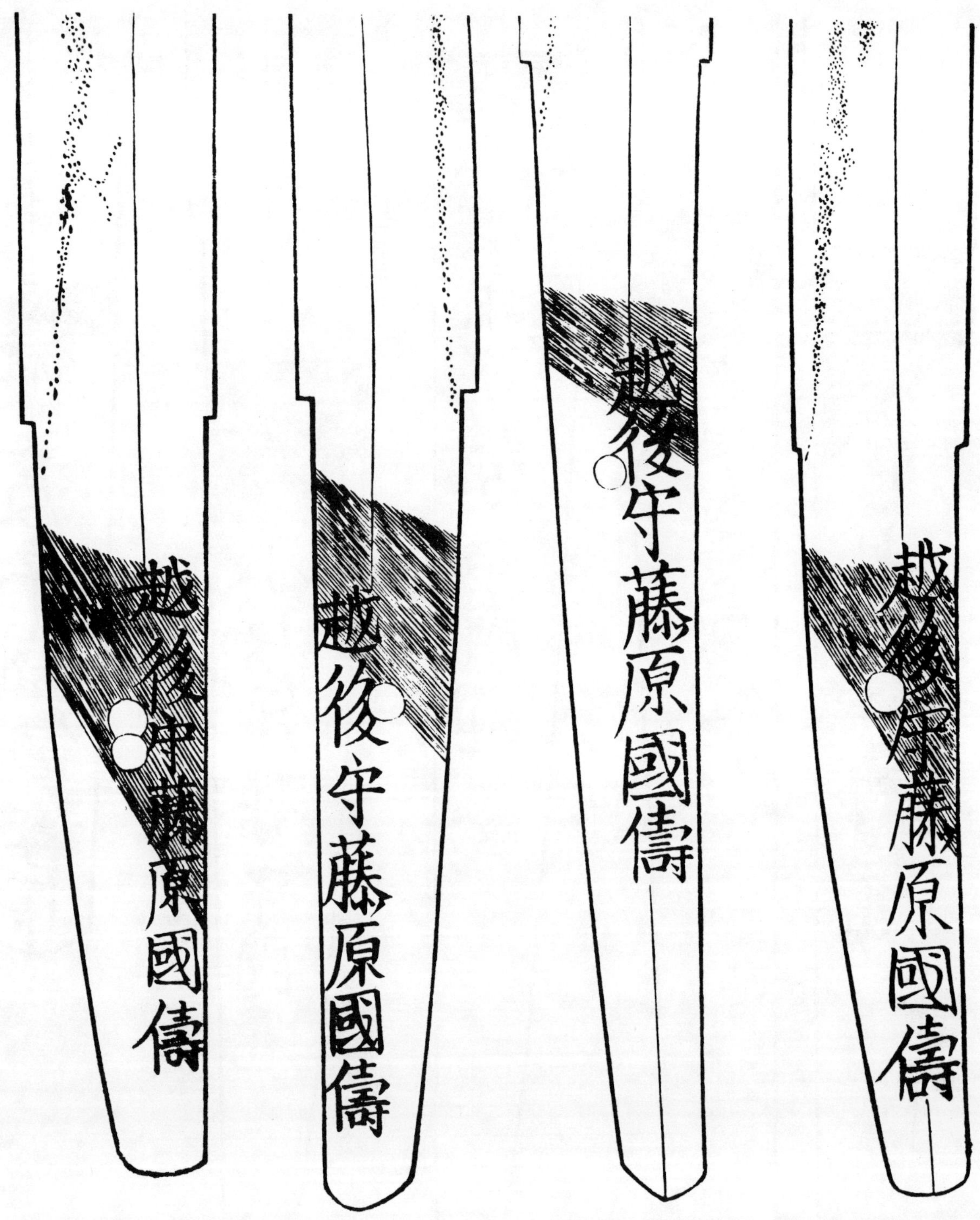

越後守藤原國儔
越後守藤原國儔
越後守藤原國儔
越後守藤原國儔

**Kunitoyo
KU 743**   Kunitsugu KU 789   Kuniyasu KU 868

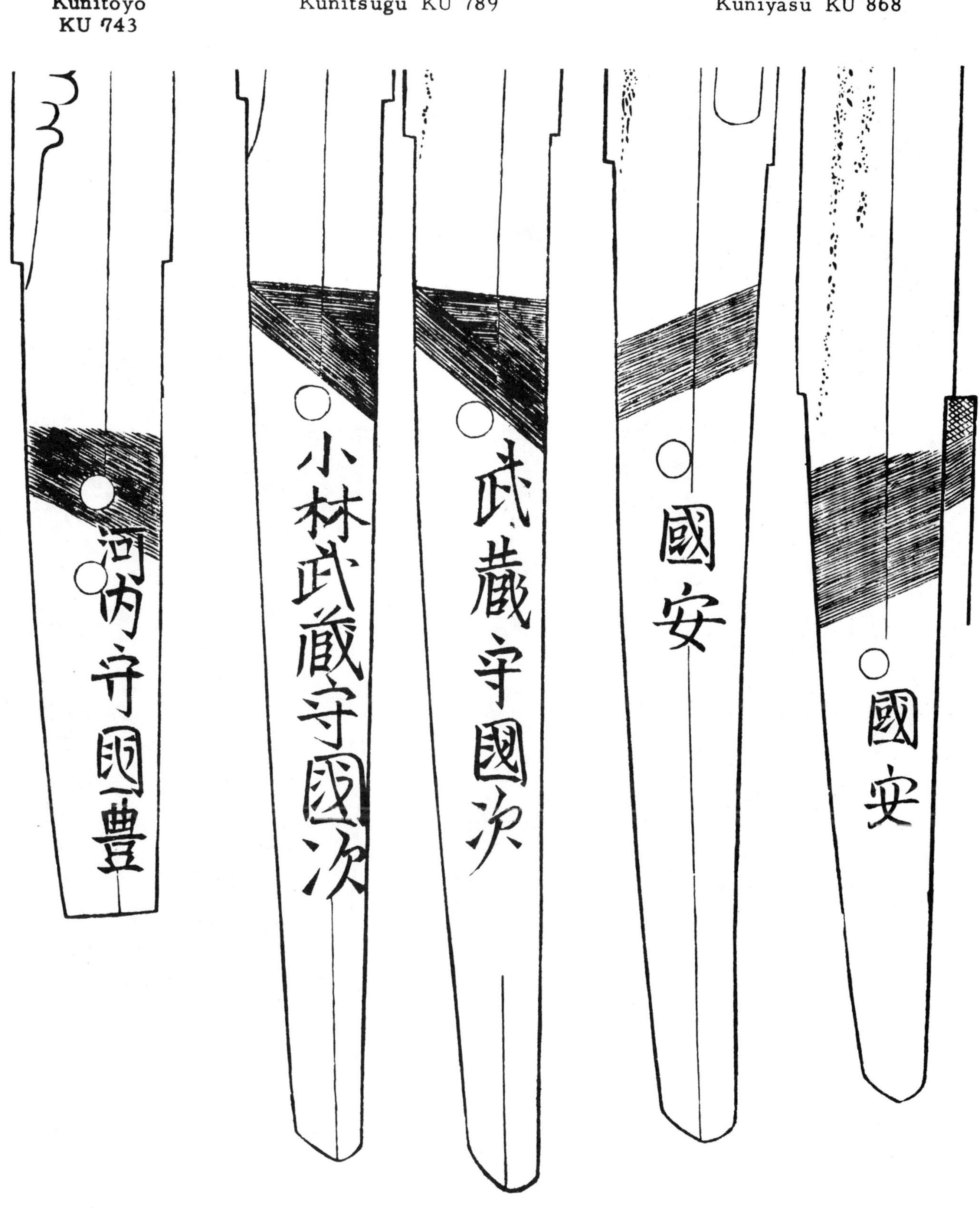

Kuniyasu KU 868　　　　　Kuniyasu
KU 873　　　　　Kuniyasu KU 885

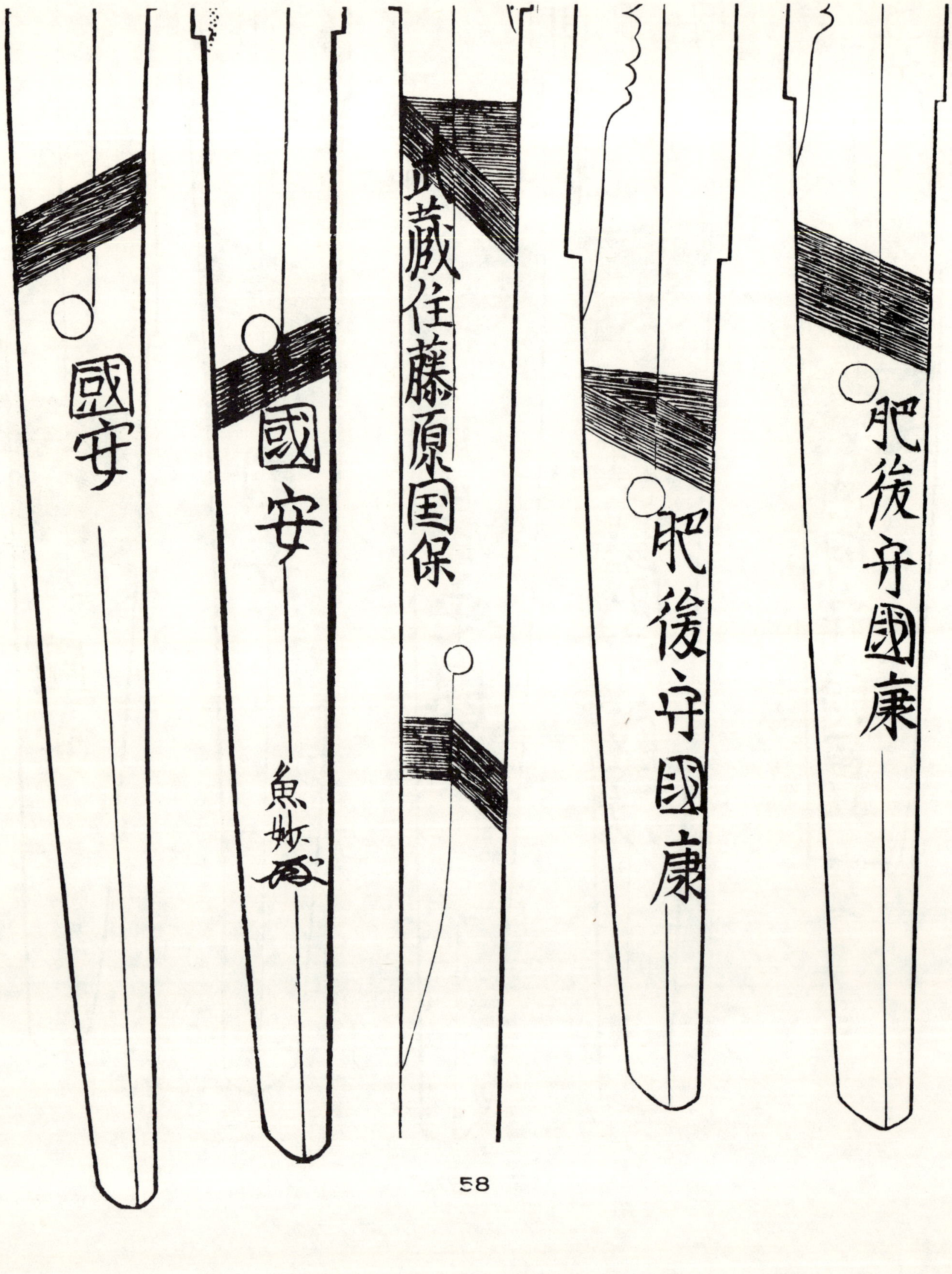

武蔵住藤原国保

國安

國安

魚妙衛

肥後守國康

肥後守國康

Kuniyoshi KU 924	Kuniyoshi KU 931	Kuniyoshi KU 948	Kuniyoshi KU 958

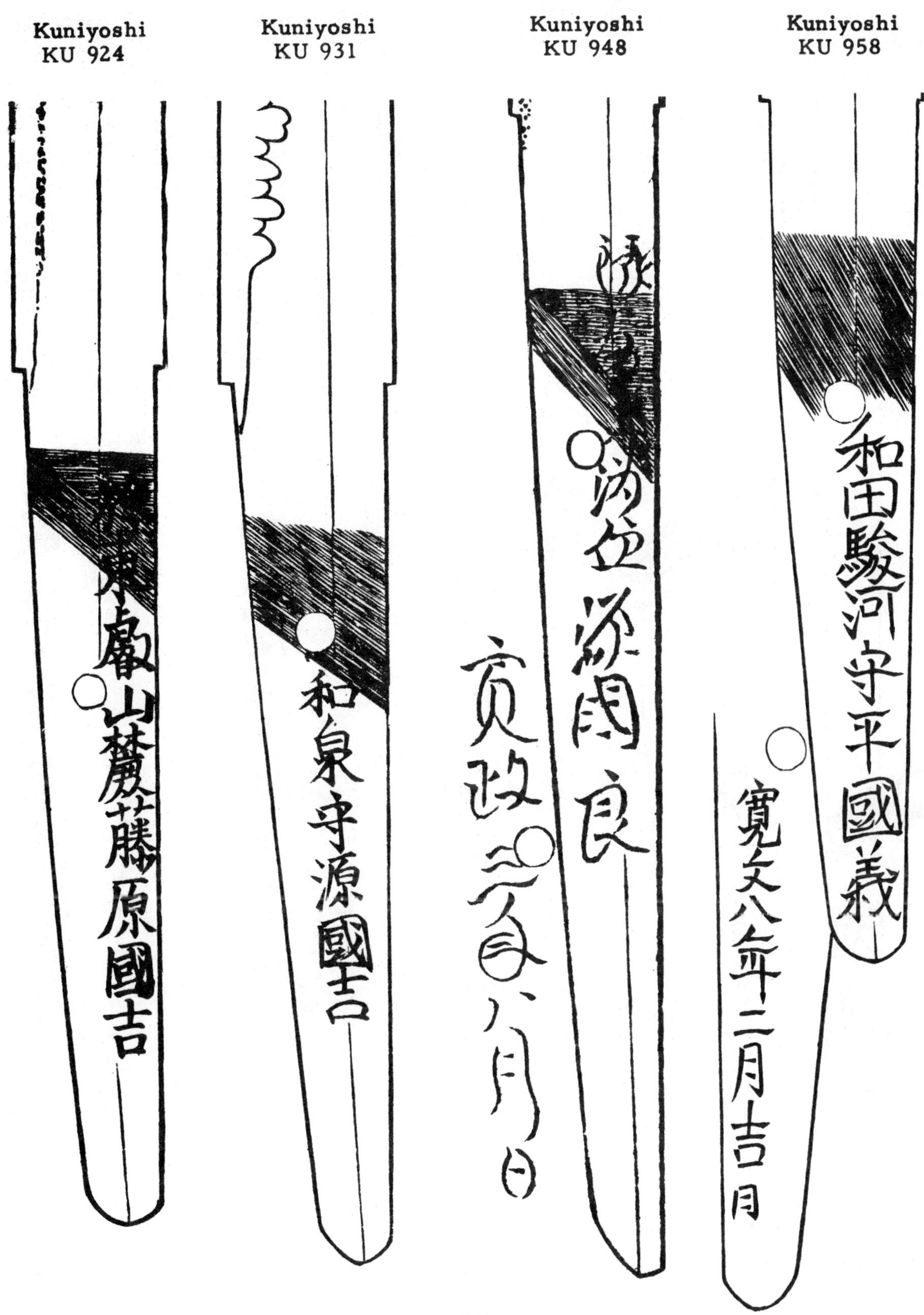

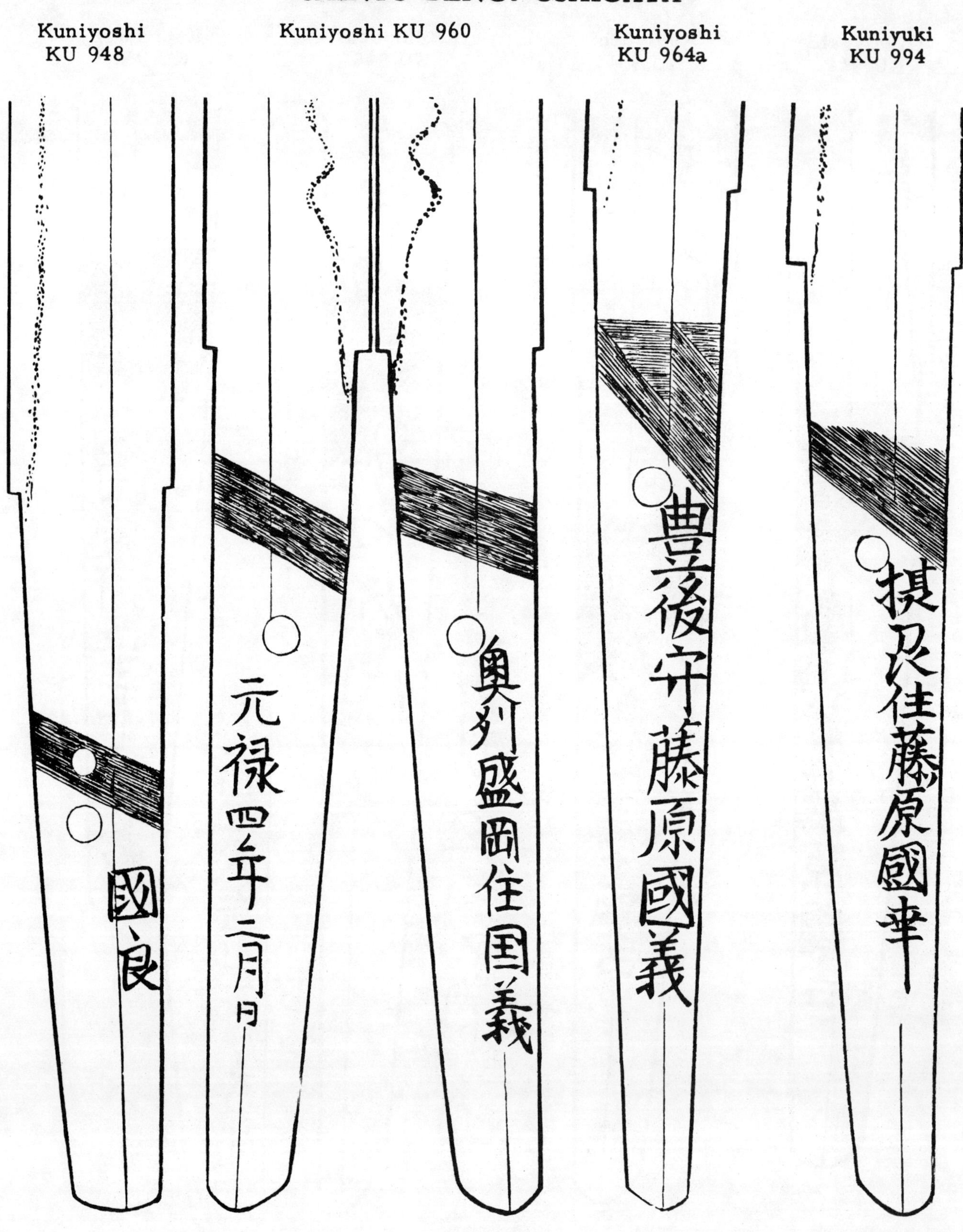
Kuniyoshi
KU 948
Kuniyoshi KU 960
Kuniyoshi
KU 964a
Kuniyuki
KU 994
國良
元禄四年二月日
奥刕盛岡住国義
豊後守藤原國義
摂刕住藤原國幸

Masayuki
MA 12

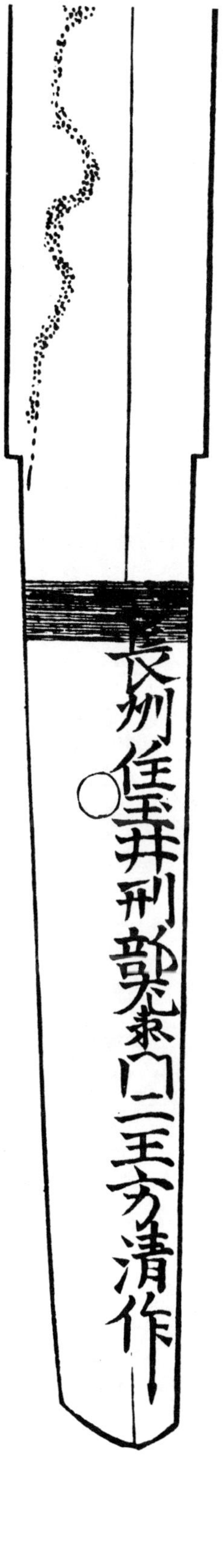

Masafusa
MA 49

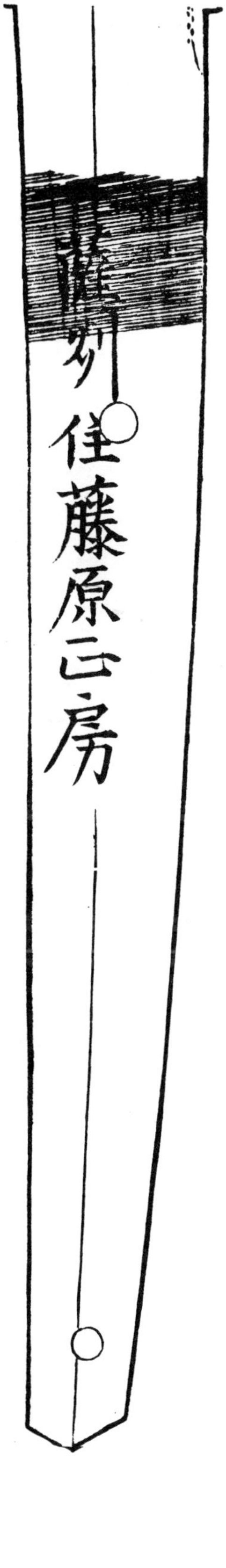

Masahiro MA 88

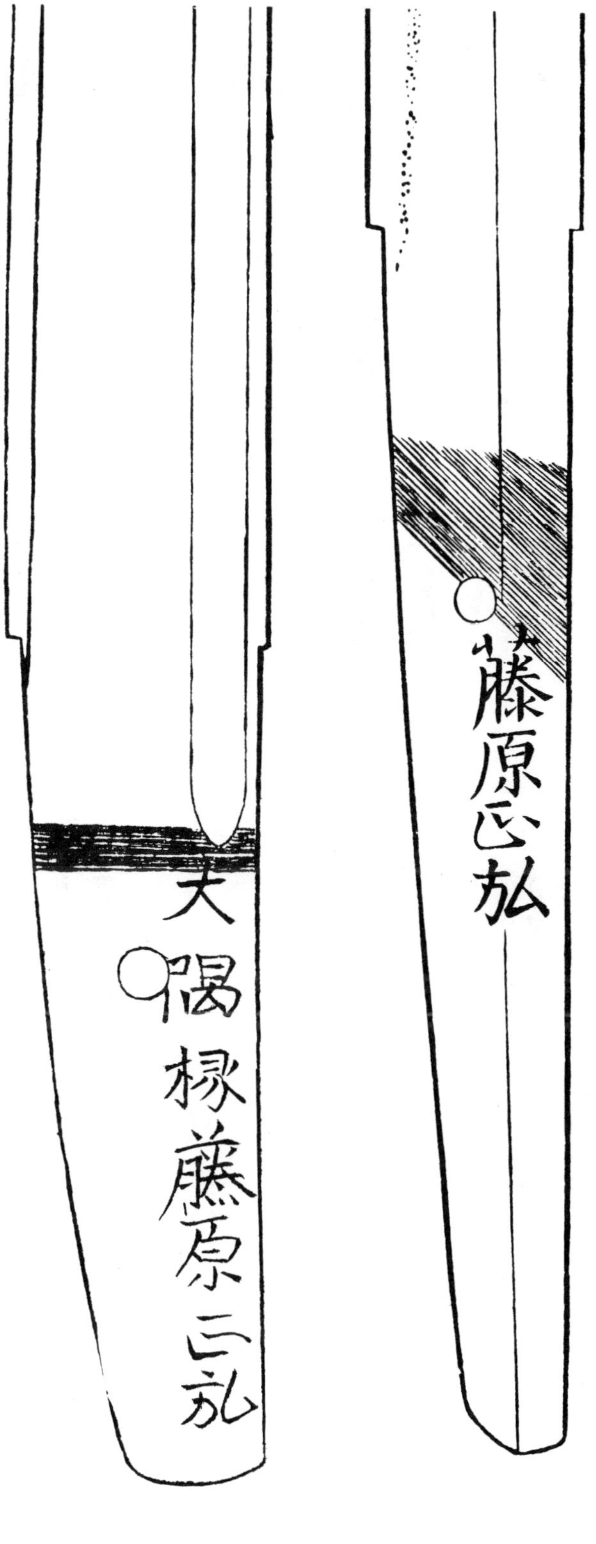

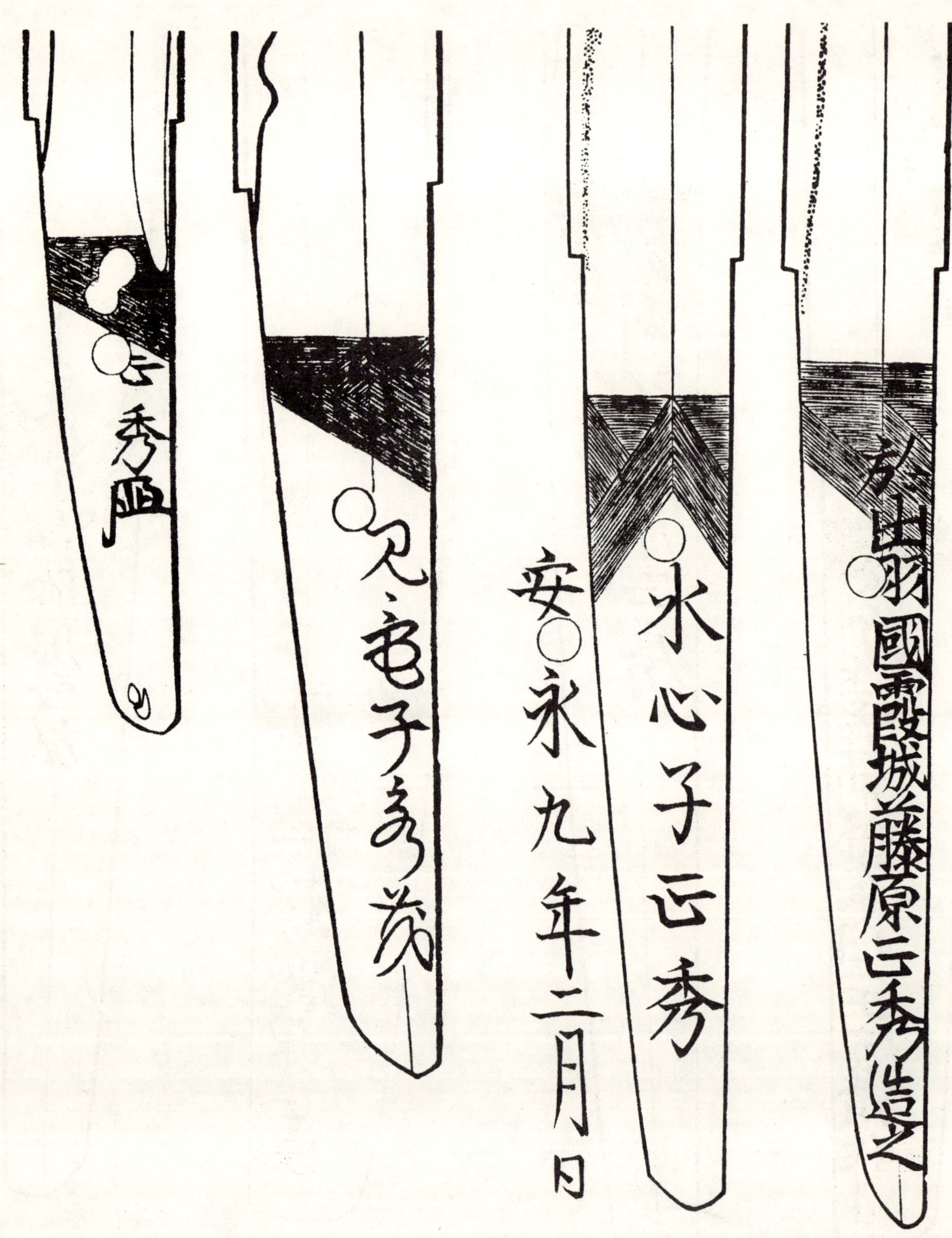
〇〇秀□

〇尺・屯子秀英

水心子正秀

安〇永九年二月日

〇出羽國〇段城主藤原正秀造之

Masahiro
MA 99

Masahiro
MA 100
Masanaga
MA 314

Masahiro
MA 100

Masahiro
MA 103

Masahisa
MA 131

肥前國河大掾藤原忠廣

肥州河大掾忠廣嫡子武藏守藤原正永

肥州河内守藤原忠廣

肥前國忠廣

肥列平戸住忠久

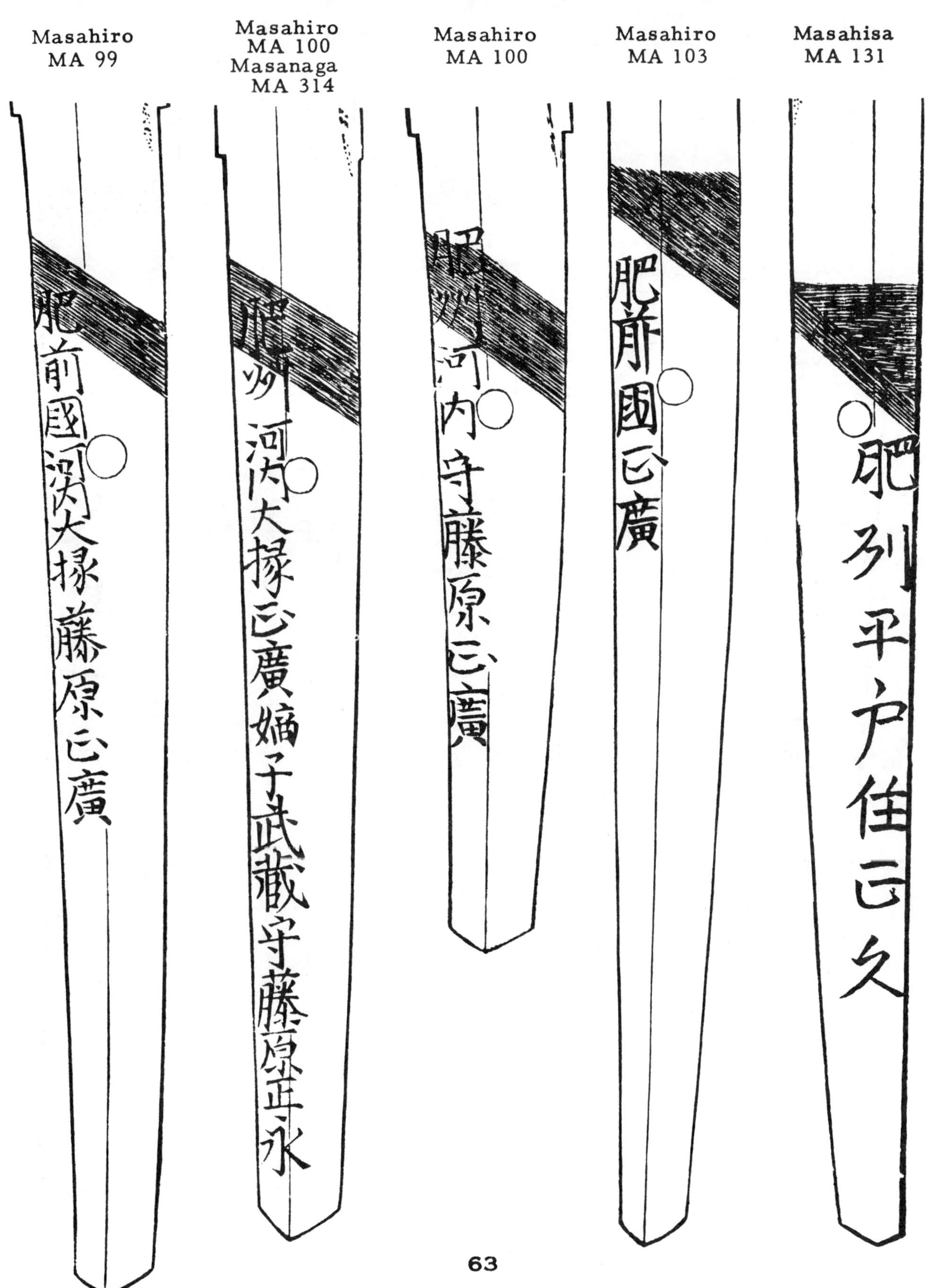

63

Masakane
MA 171

Masahisa
MA 131

Masakiyo MA 199

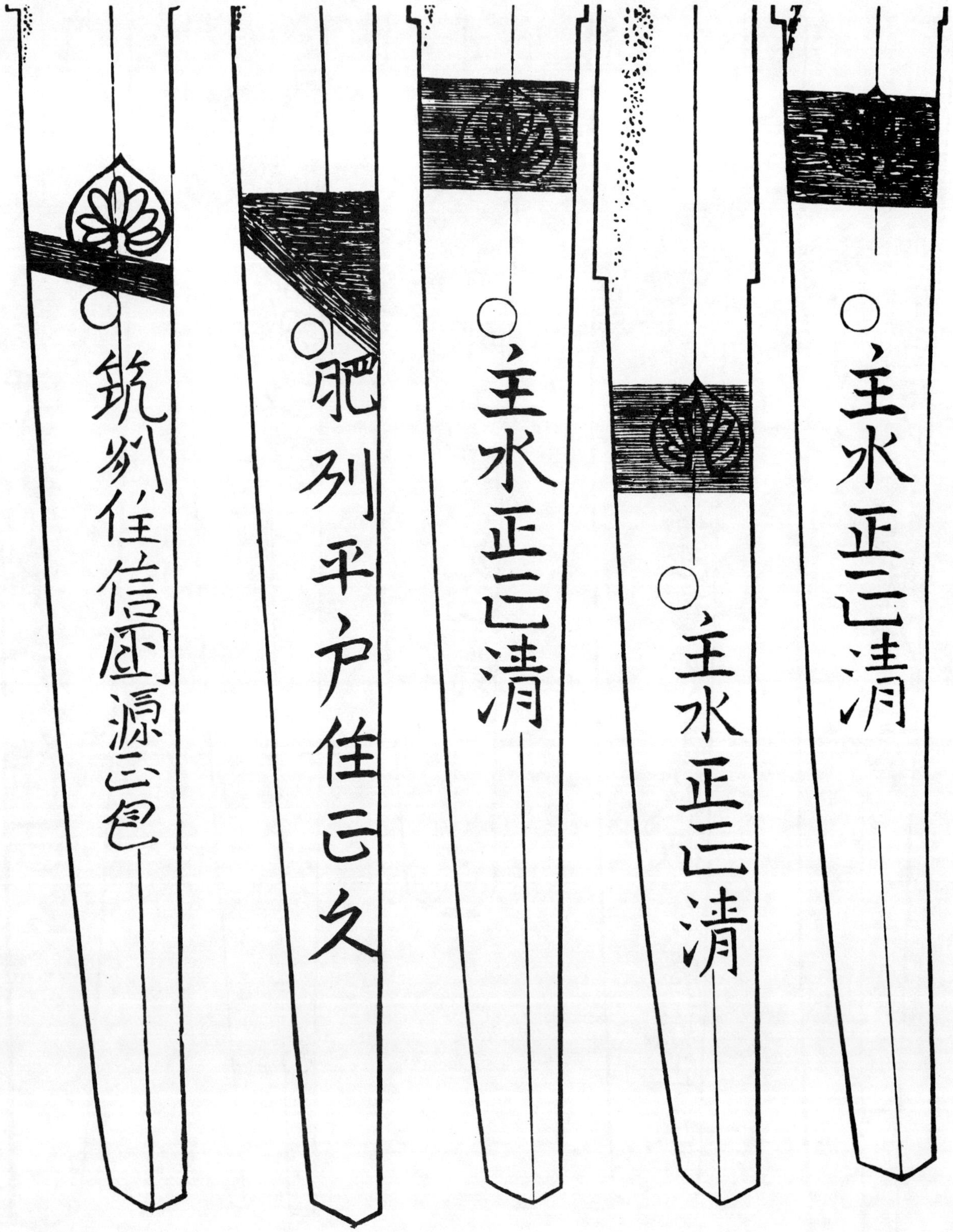

Masakiyo MA 199   Masakiyo MA 200   Masamori MA 282   Masashige MA 453

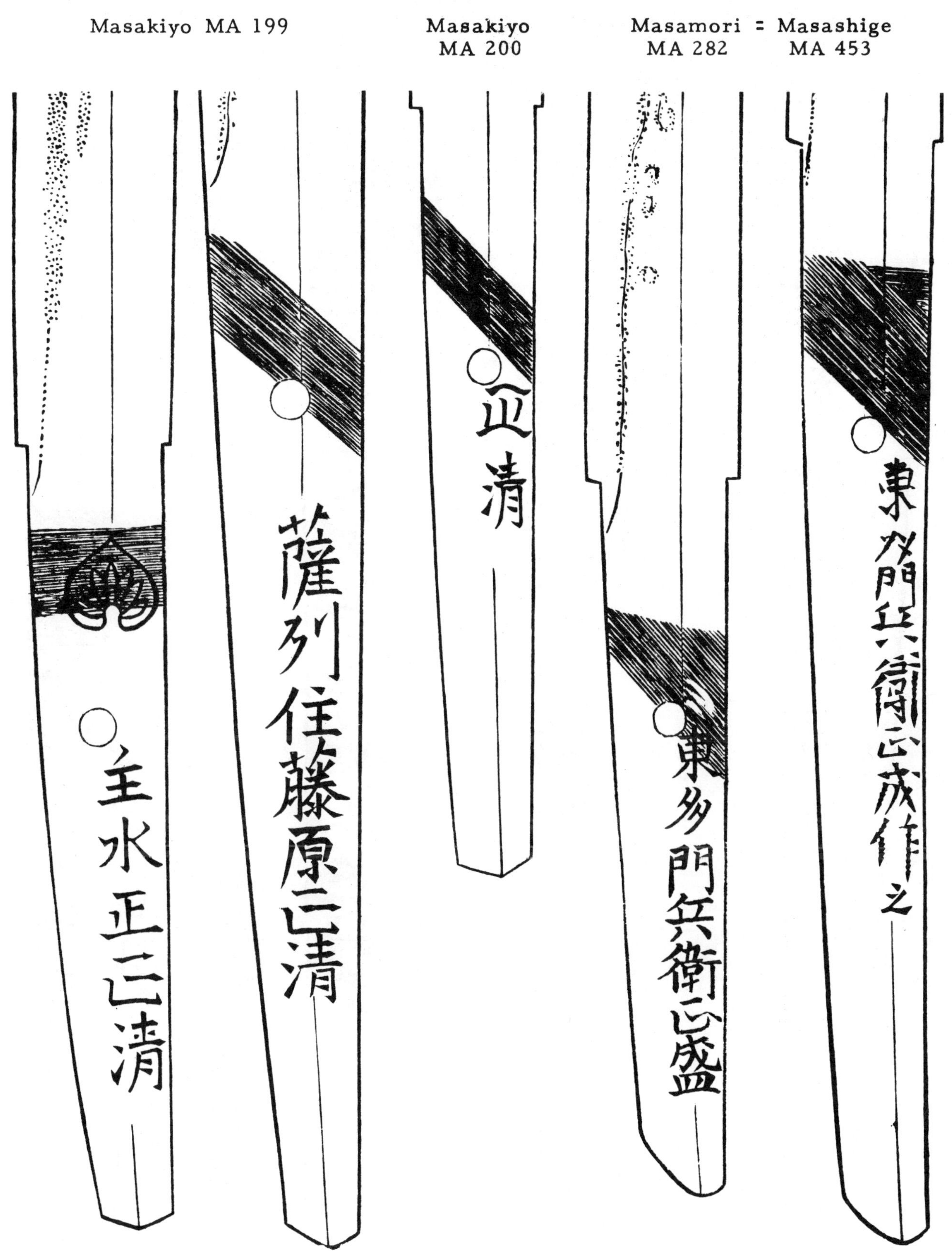

Masanao
MA 375

Masanori
MA 384

Masashige MA 484

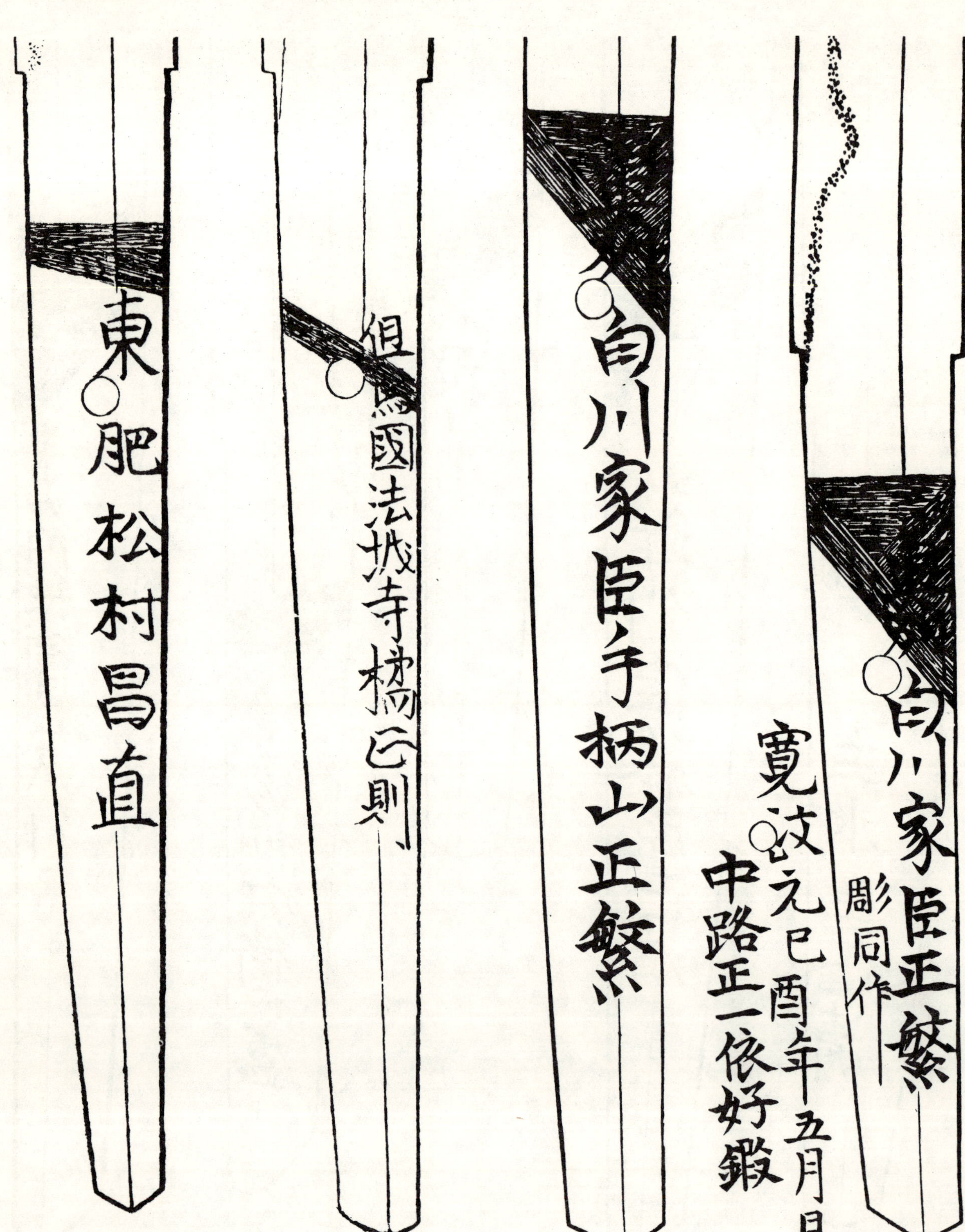

SHINTO BENGI OSHIGATA

Masashige MA 484

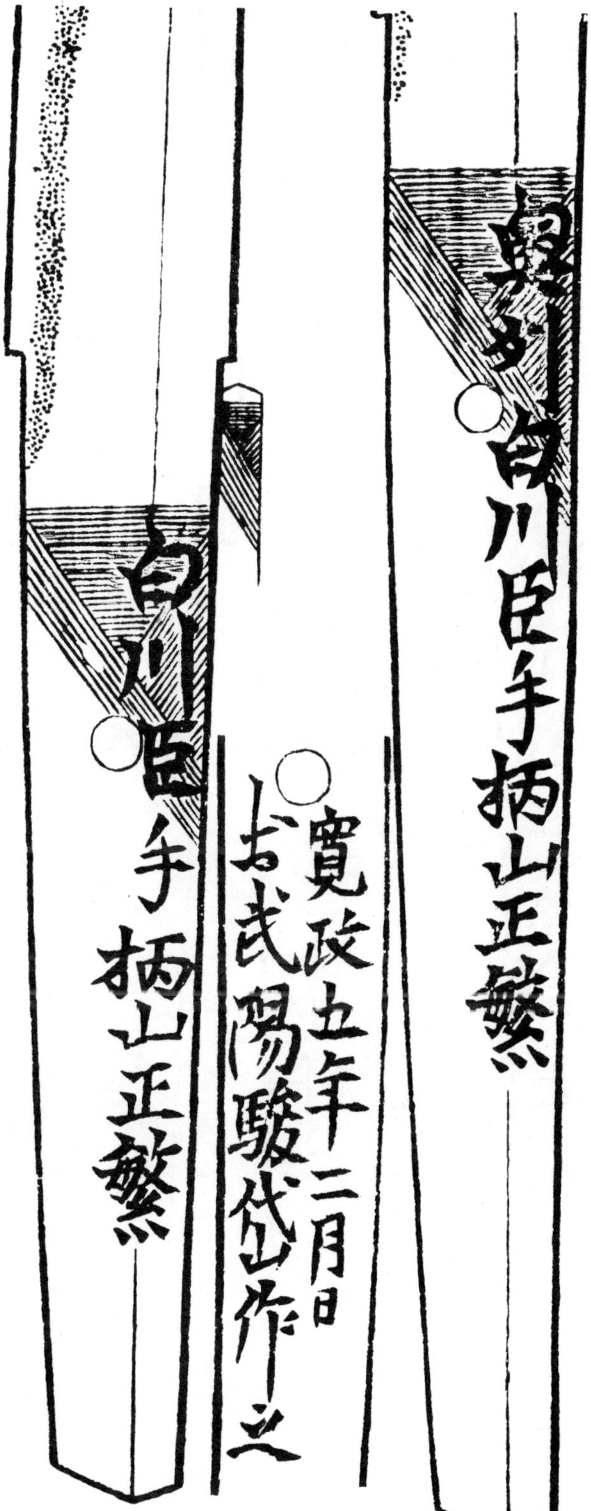

Masashige MA 466

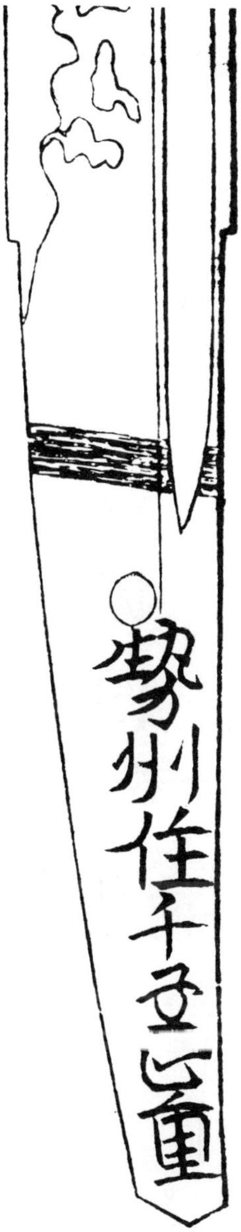

Masatake MA 504

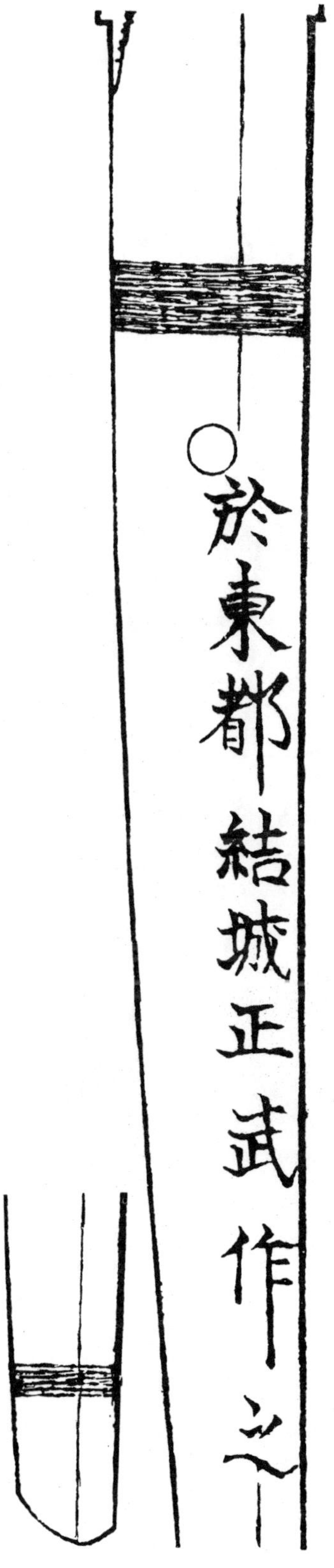

勢州住午正重

白川臣手柄山正繁

手柄山正繁

寛政五年二月日

於武陽駿代出作之

奥州白川臣手柄山正繁

於東都結城正武作之

Masatoshi MA 565

Masatoshi
MA 566

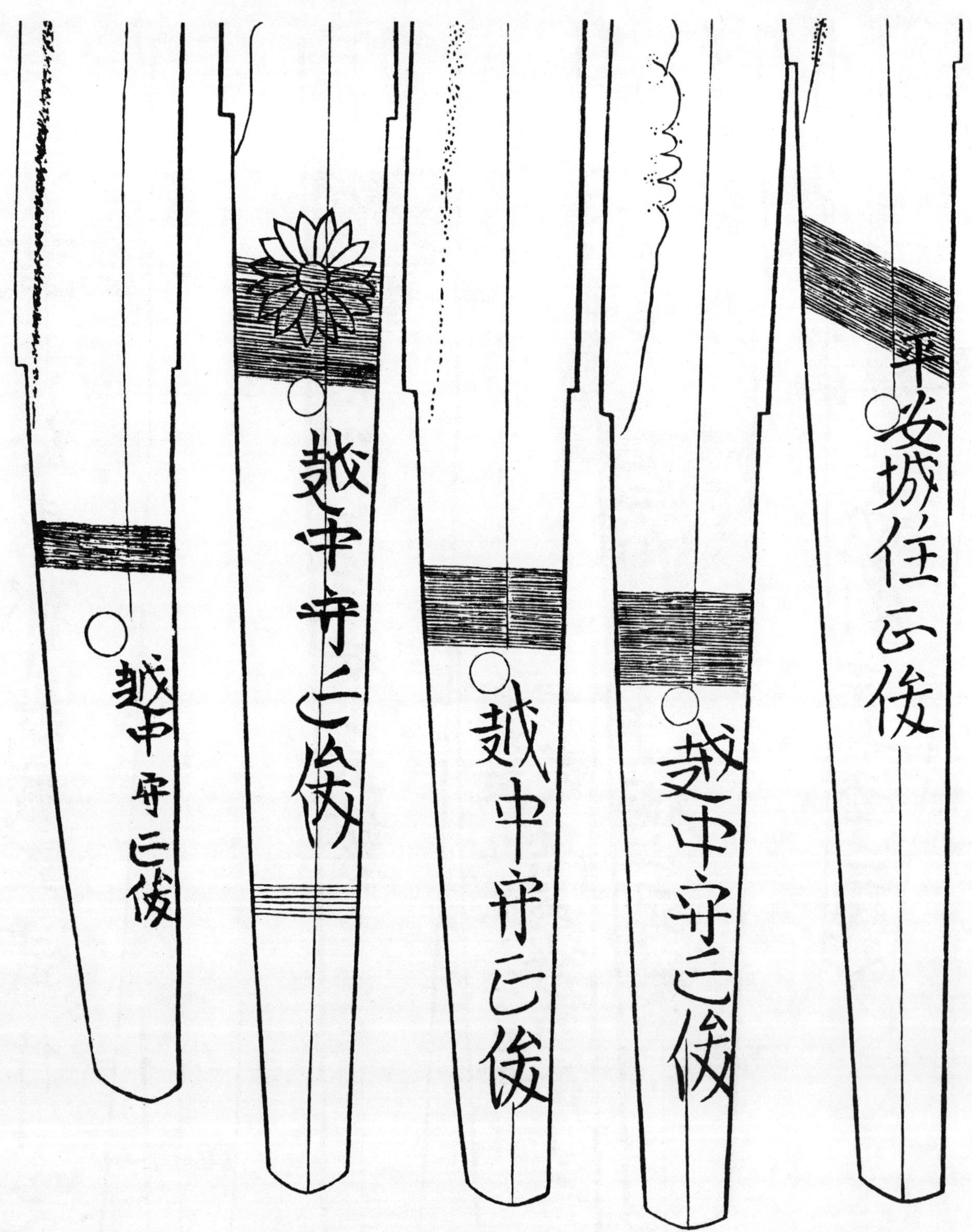

Masatsugu
MA 585

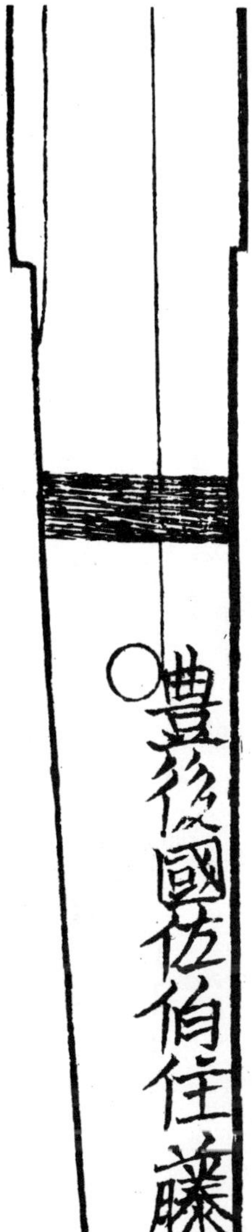

Masatsugu
MA 612

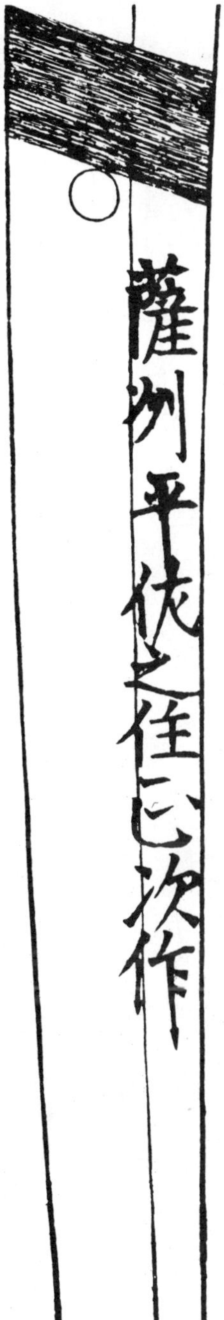

Masatsugu ＝ Tsuguhira
MA 626 TS 92

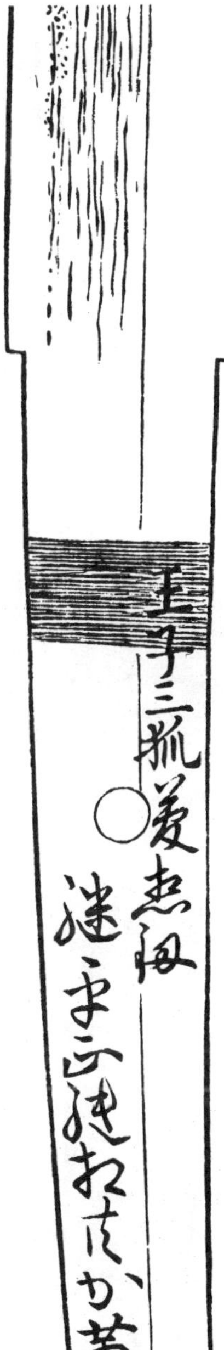

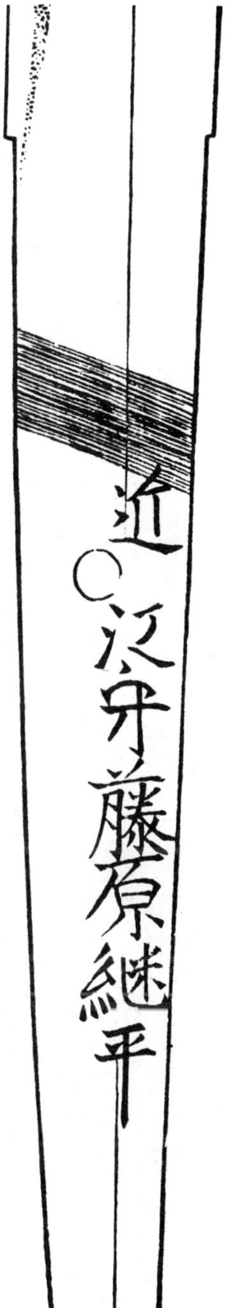

豊後國佐伯住藤原正次

薩州平伏之住正次作

土子三抓菱恵板
継ま云使われた、か黄金造

近江守藤原継平

Masayoshi MA 697

Masayuki
MA 738

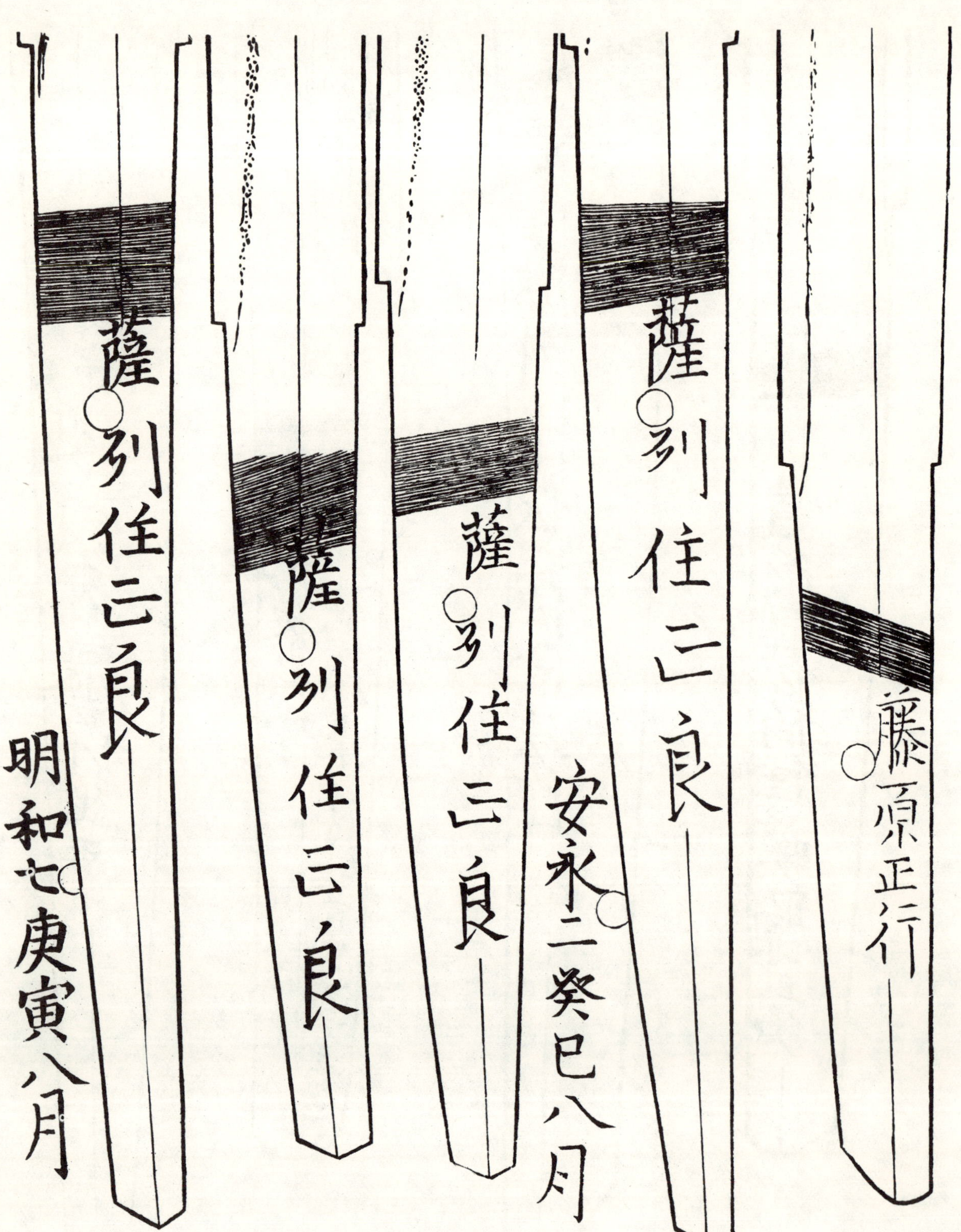

| Masakuni MA 776 | Masamitsu MA 781 | Masanari MA 906 | Masatsugu MA 837a | Masahiro MA 865 |

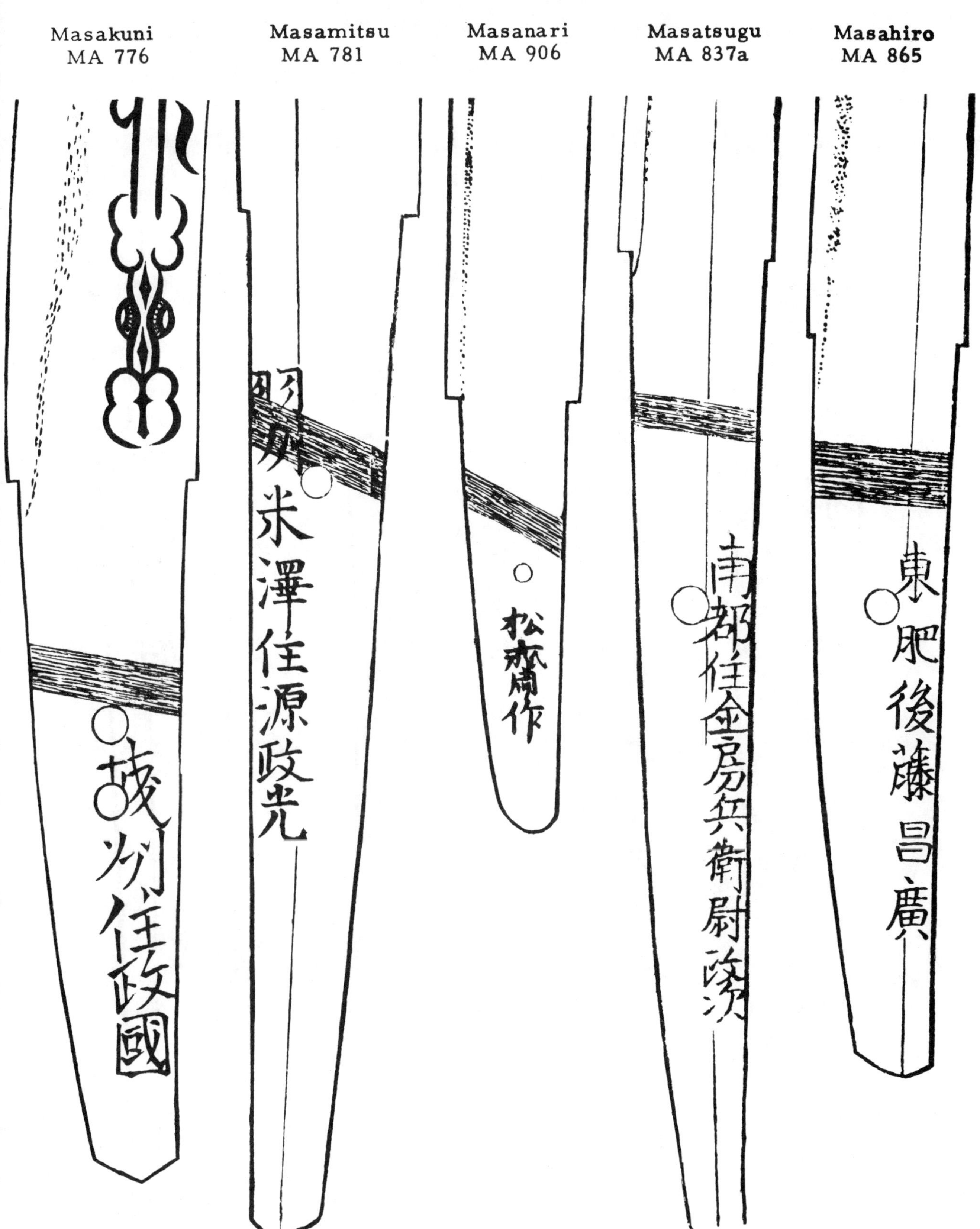

Masanao MA 875   Masatsune MA 885 / Toshimasa TO 503   Masanori MA 889

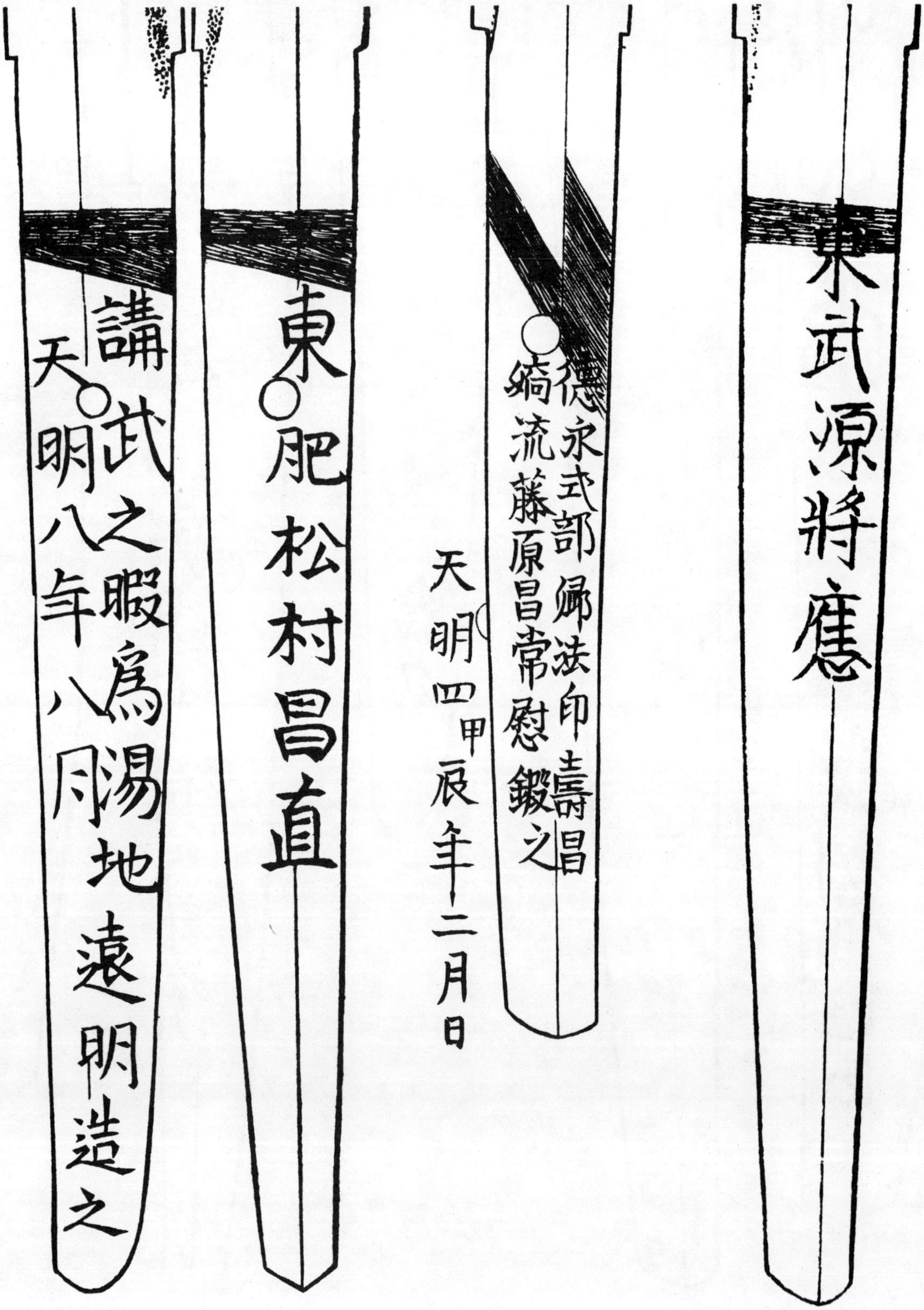

講○武之暇爲湯地遠明造之

天明八年八月

東○肥 松村昌直

德永式部婦法印壽昌

○瘸流藤原昌常慰鍛之

天明四甲辰年二月日

東武源將應

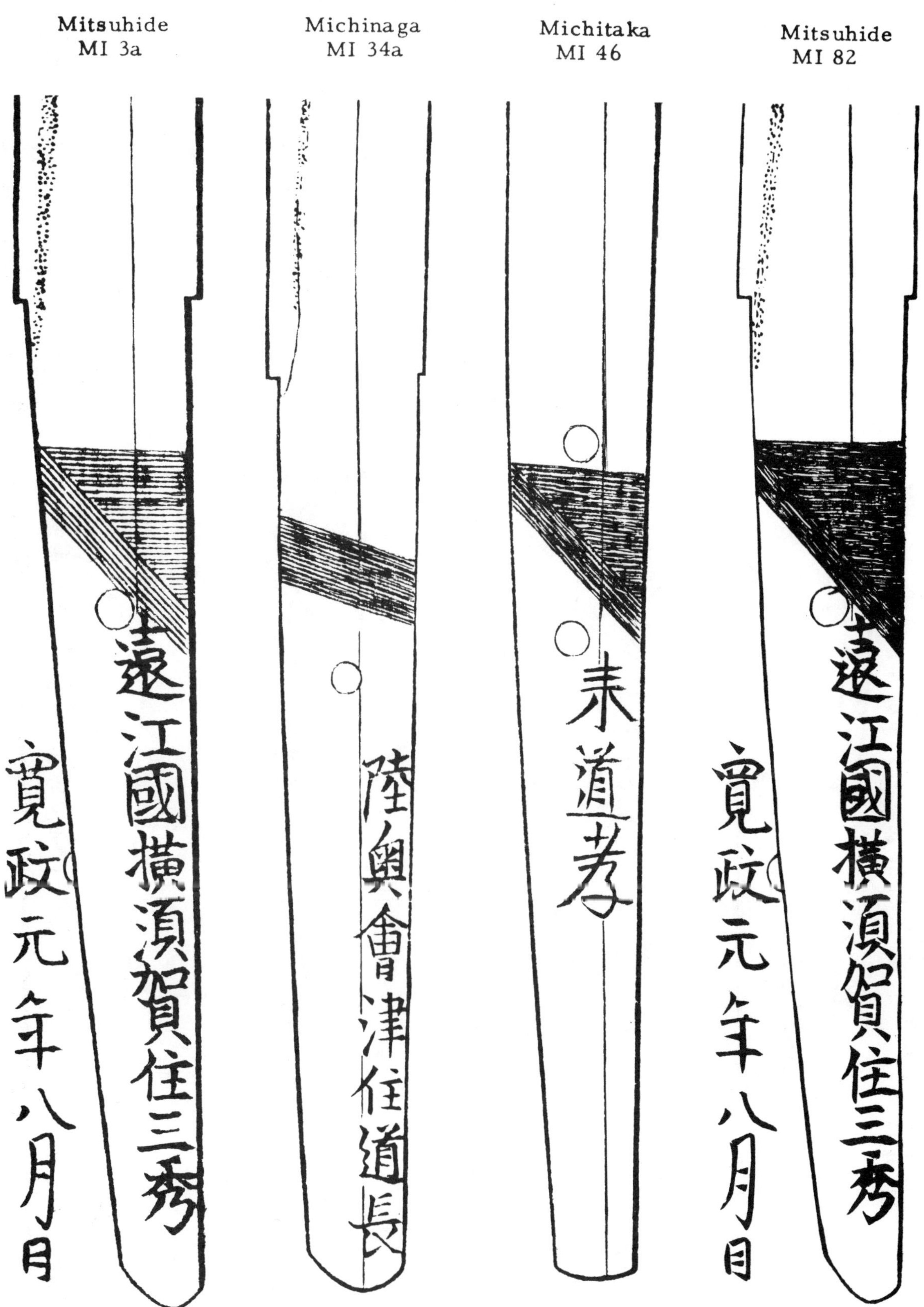

Mitsuhide
MI 3a
Michinaga
MI 34a
Michitaka
MI 46
Mitsuhide
MI 82
遠江國横須賀住三秀
寛政元年八月日
陸奥會津住道長
未道芳
遠江國横須賀住三秀
寛政元年八月日

Mitsumasa MI 143	Mitsumasa MI 145	Morikuni MO 351	Morinaga MO 398

煉拾八幡燈　淬於釜割泉　三郎兵衛光忠造

○安永八年冬廣

信圓光昌造

安永○六子八月日

和泉守来院盛國作

○相摸守藤原盛永

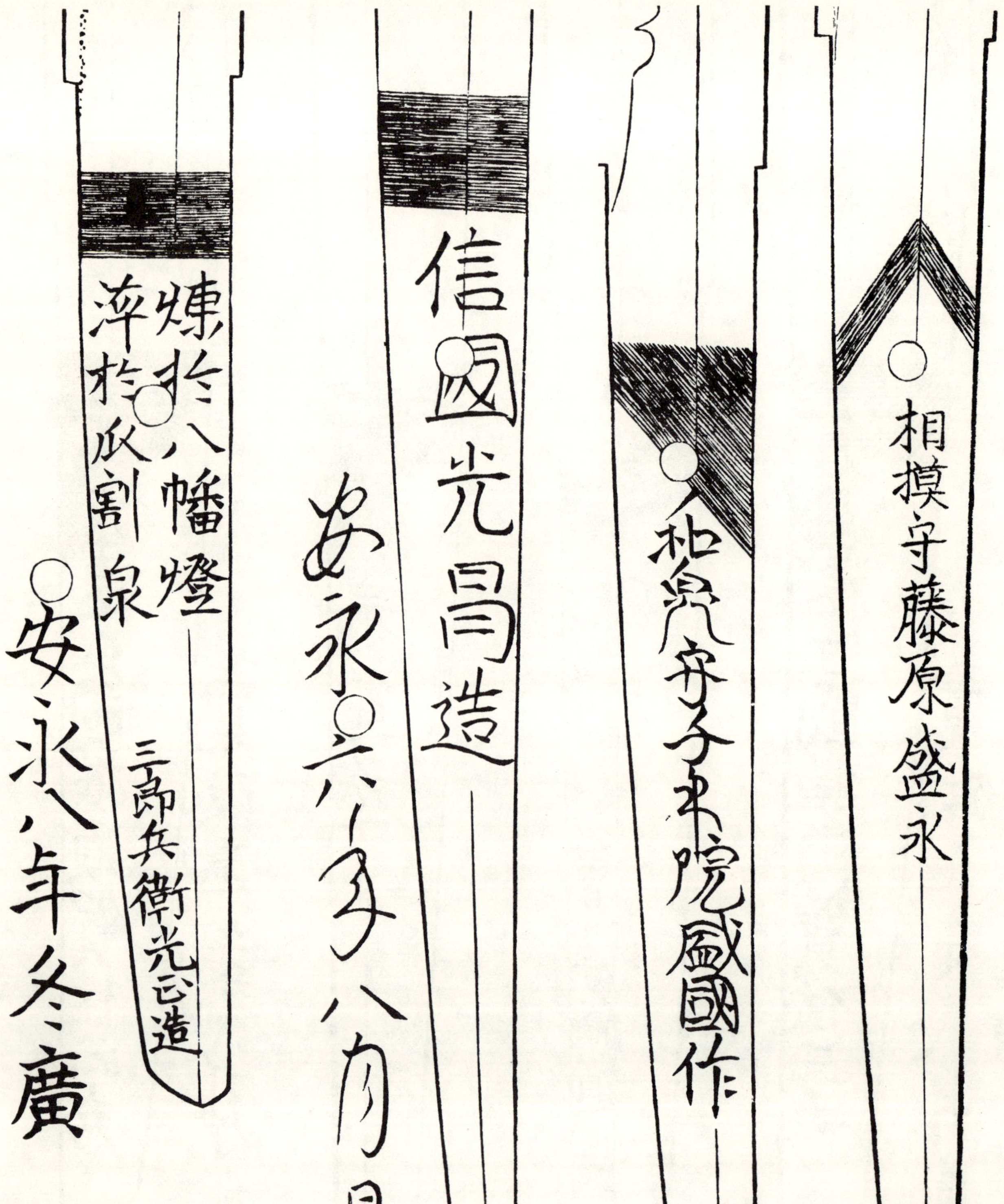

Moritsuna MO 514	Moriyoshi MO 531	Moriyuki MO 547	Motohira MO 586

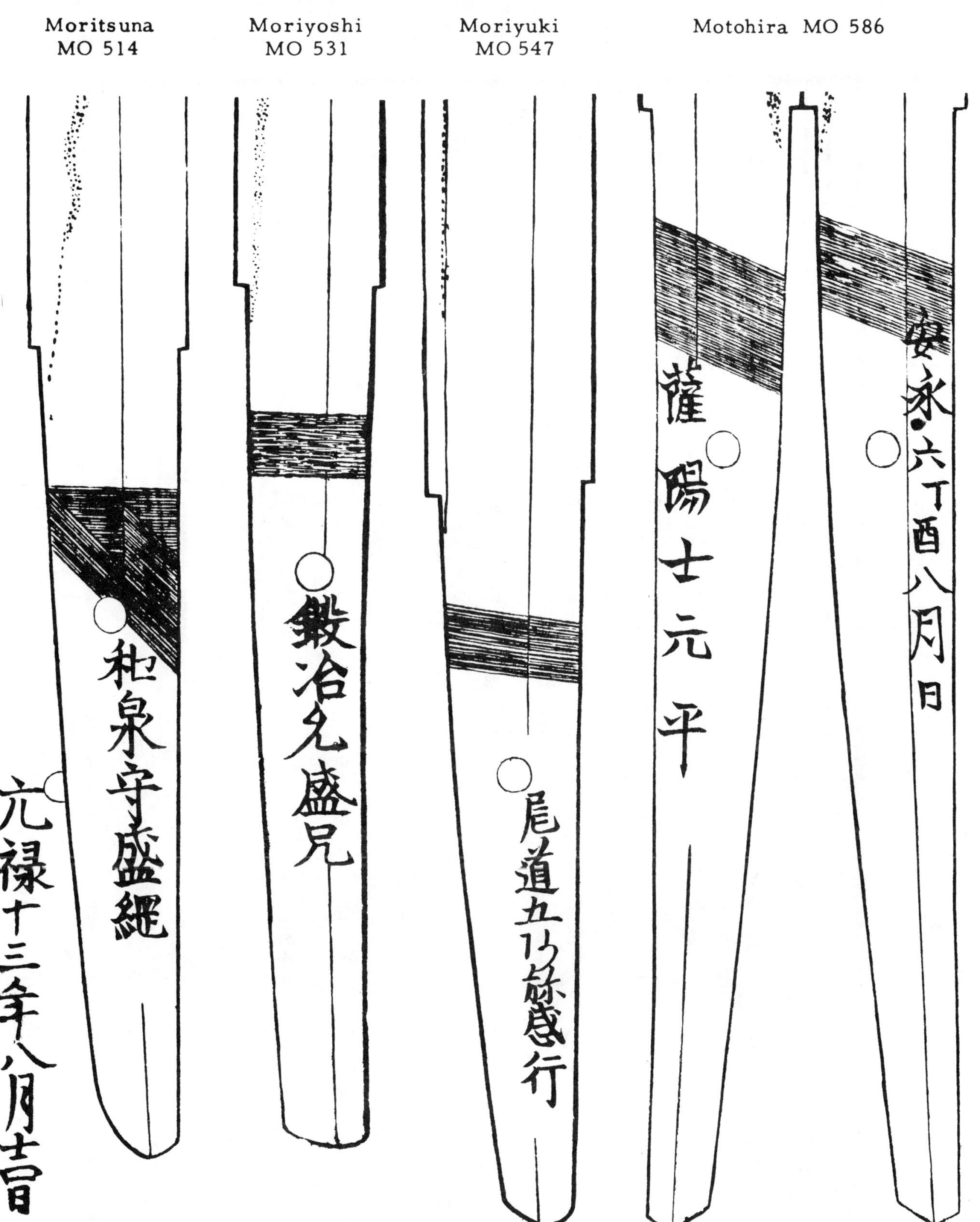

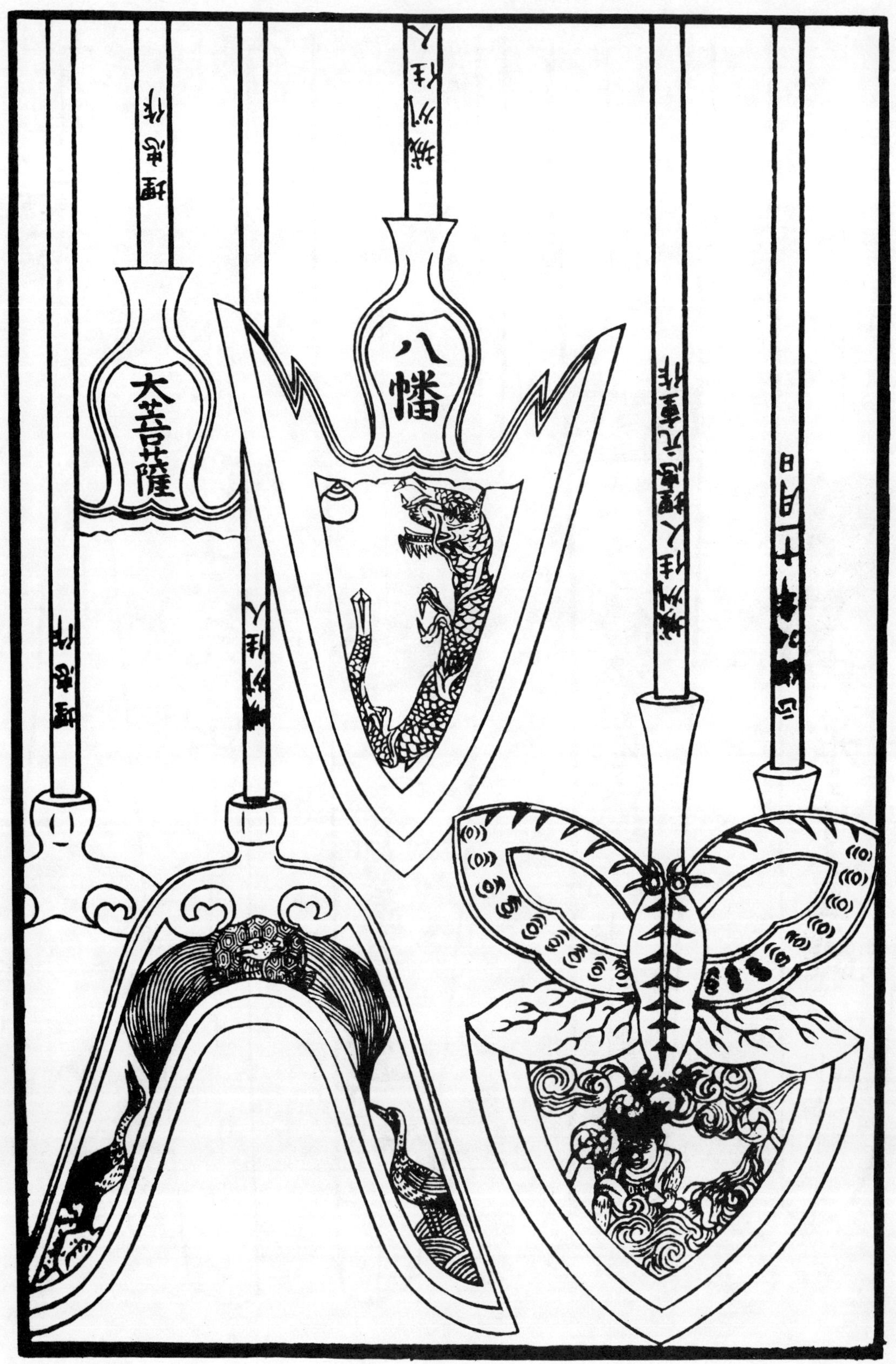

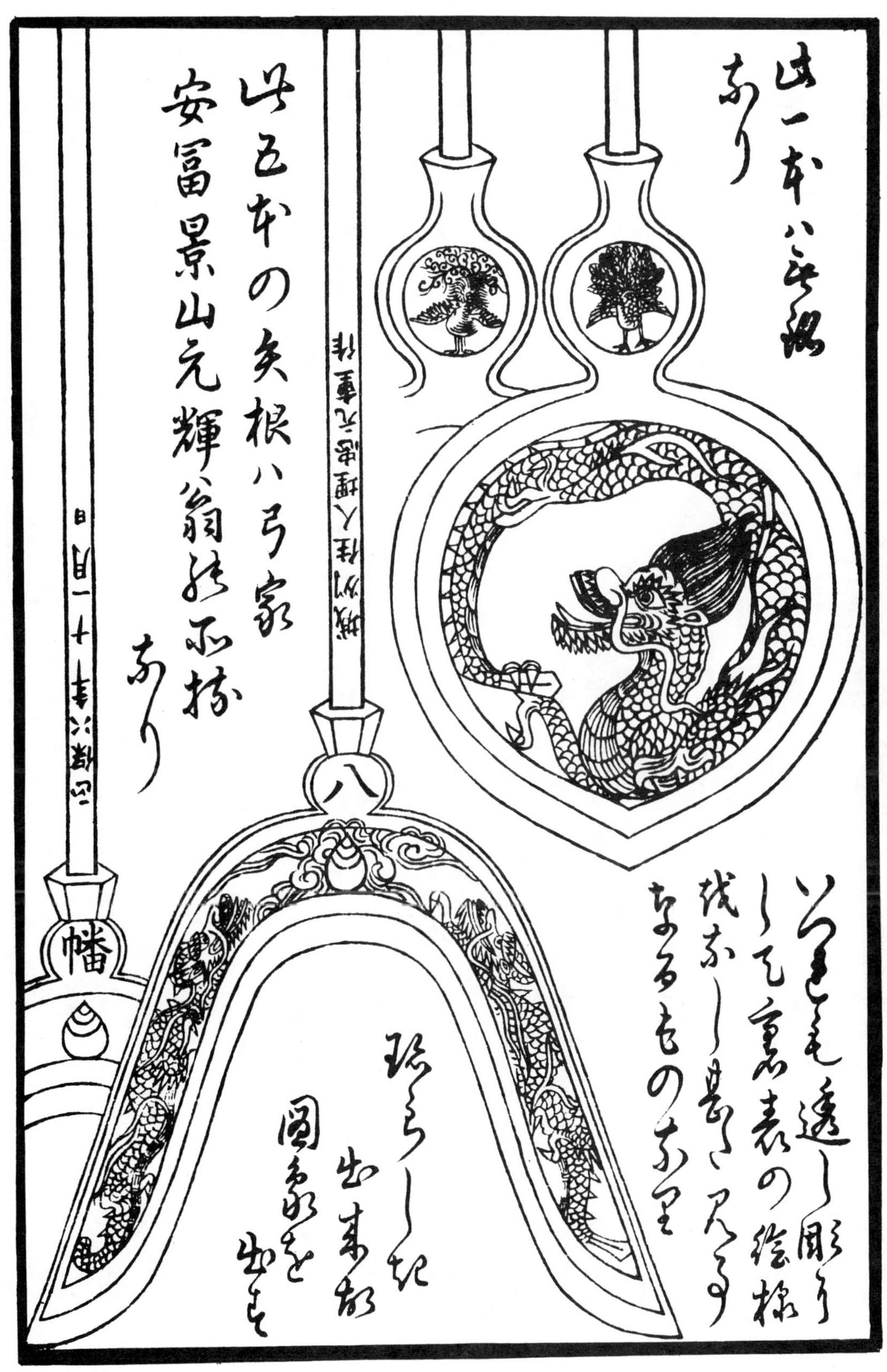

Motohira MO 586   Motonao MO 624   Motoyasu MO 664

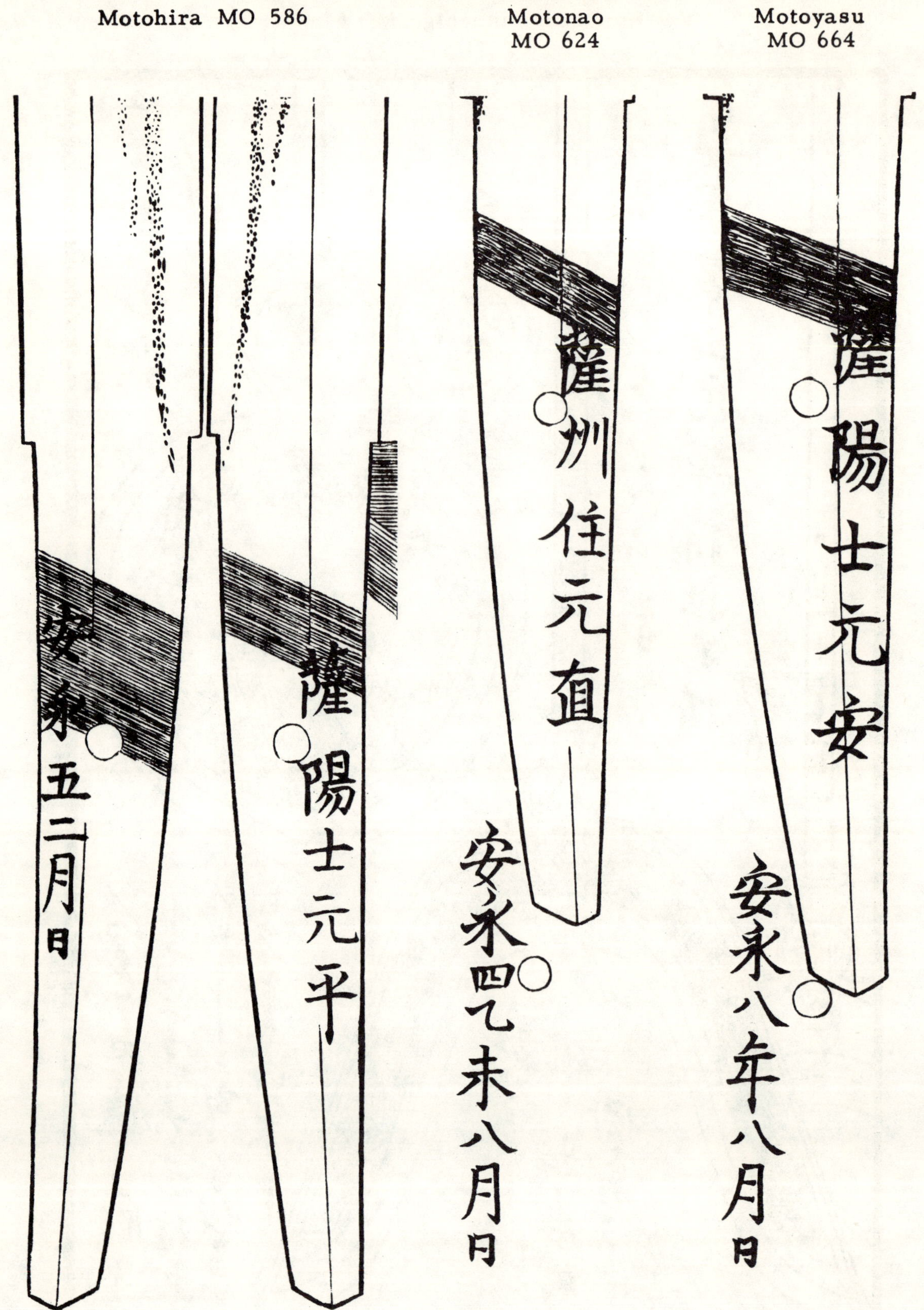

Munenaga
MU 147 — 常州住藤原宗永

常陸守宗重

Muneshige MU 203 — 常陸守宗重

常陸大掾宗重

Munetoshi
MU 234 — 常州近藤宗利

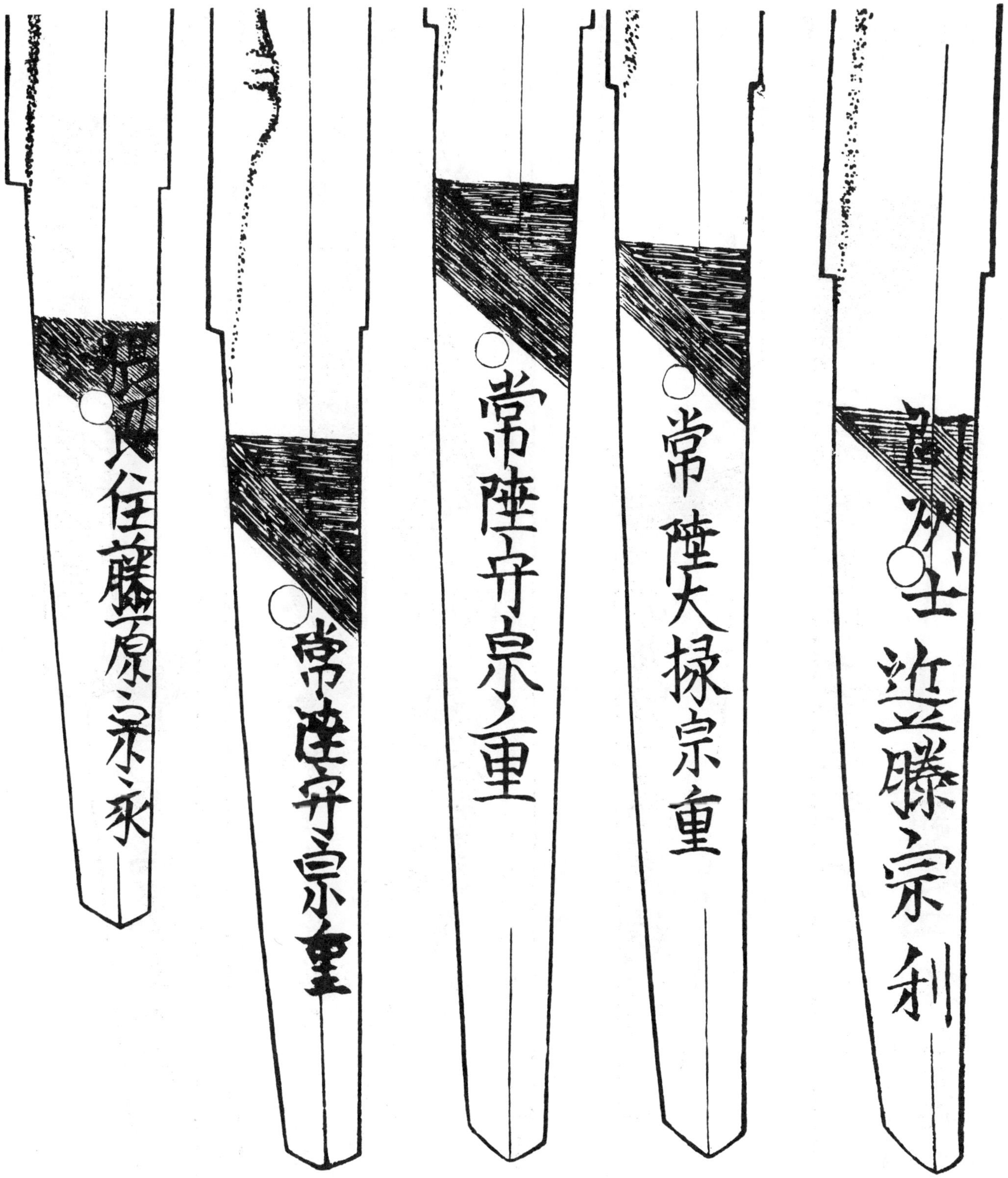

Munetsugu
MU 278

Muneyuki
MU 379

Umetada Myoju MY 2

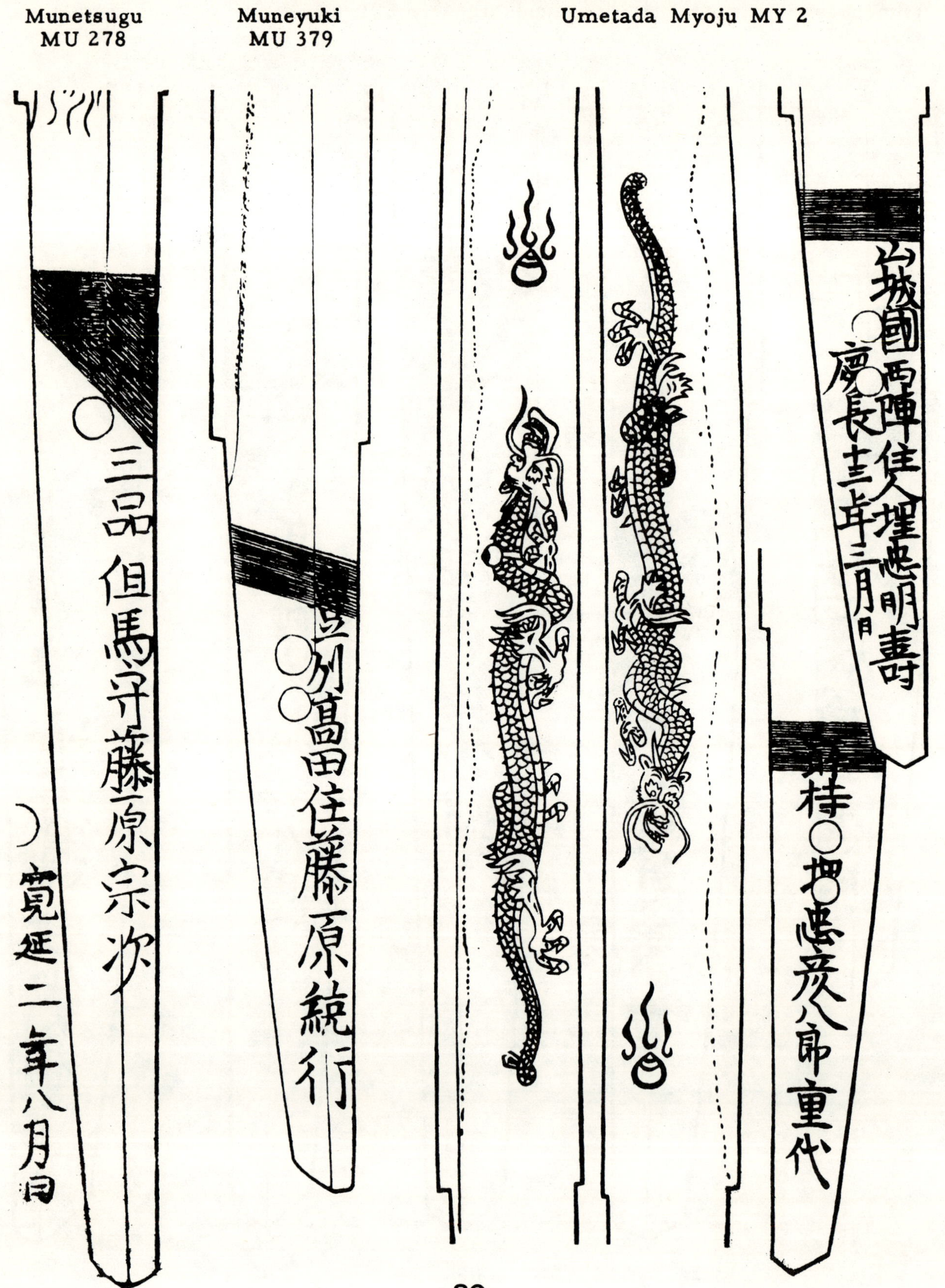

山城國西陳住埋忠明壽作

埋忠明壽

刻物埋忠七左

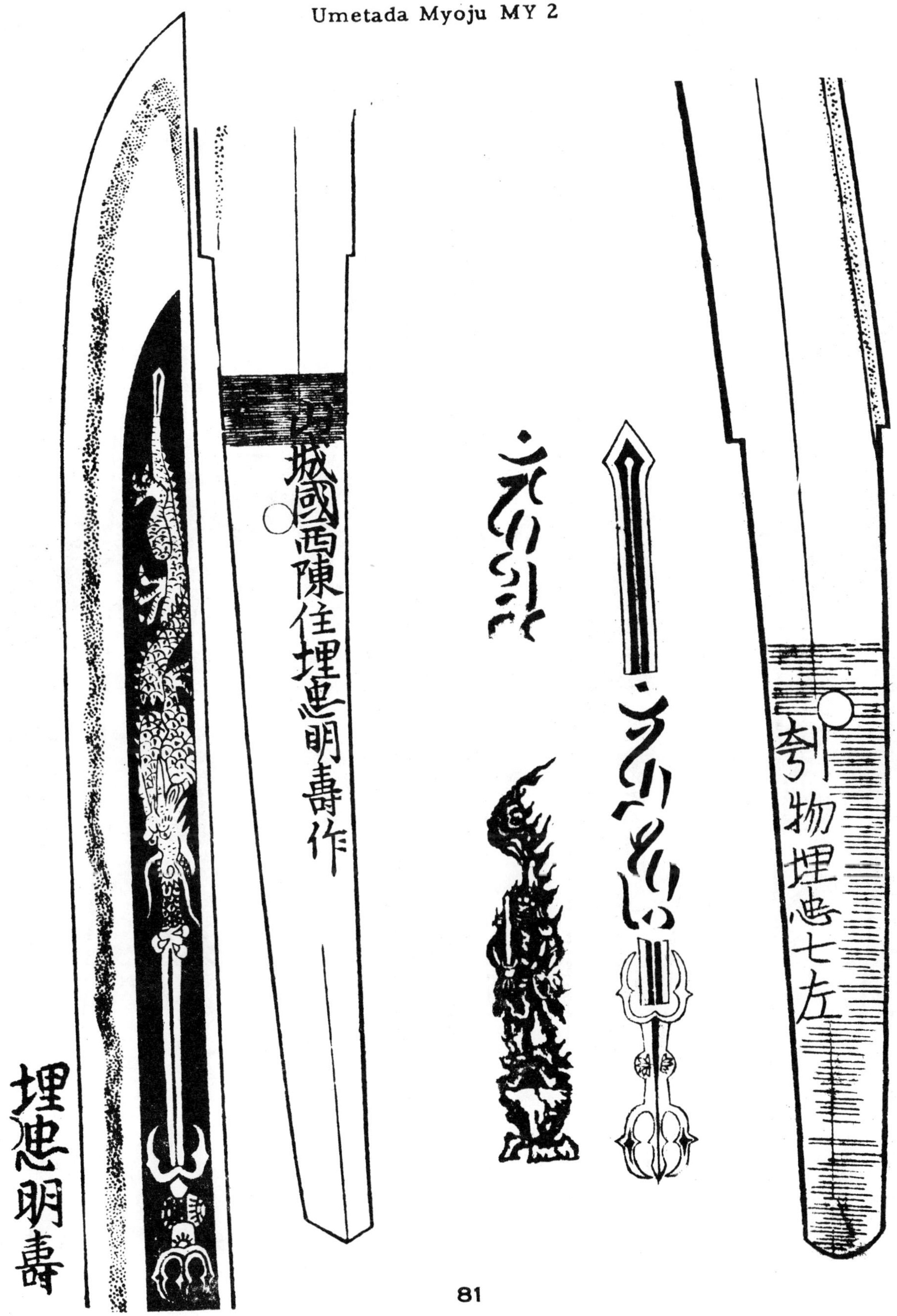

Nagakuni NA 21   Nagamichi NA 28   Nagashige NA 56 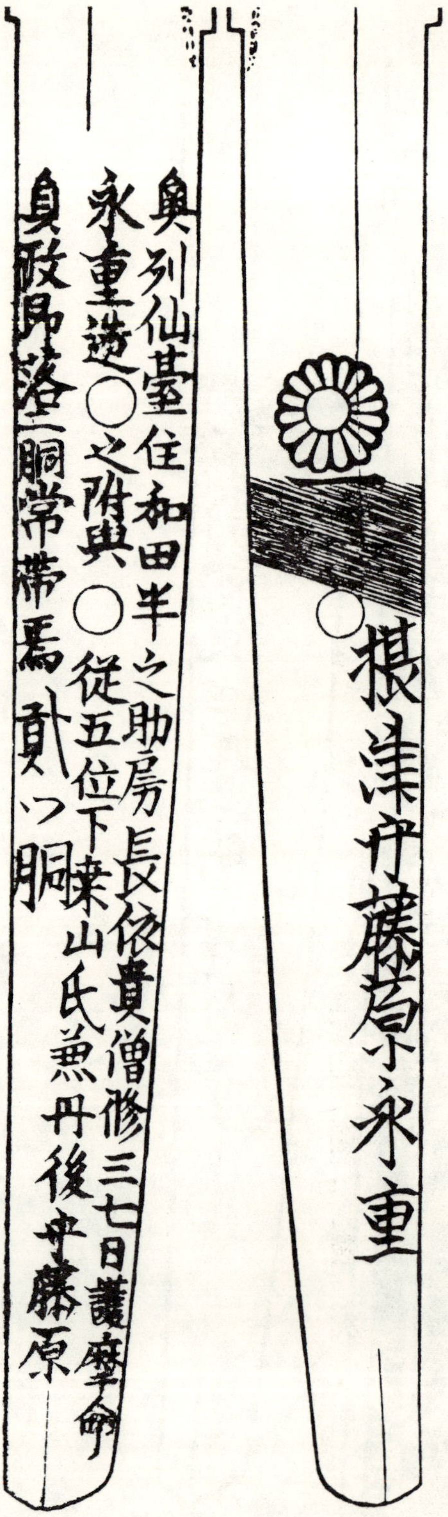   Nagashige NA 57

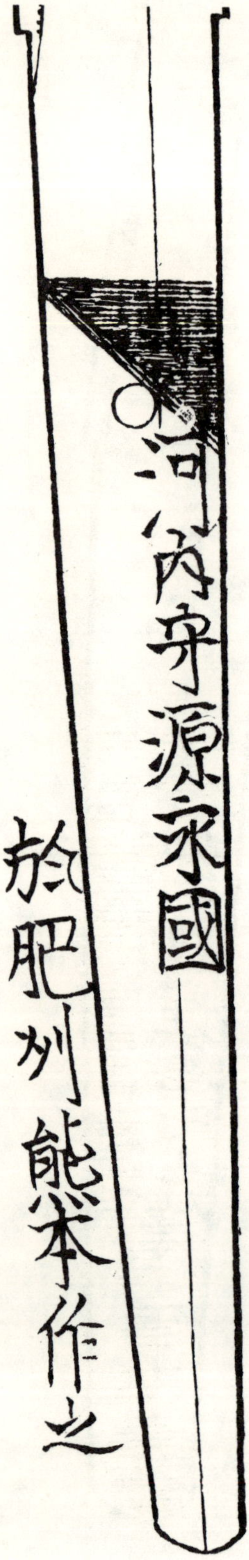

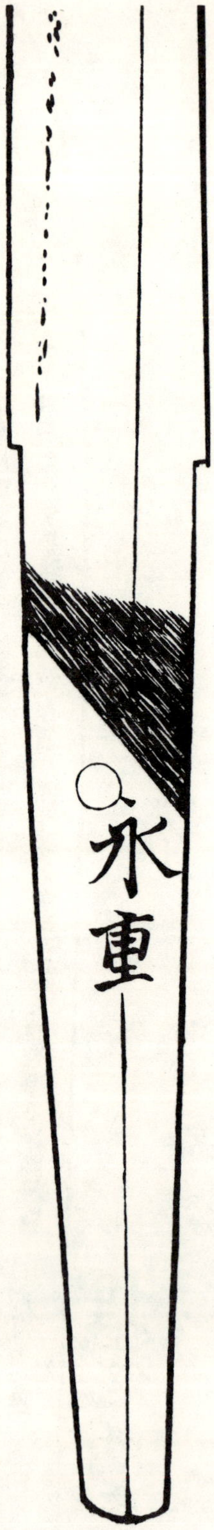

河内守源永國
於肥州熊本作之

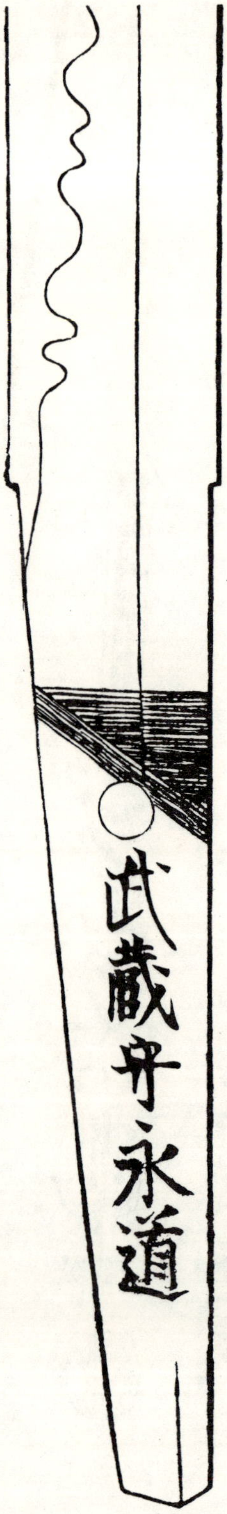

武蔵守永道

奥列仙臺住和田半之助房長依貞僧修三七日護摩○命
永重造○之附與○従五位下棘山氏薫丹後平藤原
貞政所落一胴常帶焉貮つ胴

摂津守藤原永重

永重

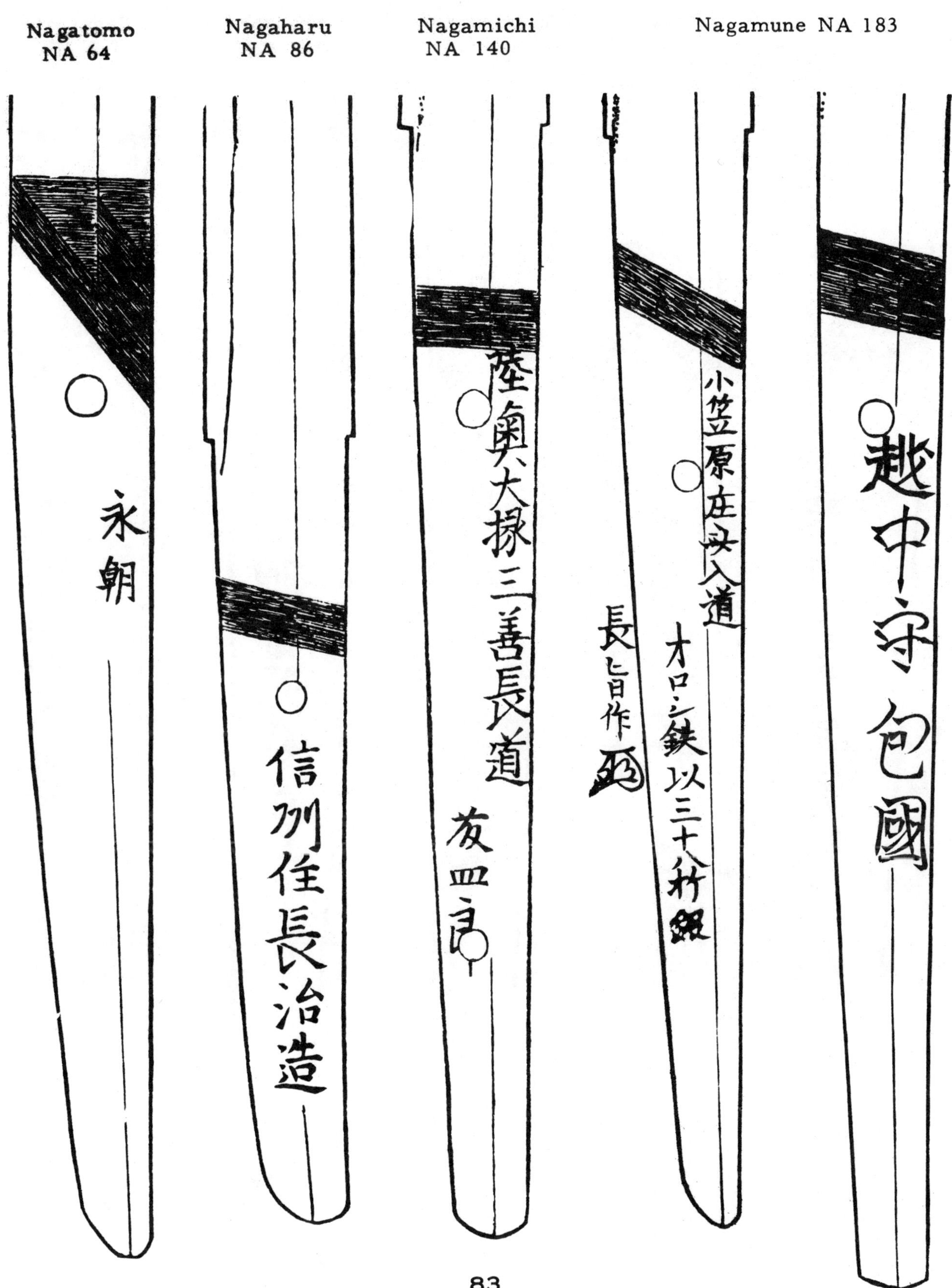
Nagatomo
NA 64
Nagaharu
NA 86
Nagamichi
NA 140
Nagamune NA 183
永朝
信州住長治造
陸奥大掾三善長道
友皿良
小笠原庄頭入道
オロシ鉄以三十八貫鍛
長旨作
越中守包國

Naganobu NA 198	Nagatsuna & Tadatsuna NA 248 TA 129	Nagayoshi NA 276	Nagayoshi NA 283

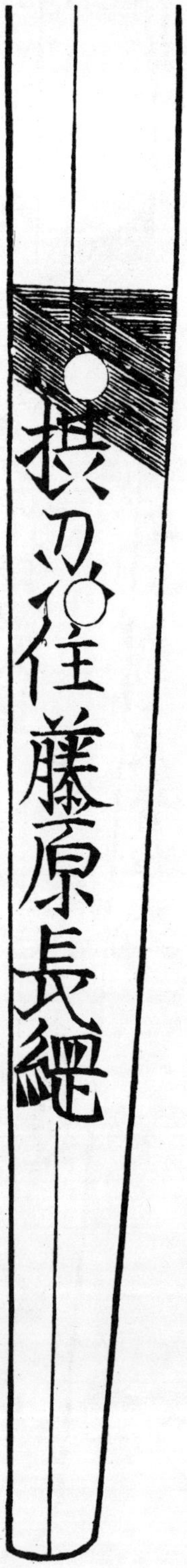

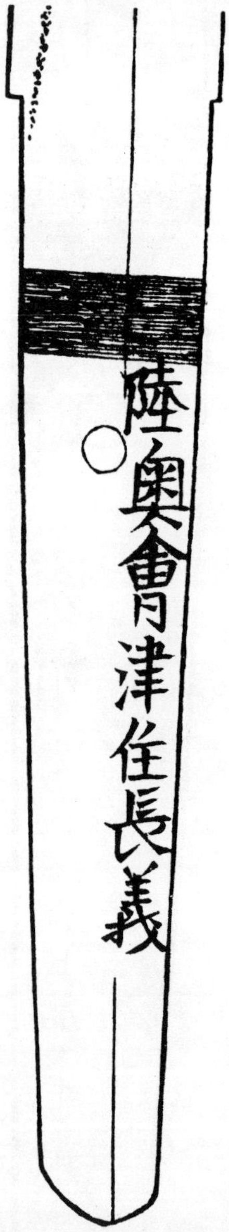

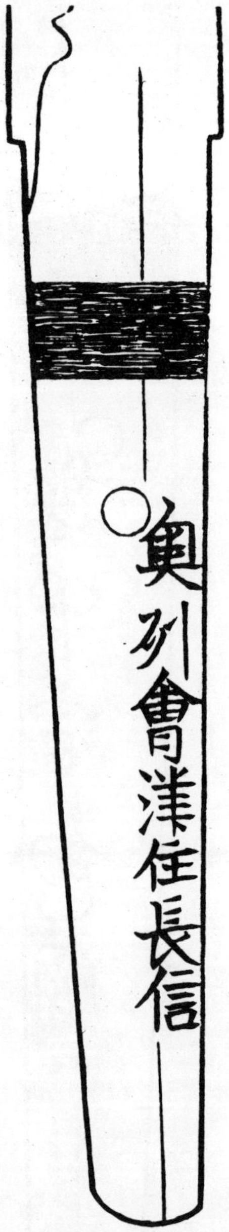

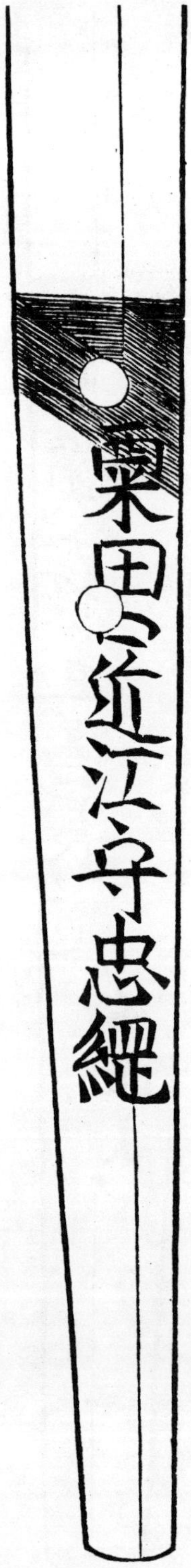

奥州會津住長信

摂刀住藤原長繩

粟田近江守忠繩

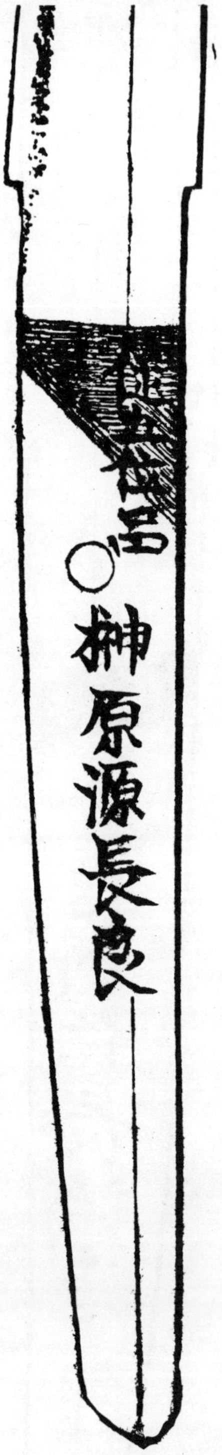

榊原源長良

陸奥會津住長義

Nagayuki
NA 292

Naomichi
NA 346

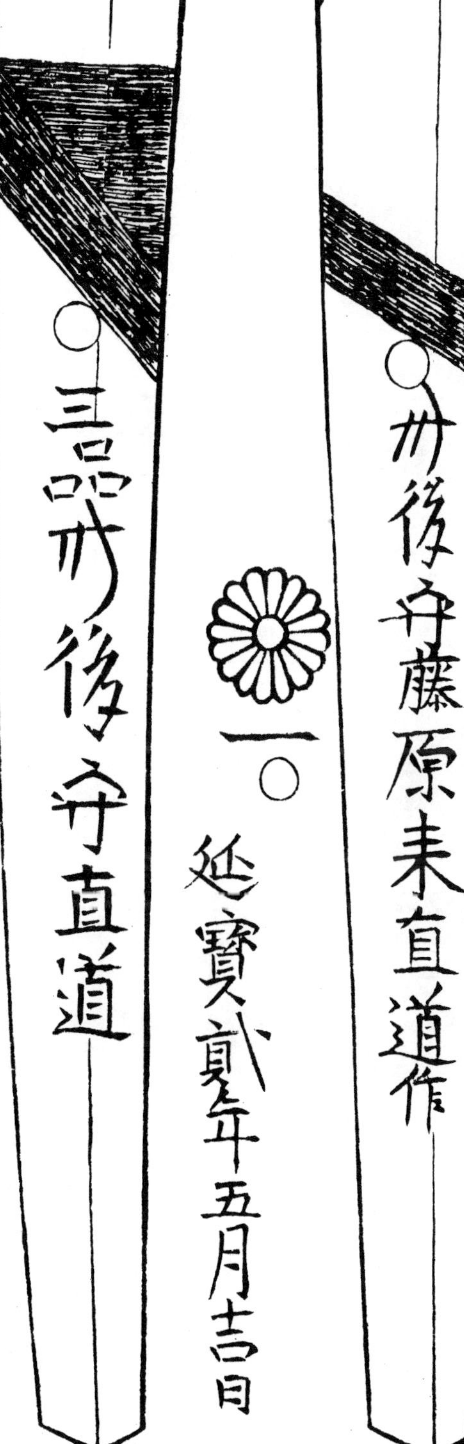

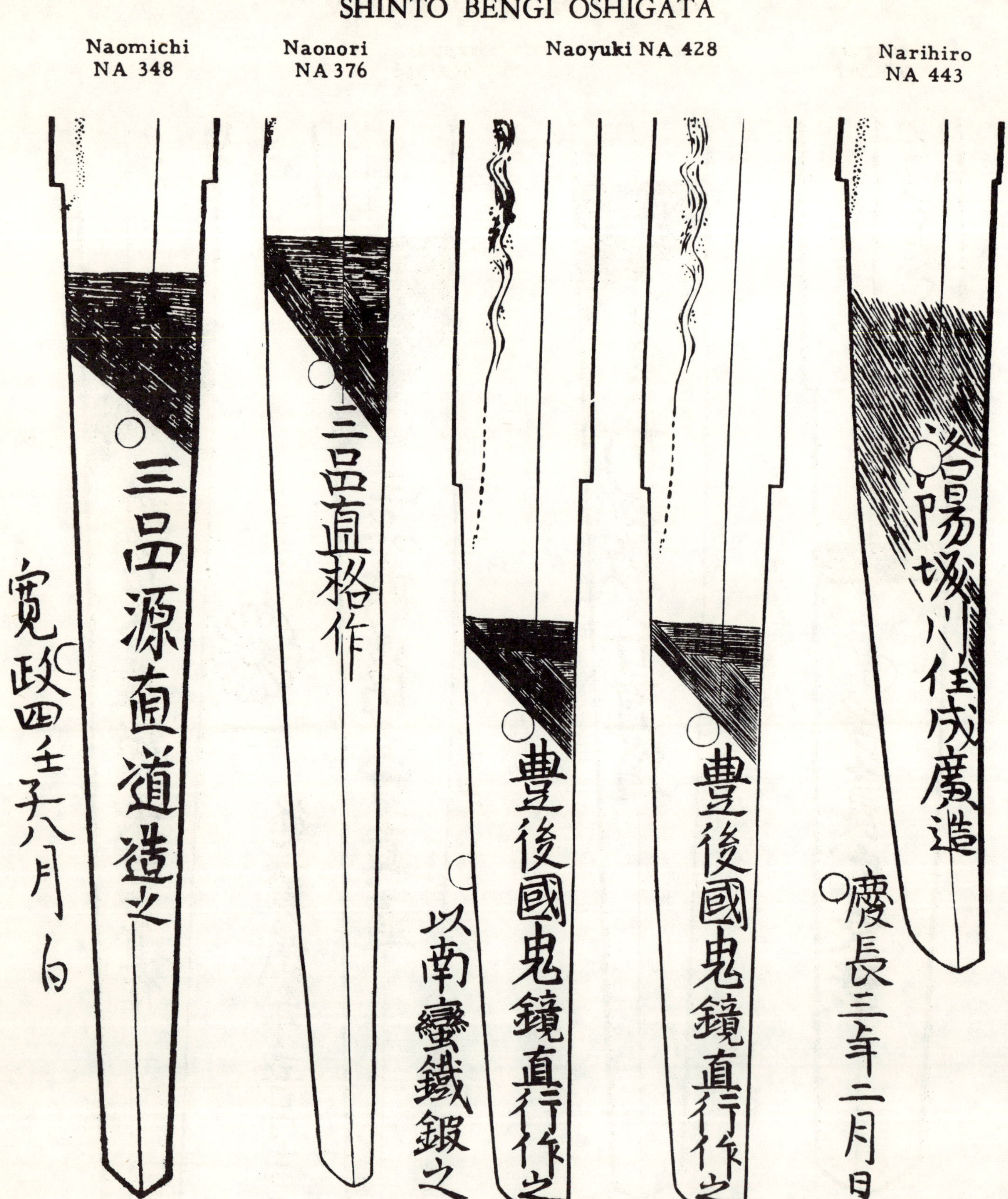
Naomichi
NA 348
Naonori
NA 376
Naoyuki NA 428
Narihiro
NA 443
三品源直道造之
寛政四壬子八月日
三品直裕作
豊後國鬼鏡直行作之
以南蠻鐵鍛之
豊後國鬼鏡直行作之
洛陽城川住戌廣造
慶長三年二月日

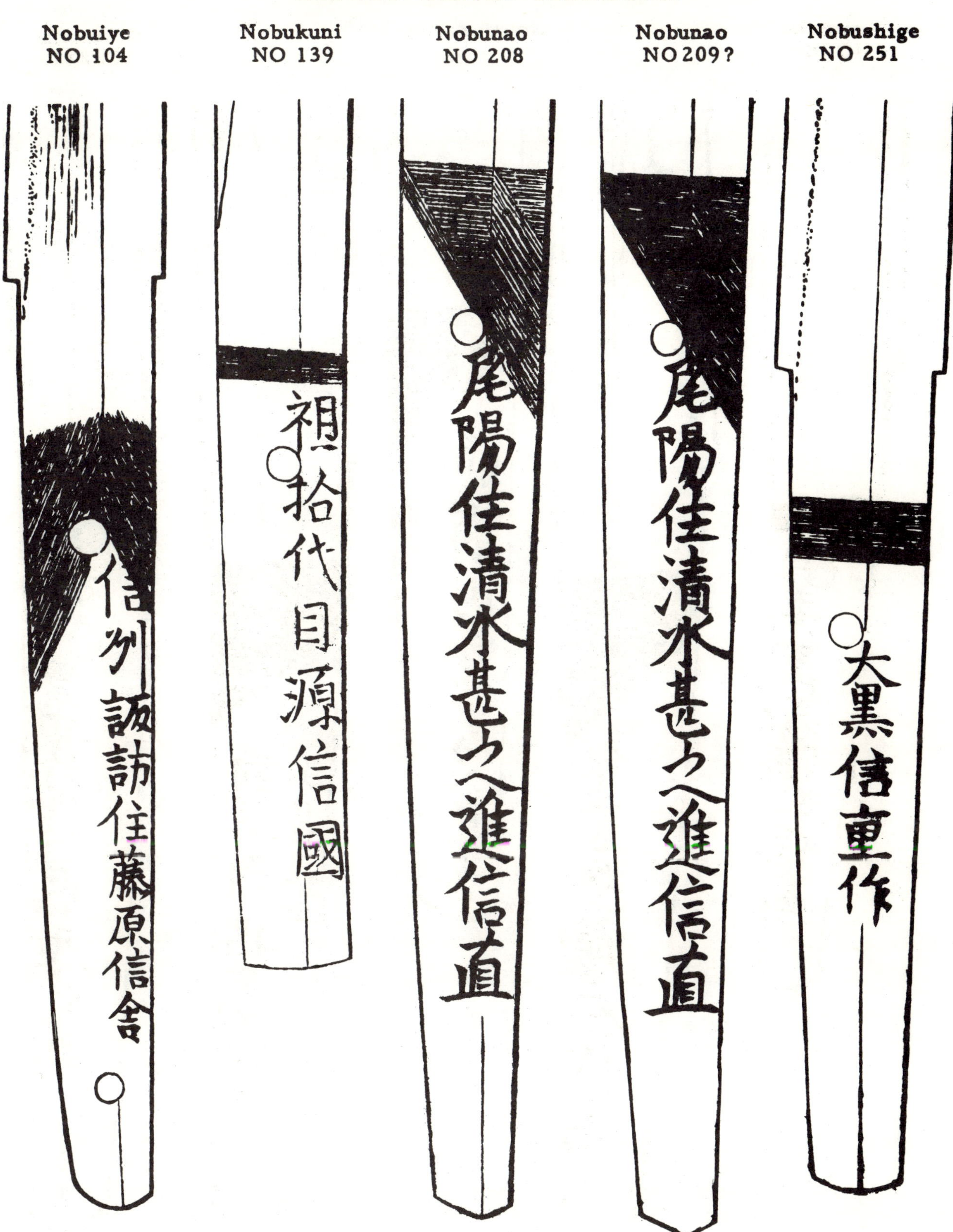

Nobuiye
NO 104
信州諏訪住藤原信舎
Nobukuni
NO 139
祖拾代目源信國
Nobunao
NO 208
尾陽住清水甚ろ〳進信直
Nobunao
NO 209?
尾陽住清水甚ろ〳進信直
Nobushige
NO 251
大黒信重作

**Nobutaka
NO 259**

Nobutaka NO 260

**Nobutoshi
NO 289**

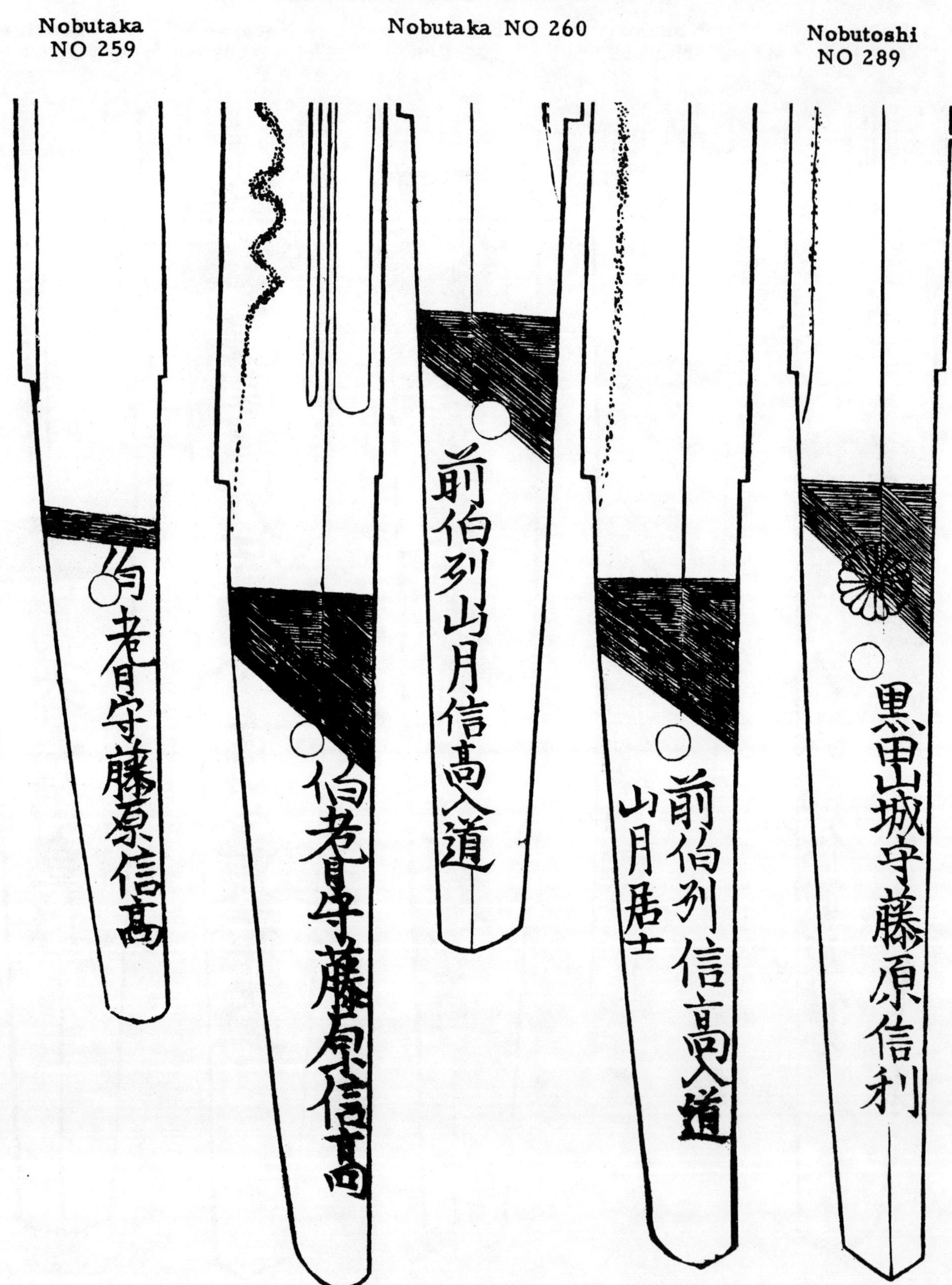

Nobuyoshi & Kuniyoshi
NO 317   KU 964

Nobuyoshi NO 317

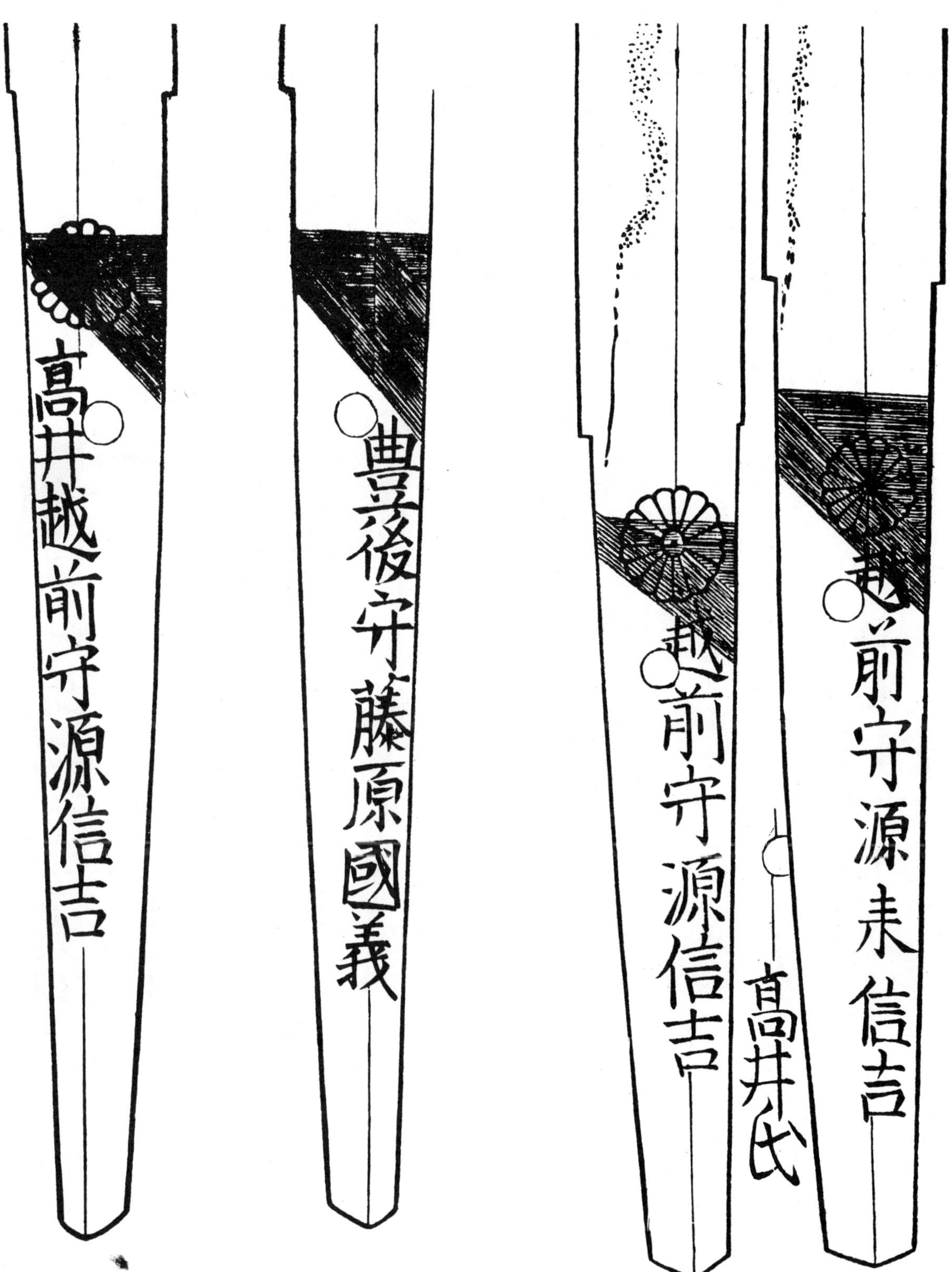

Nobuyoshi NO 317

Nobuyoshi
NO 321

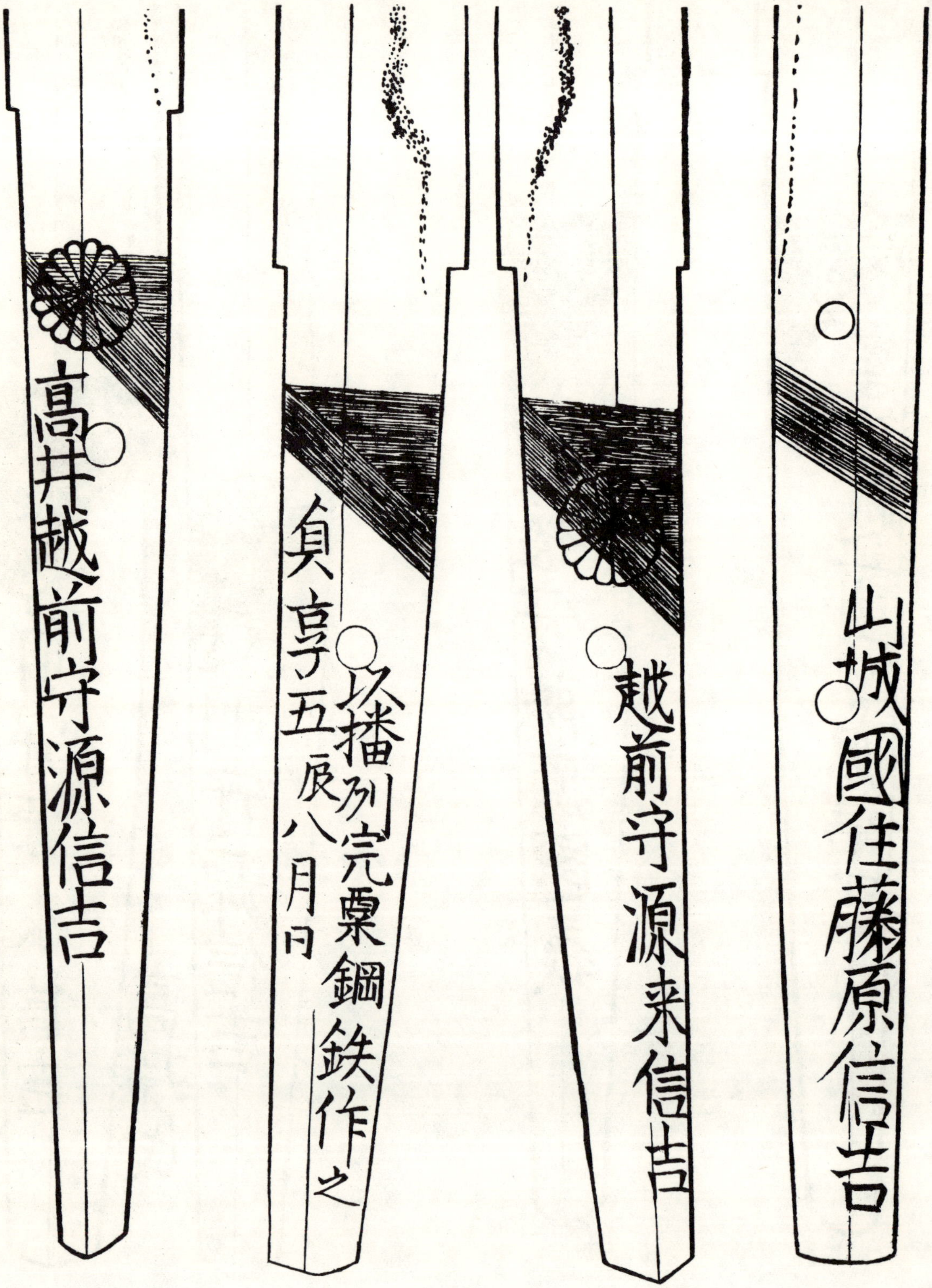

高井越前守源信吉

貞享五辰八月日
以播列完栗鋼鉄作之

越前守源来信吉

山城國住藤原信吉

Nobuyoshi	Nobuyuki	Norifusa	Norihiro
NO 321	NO 365	NO 394	NO 413a

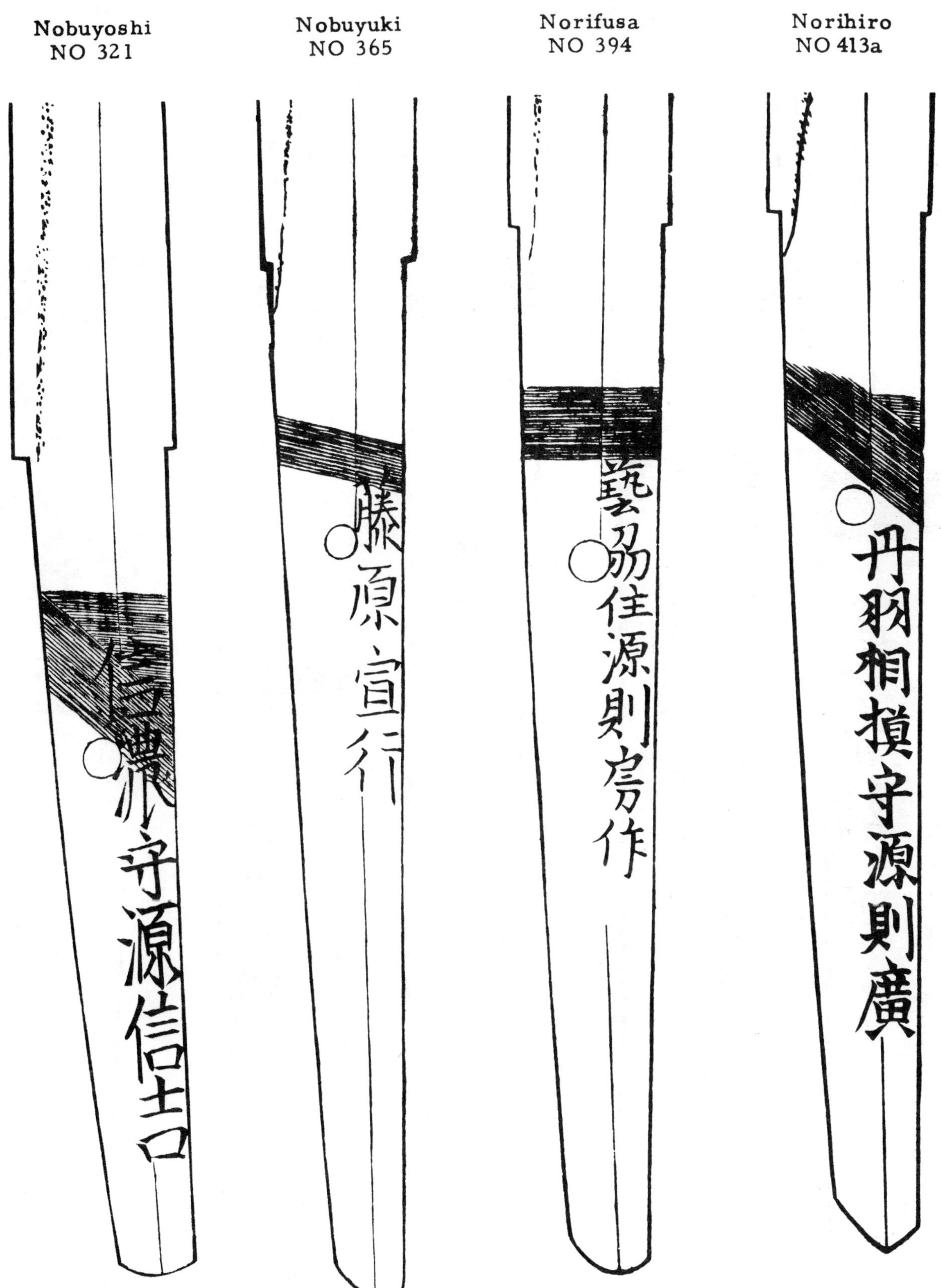

SHINTO BENGI OSHIGATA

Okimasa OK 3

Okisato
OK 5

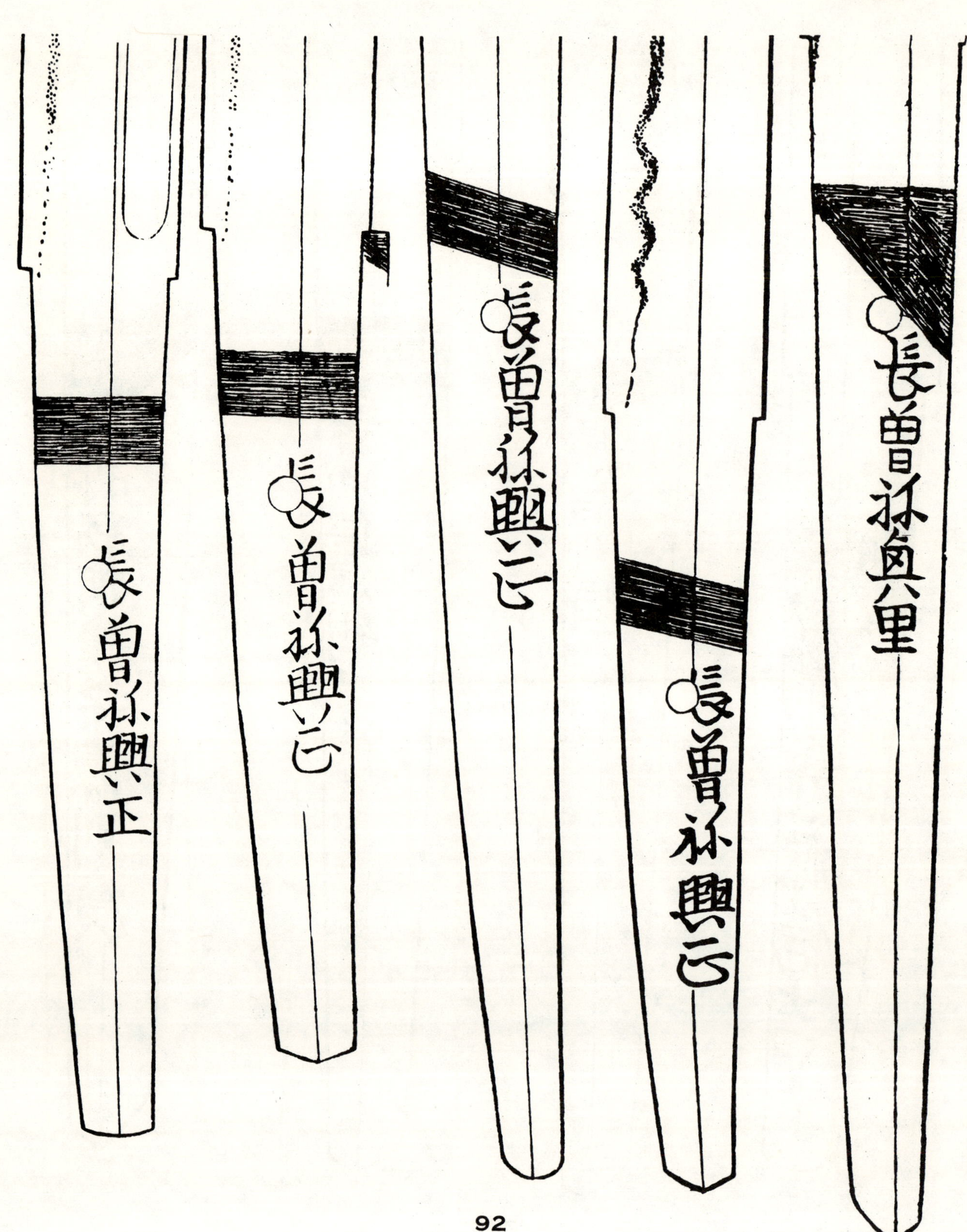

Sadamichi
SA 49

Sadahira
SA 176

Sadahiro SA 183

Sadakuni
SA 227

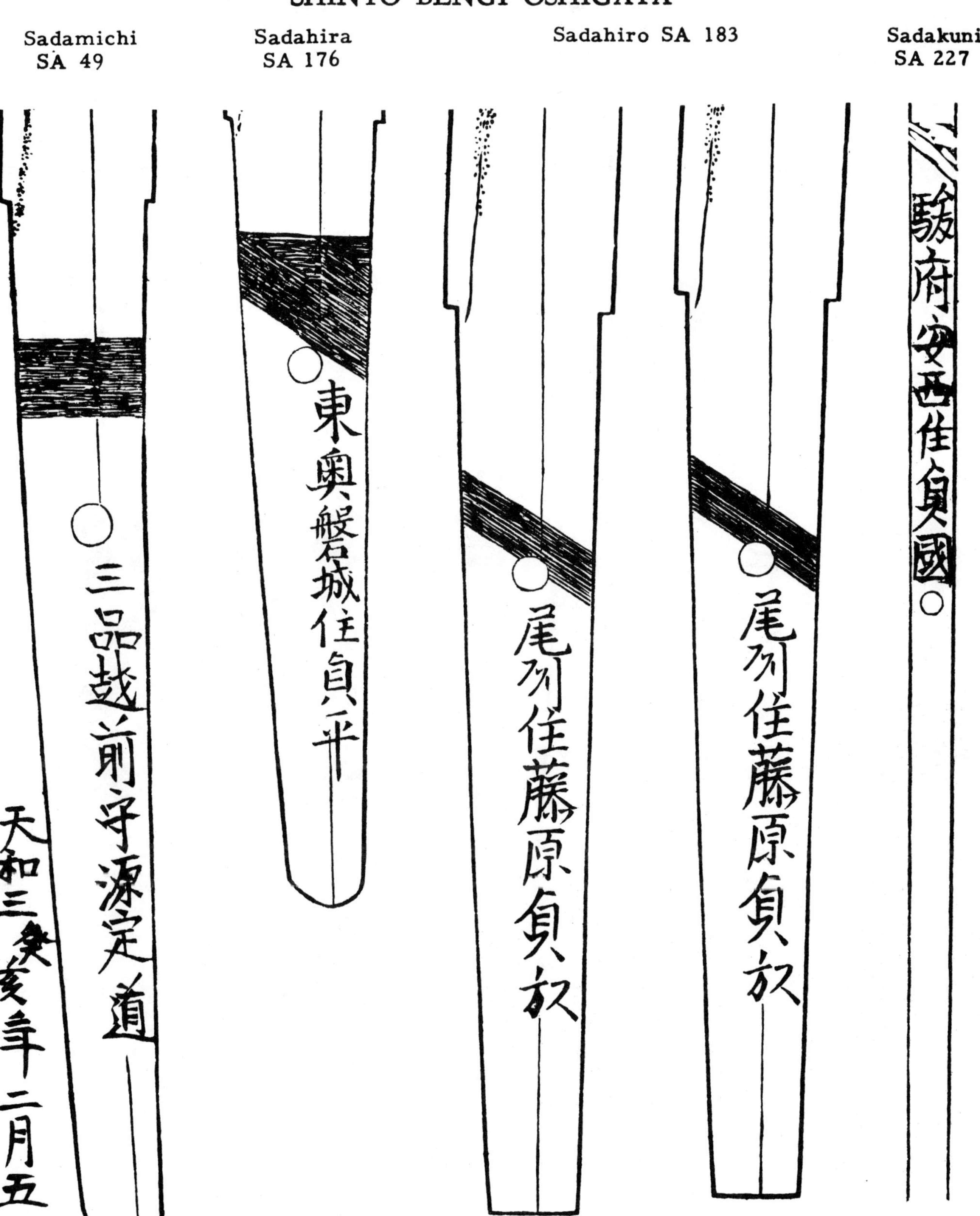

Sadamichi
SA 233

Sadanori SA 299

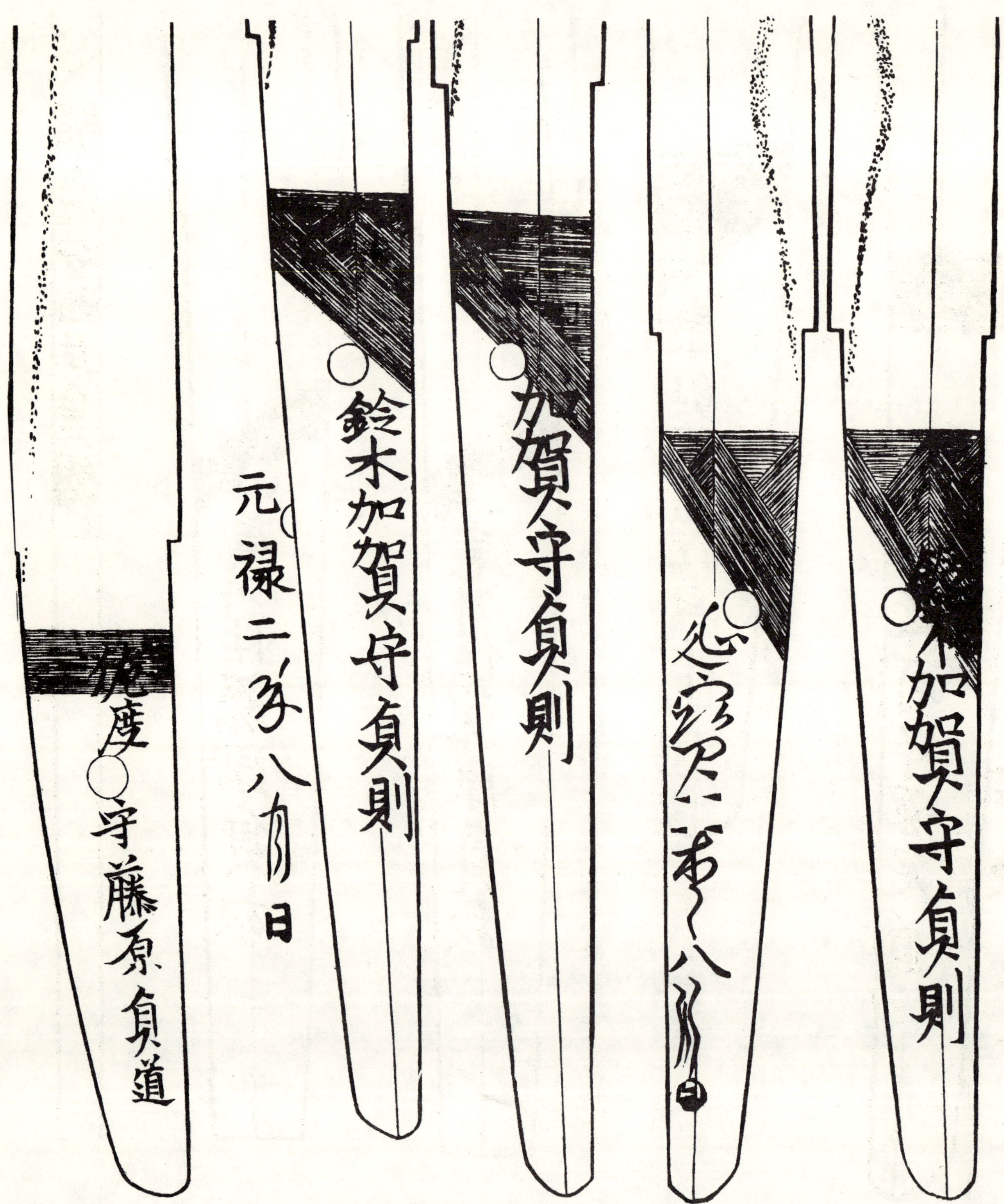

Sadanori SA. 299 Sadatoshi SA 344 Sadatsugu SA 375 Sadayuki SA 446

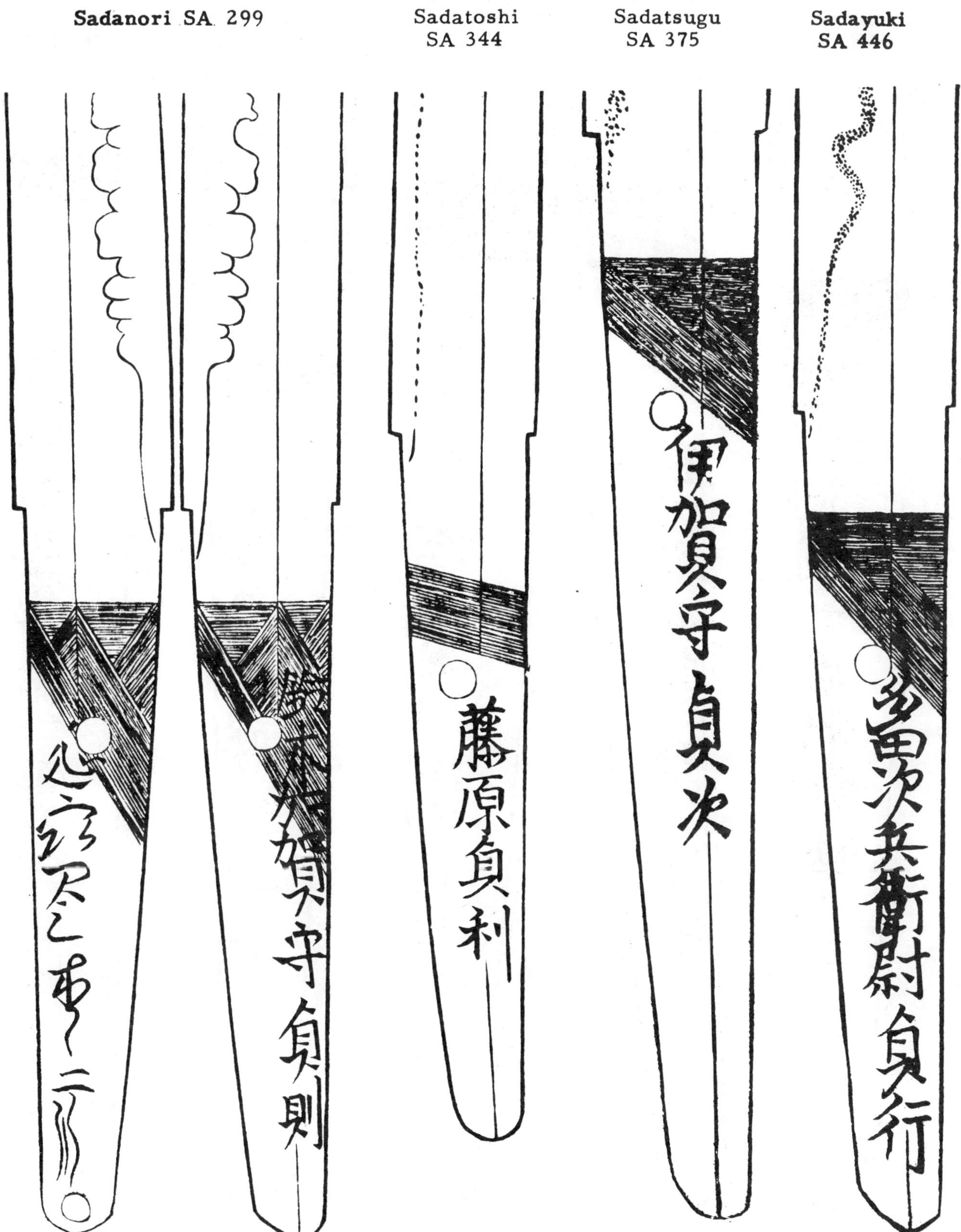

Sadayuki
SA 449

Sanesumi SA 703

Senriki
SE 17

Shigekuni
SH 95

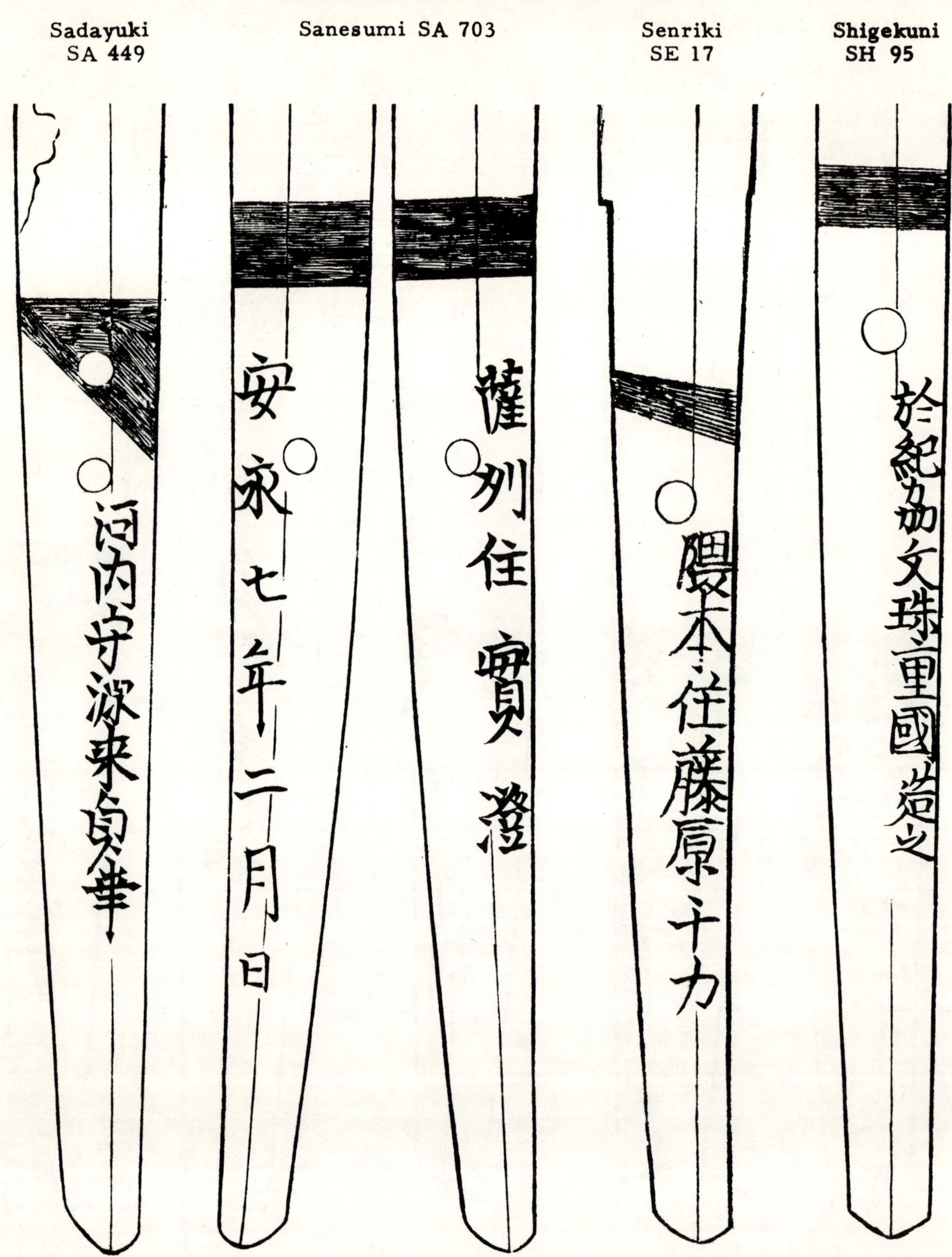

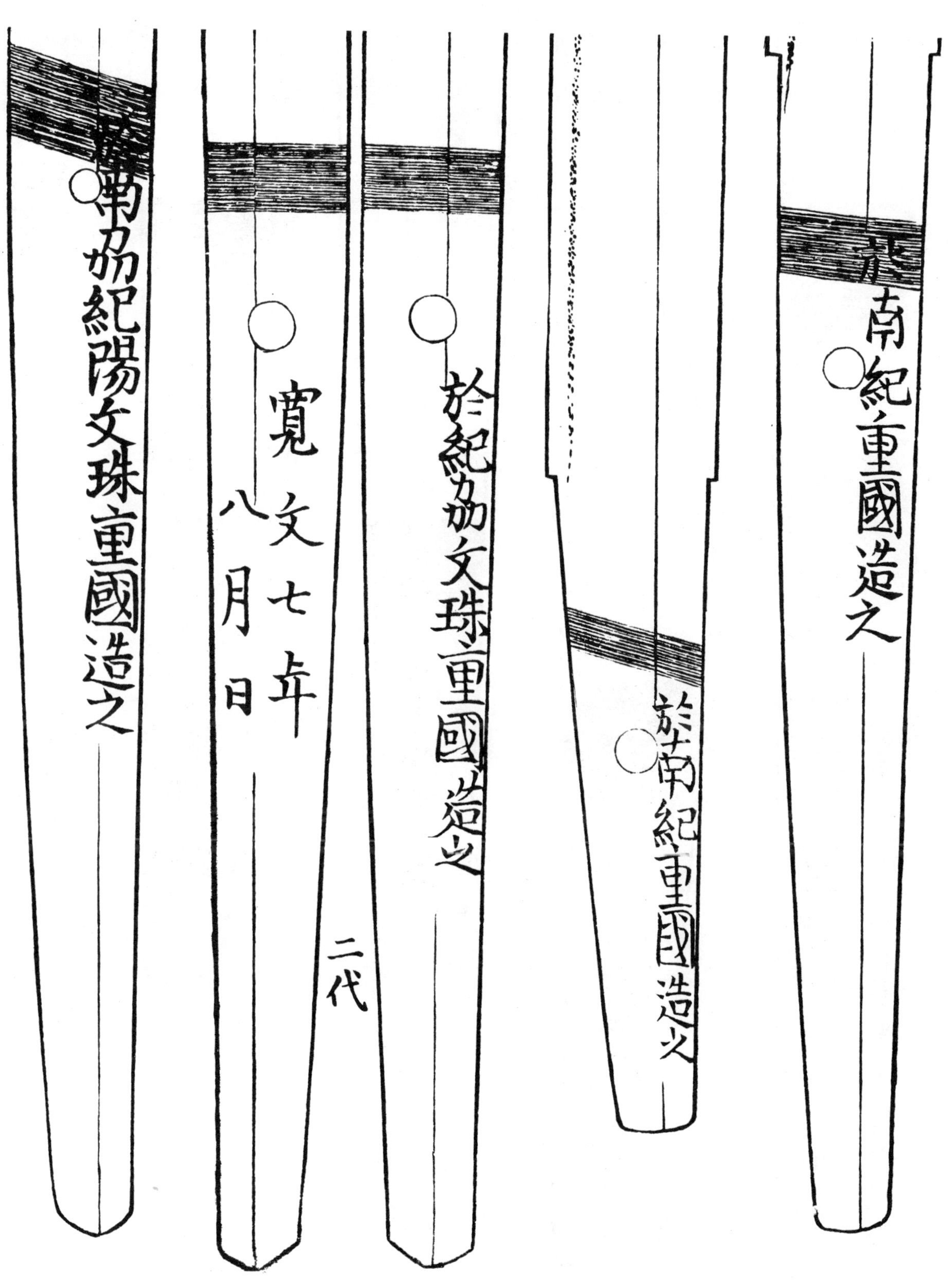

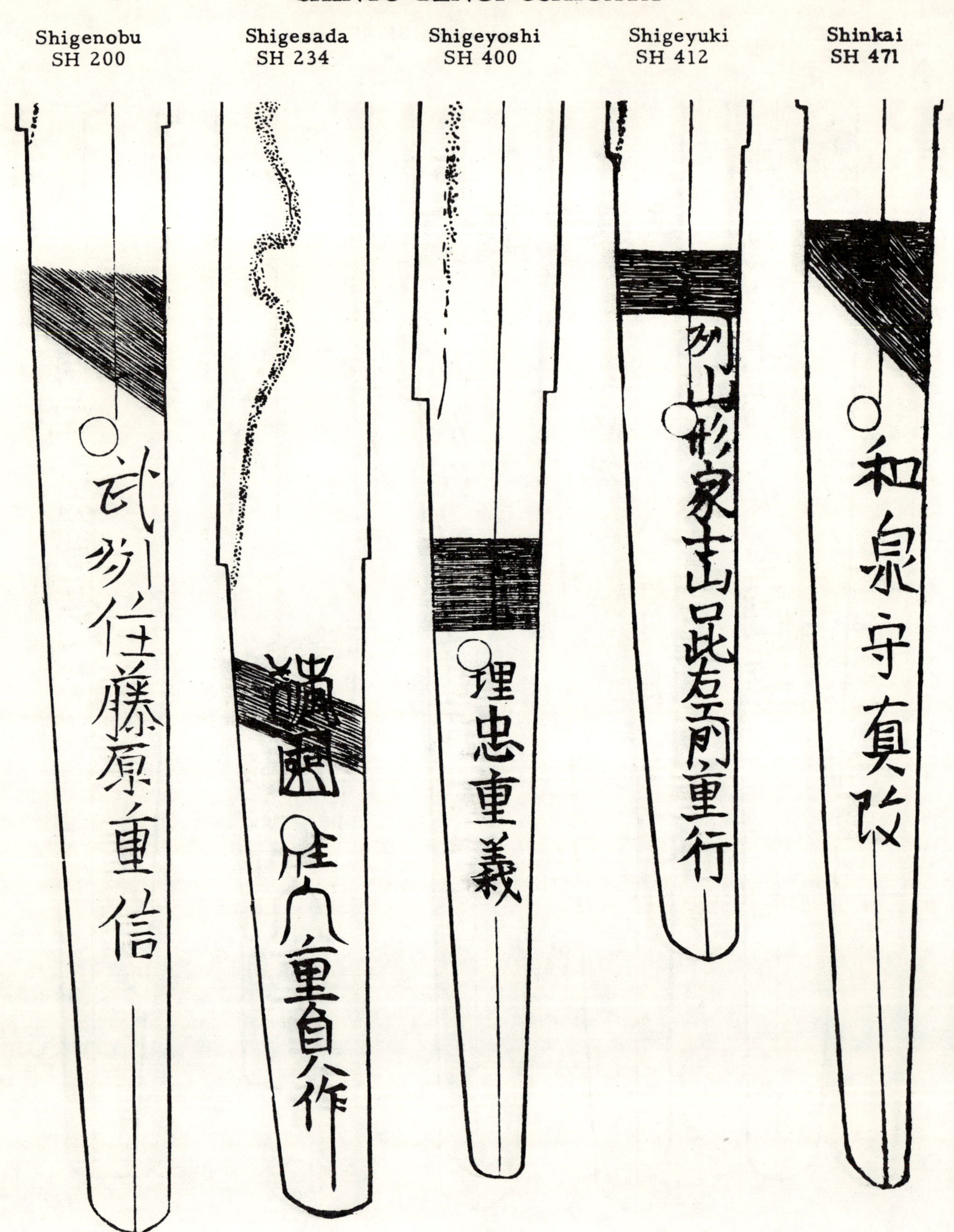

Shigenobu
SH 200
Shigesada
SH 234
Shigeyoshi
SH 400
Shigeyuki
SH 412
Shinkai
SH 471

Shinkai SH 471

Shinkai & Sukehiro
SH 471   SU 70

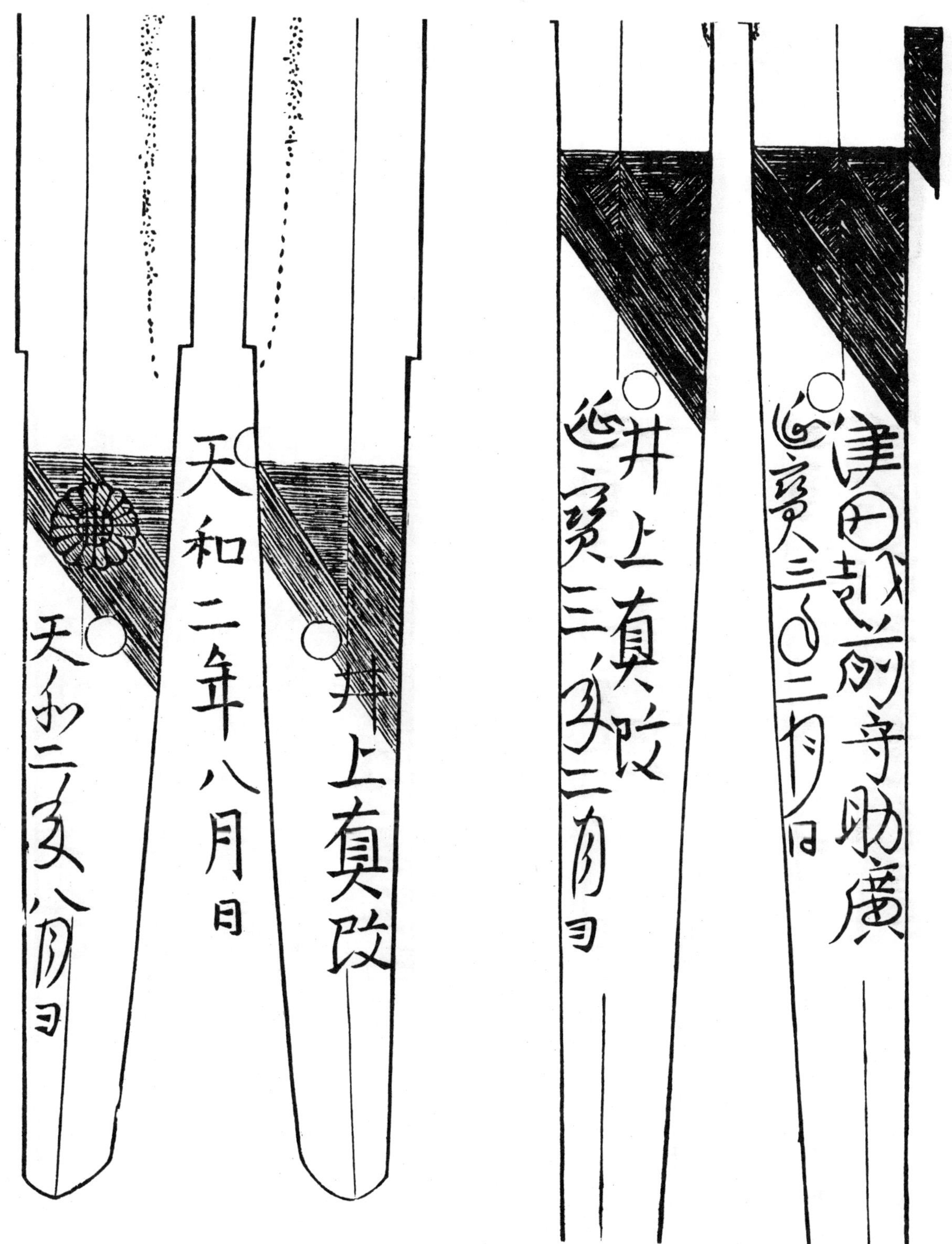

SHINTO BENGI OSHIGATA

Shinkai SH 471

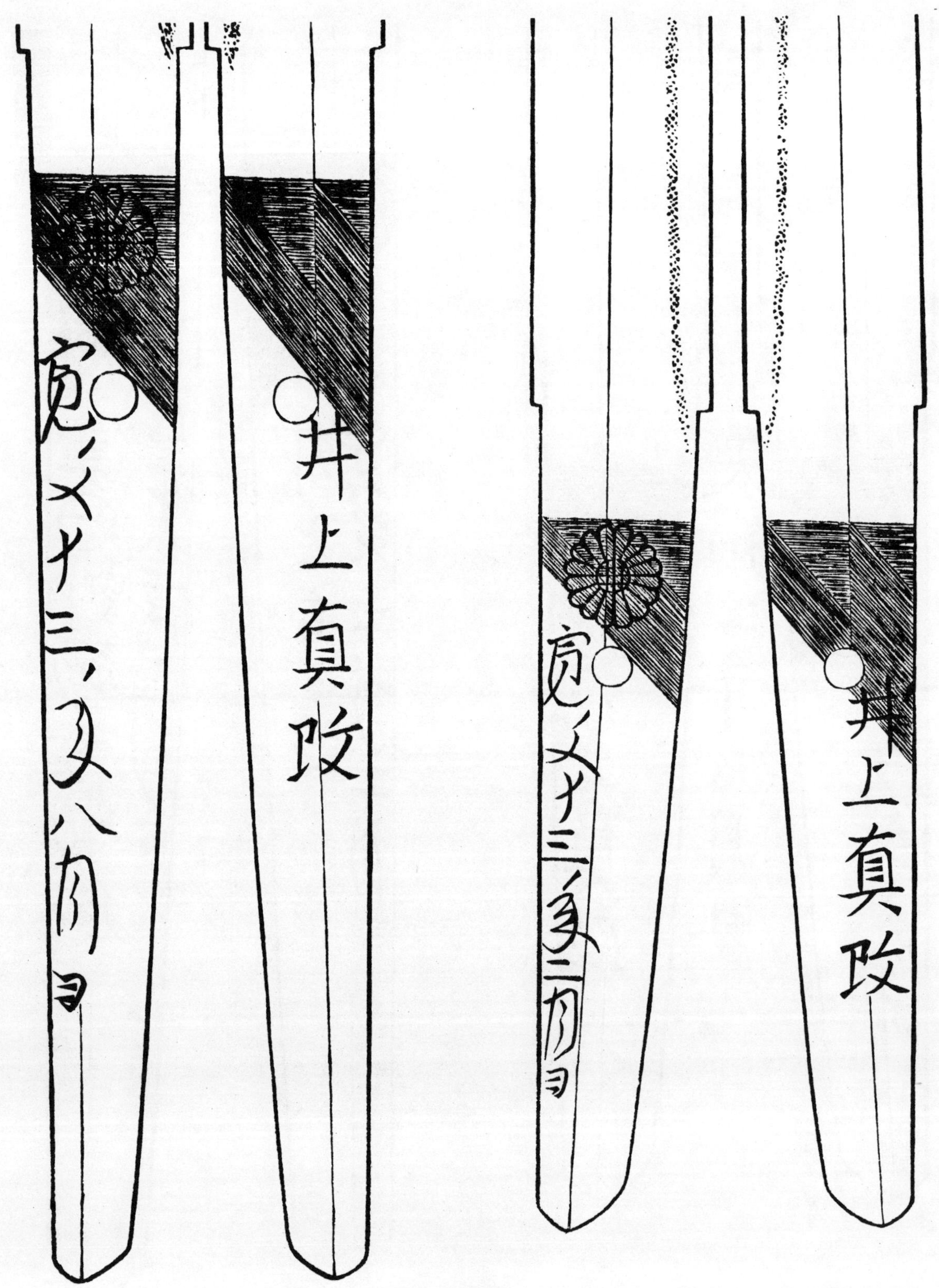

SHINTO BENGI OSHIGATA

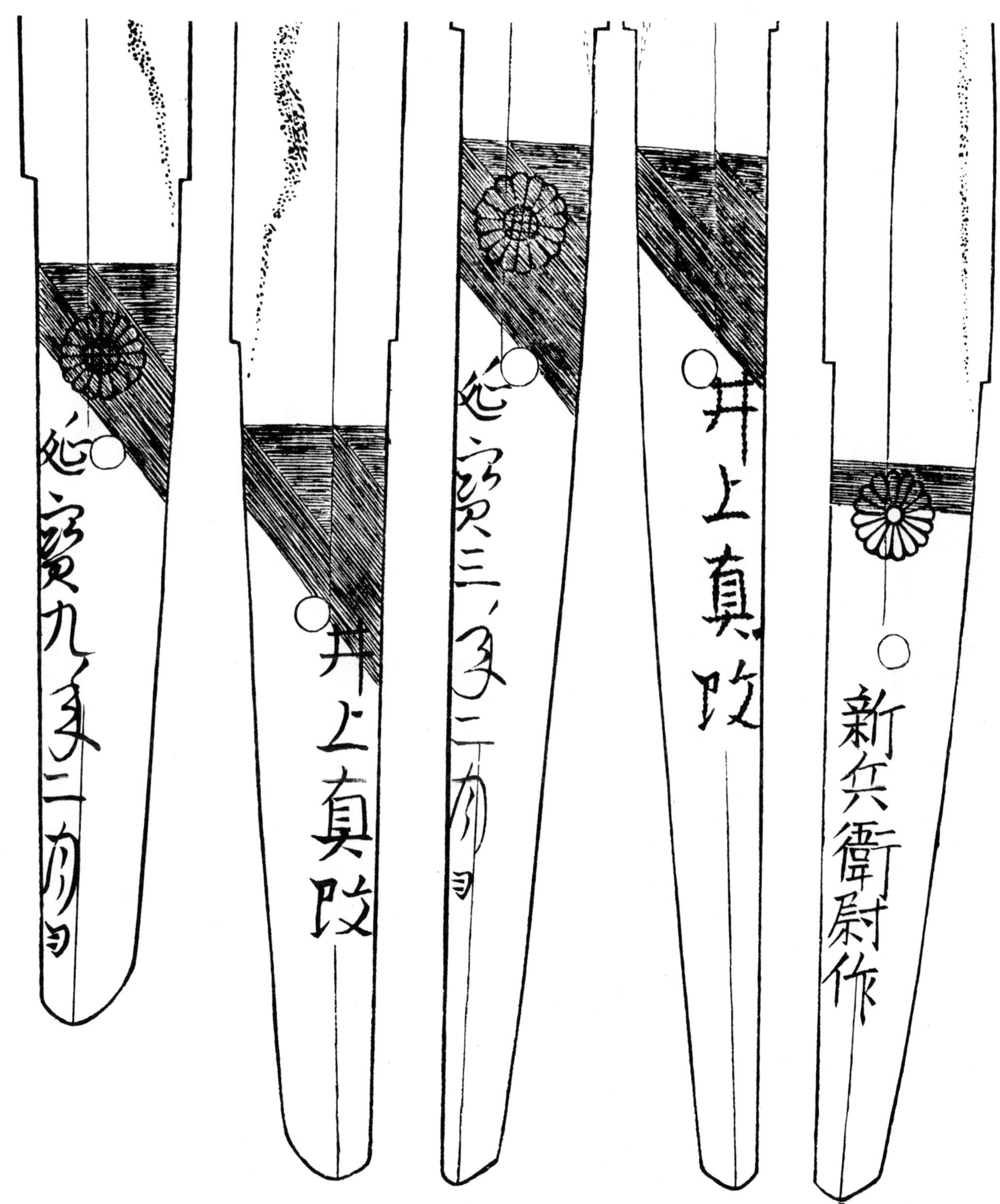

Shinryō SH 474   Shinbe SH 483   Shin SH 491

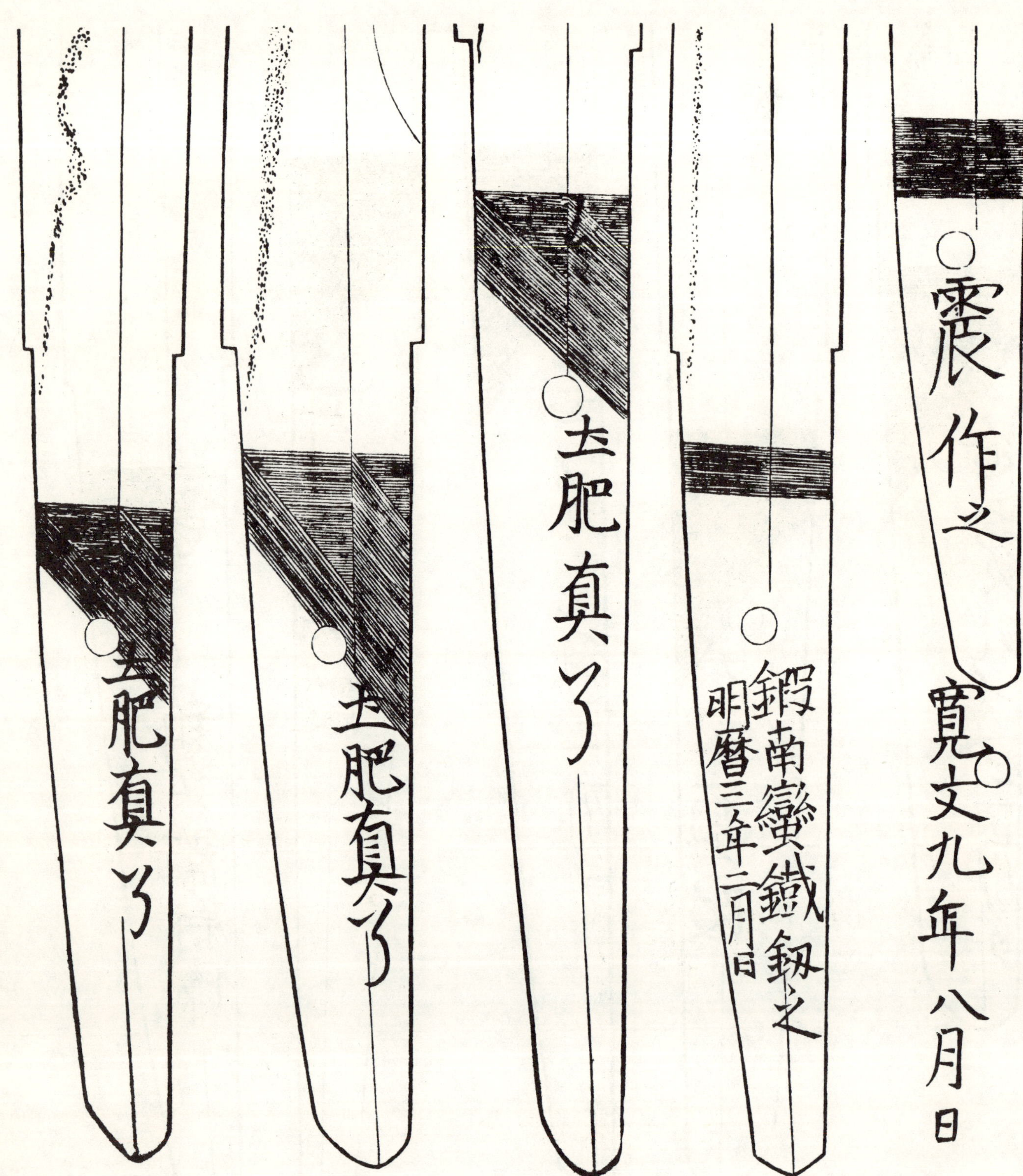

Soei (Muneyoshi MU 349)   Sukehiro SU 69 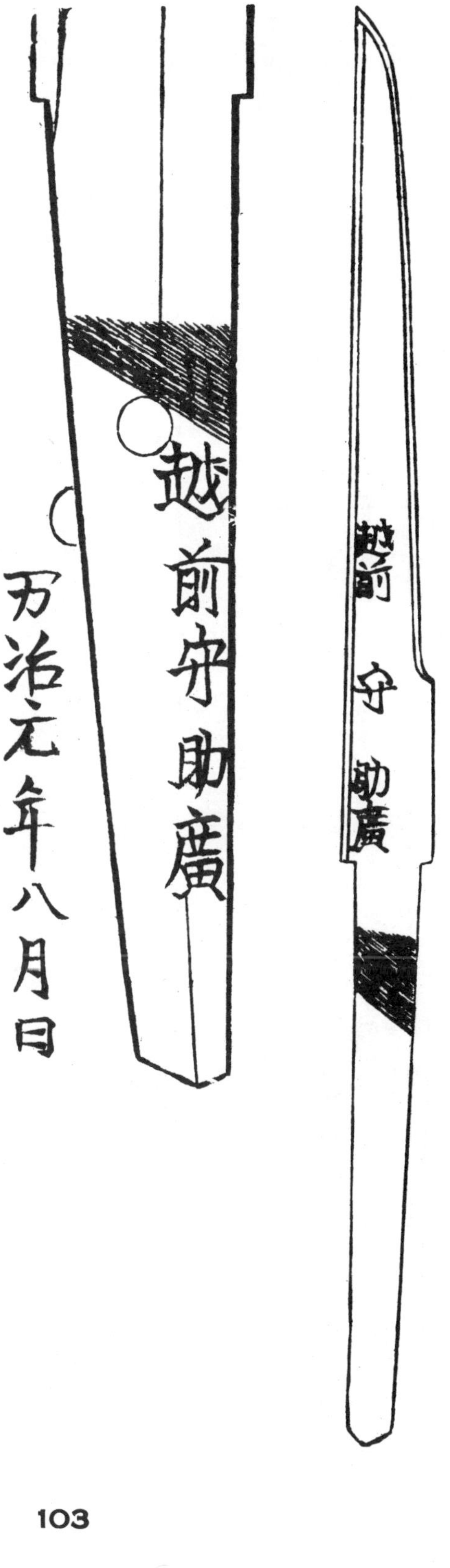   Sukehiro
SU 70

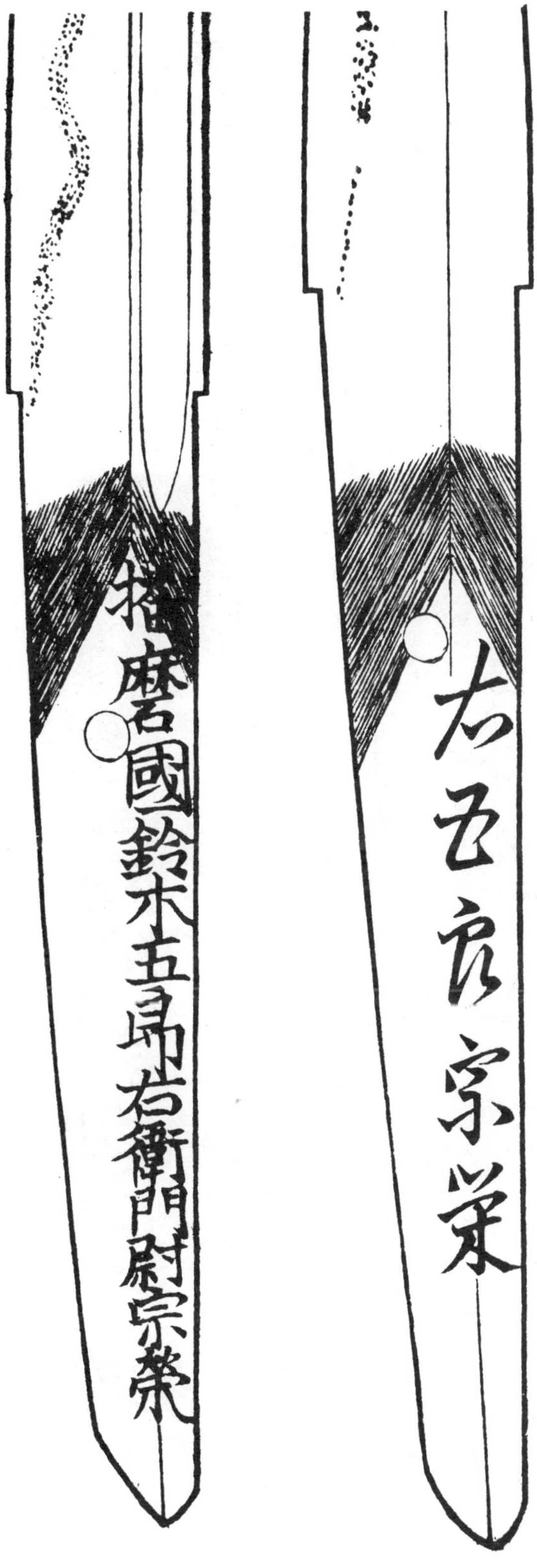

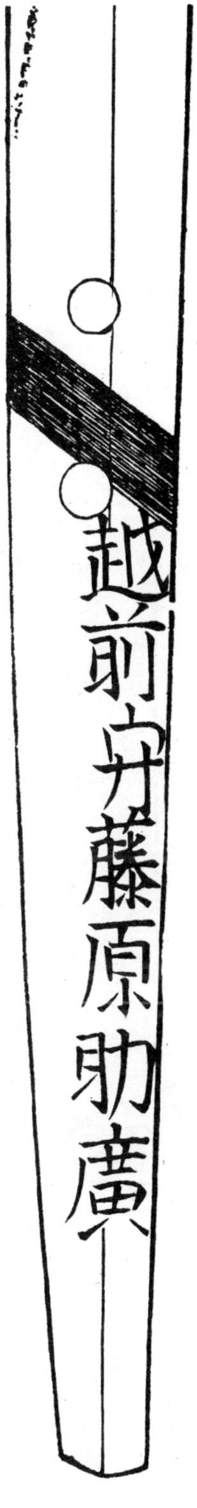

播磨國鈴木五郎右衛門尉宗榮

右玉店宗榮

万治元年八月日

越前守助廣

越前守助廣

越前守藤原助廣

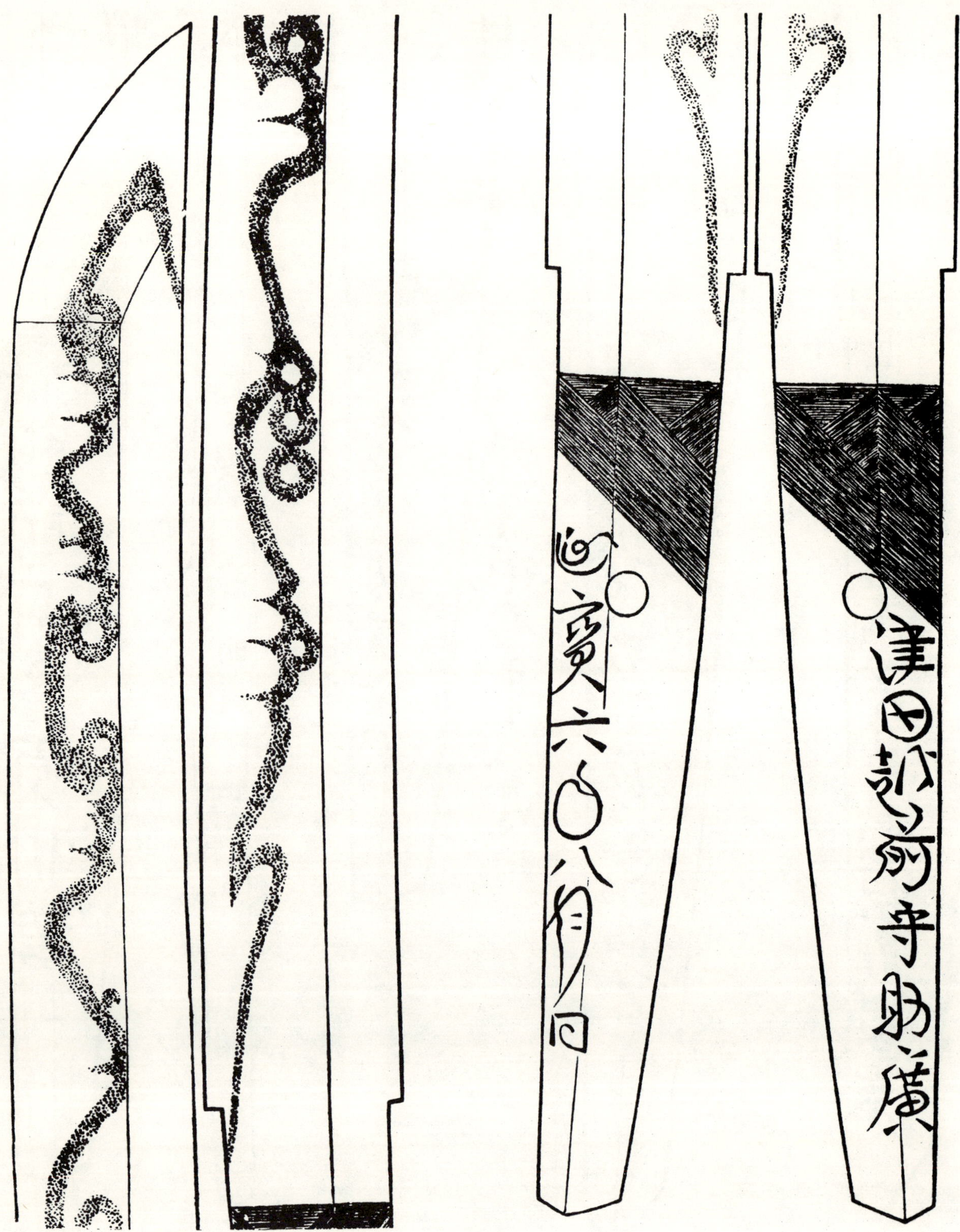

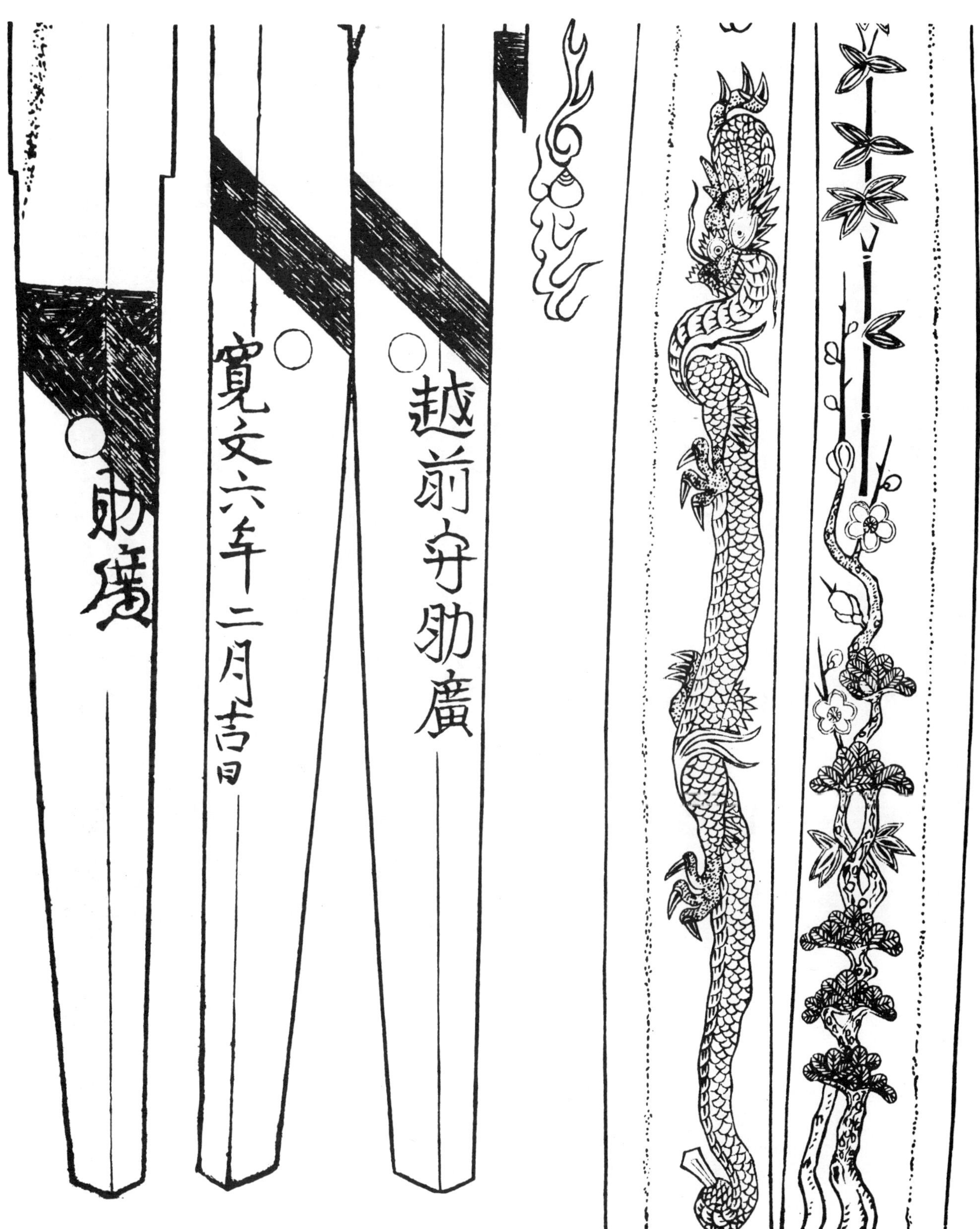

助廣
寛文六年二月吉日
越前守助廣

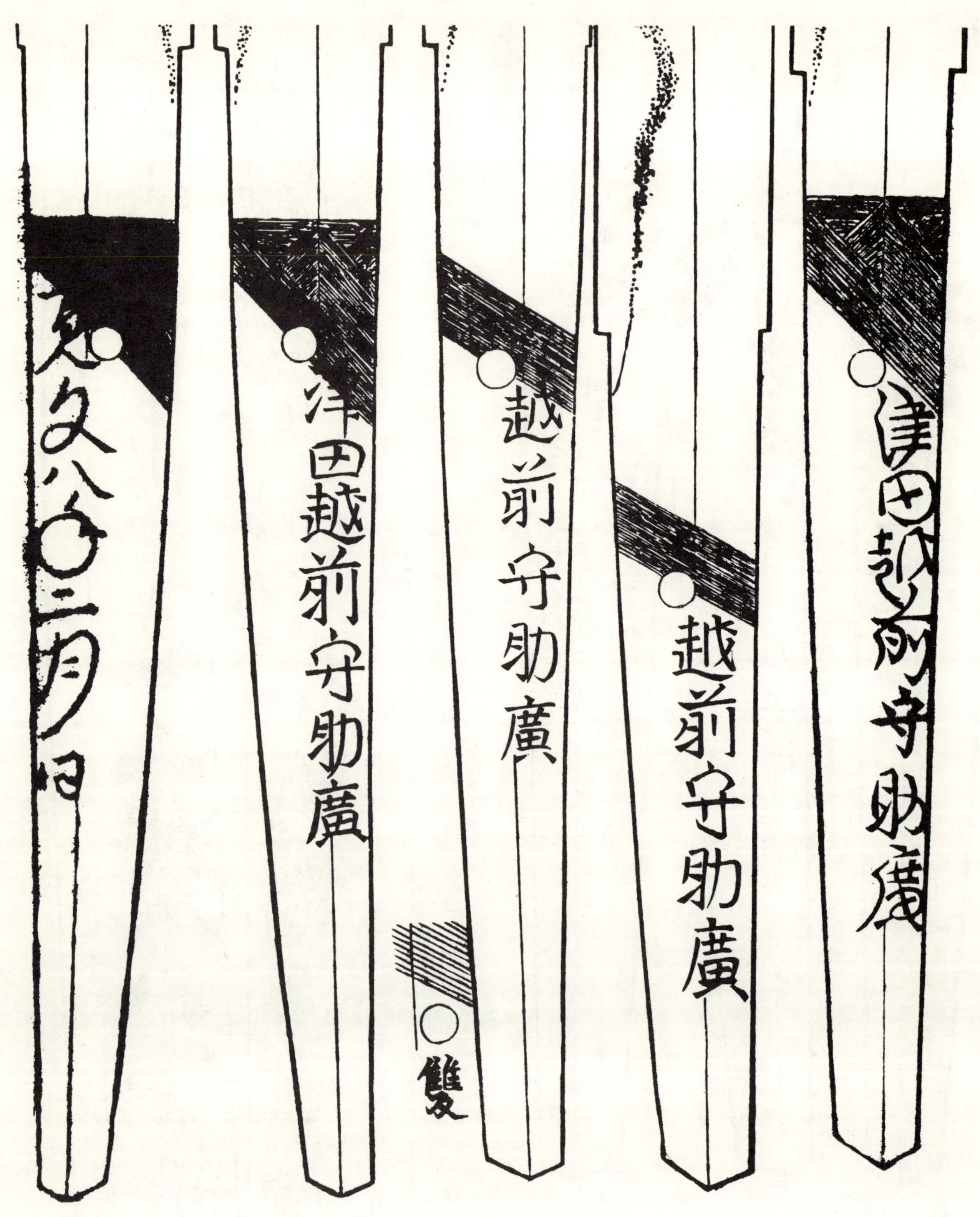

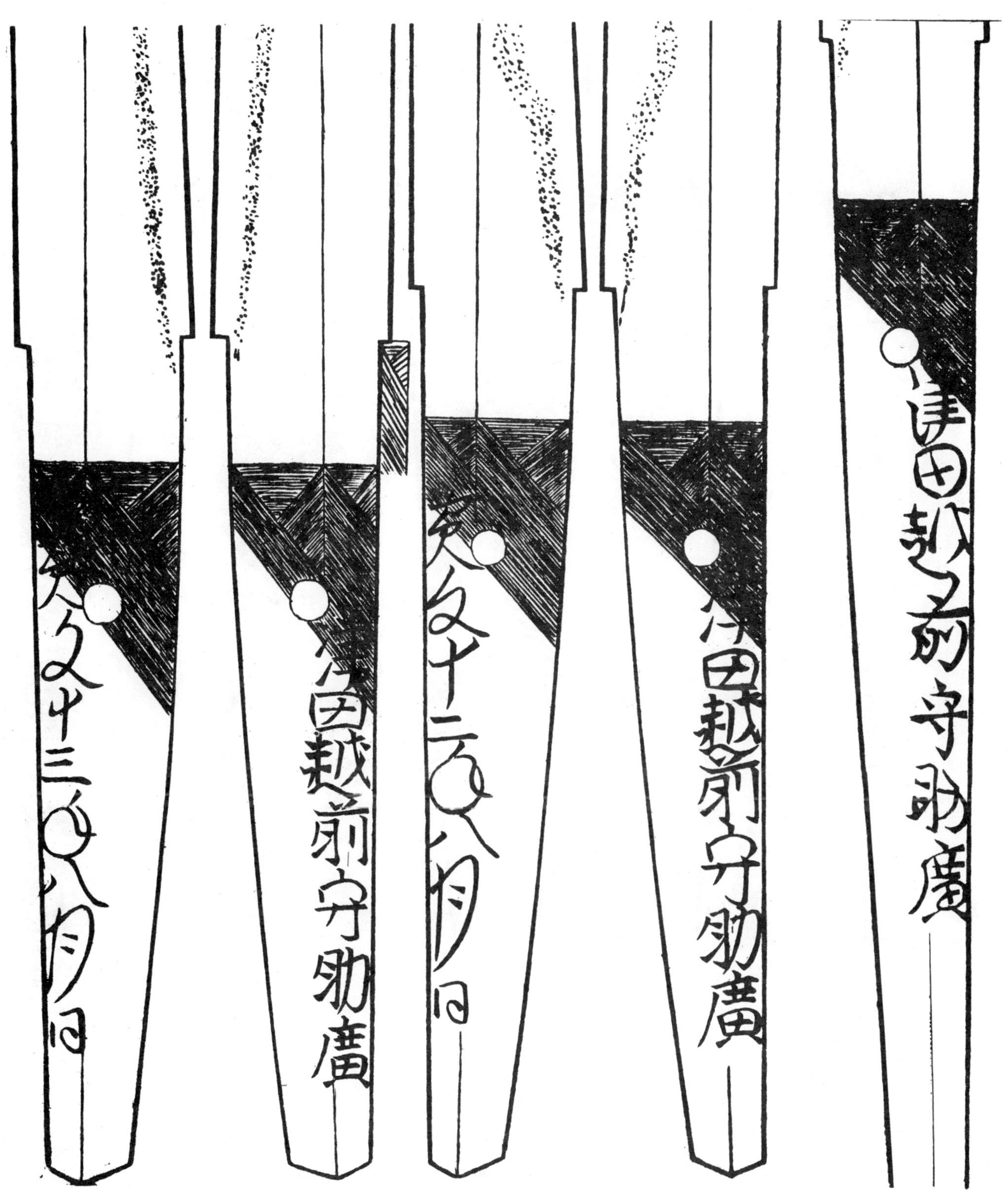

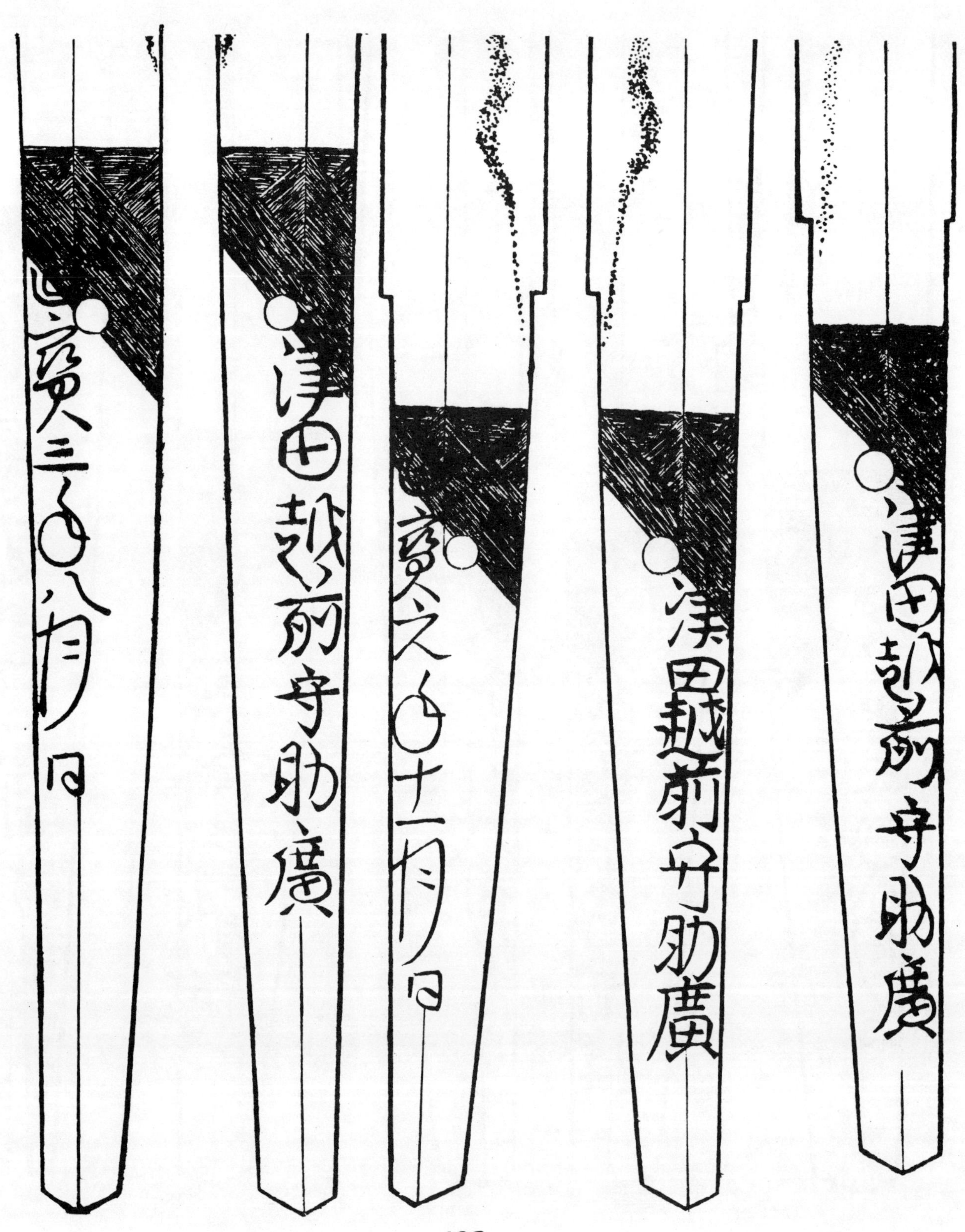

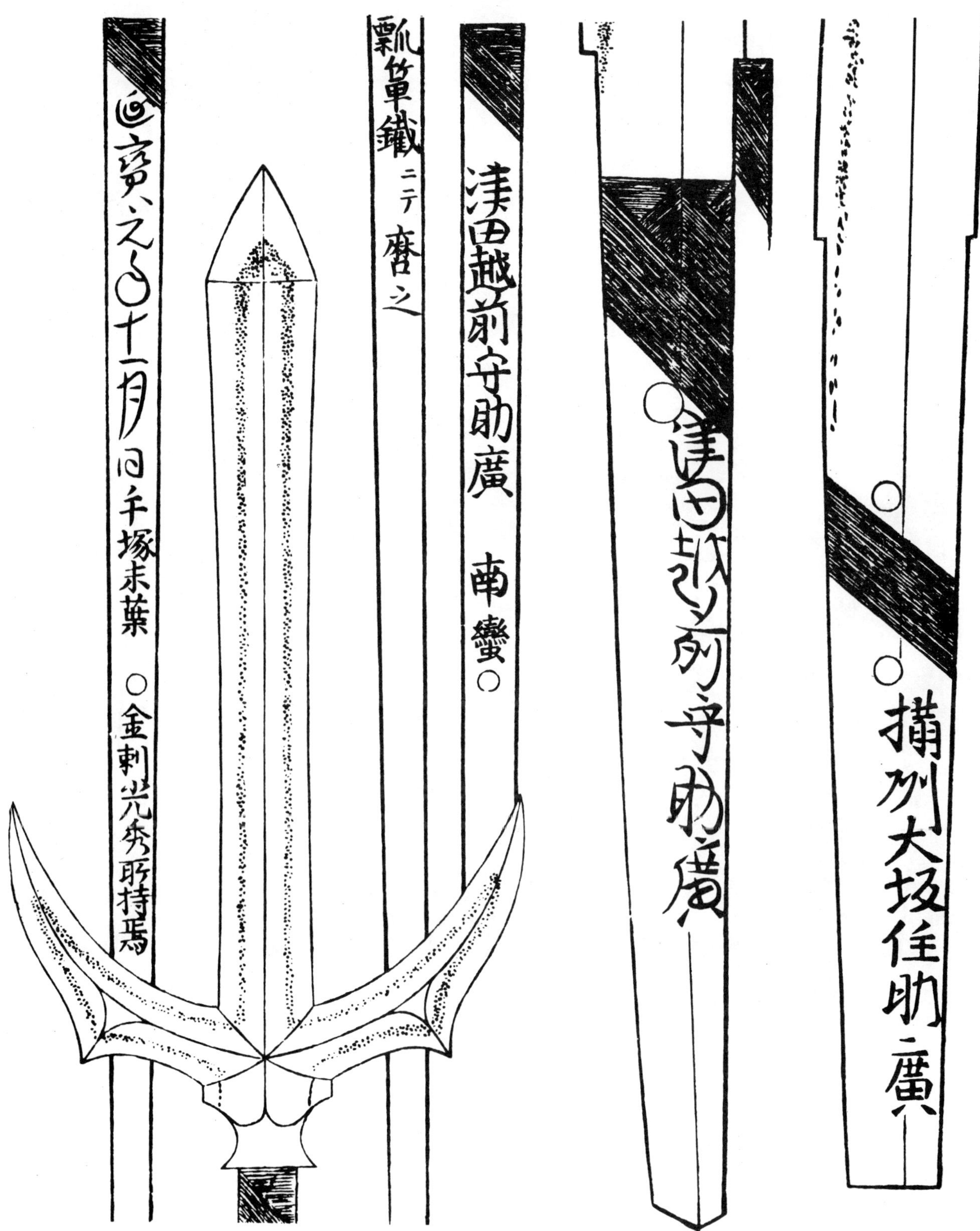

Sukehiro SU 74a   Sukekane   Sukemasa SU 112
SU 92

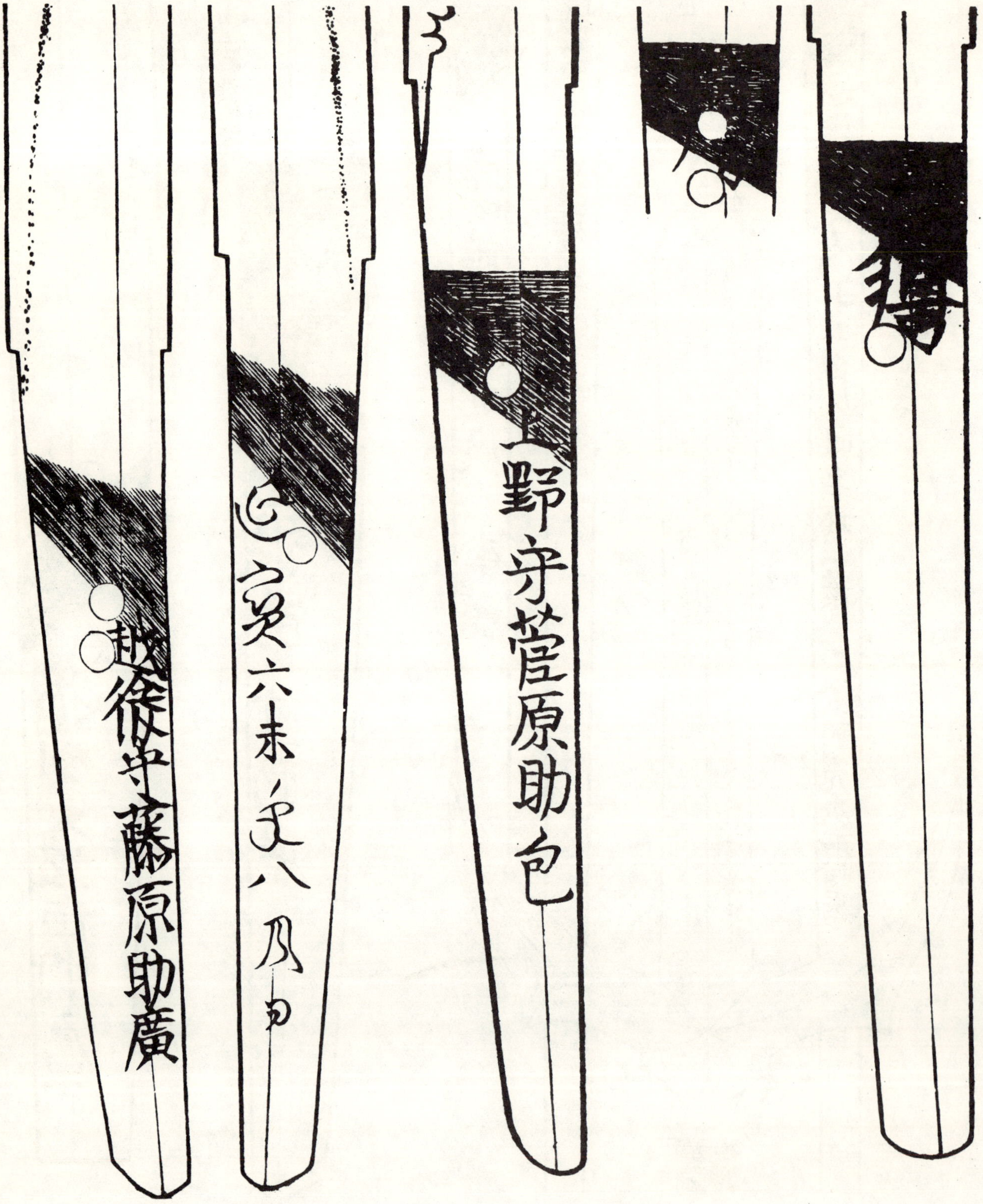

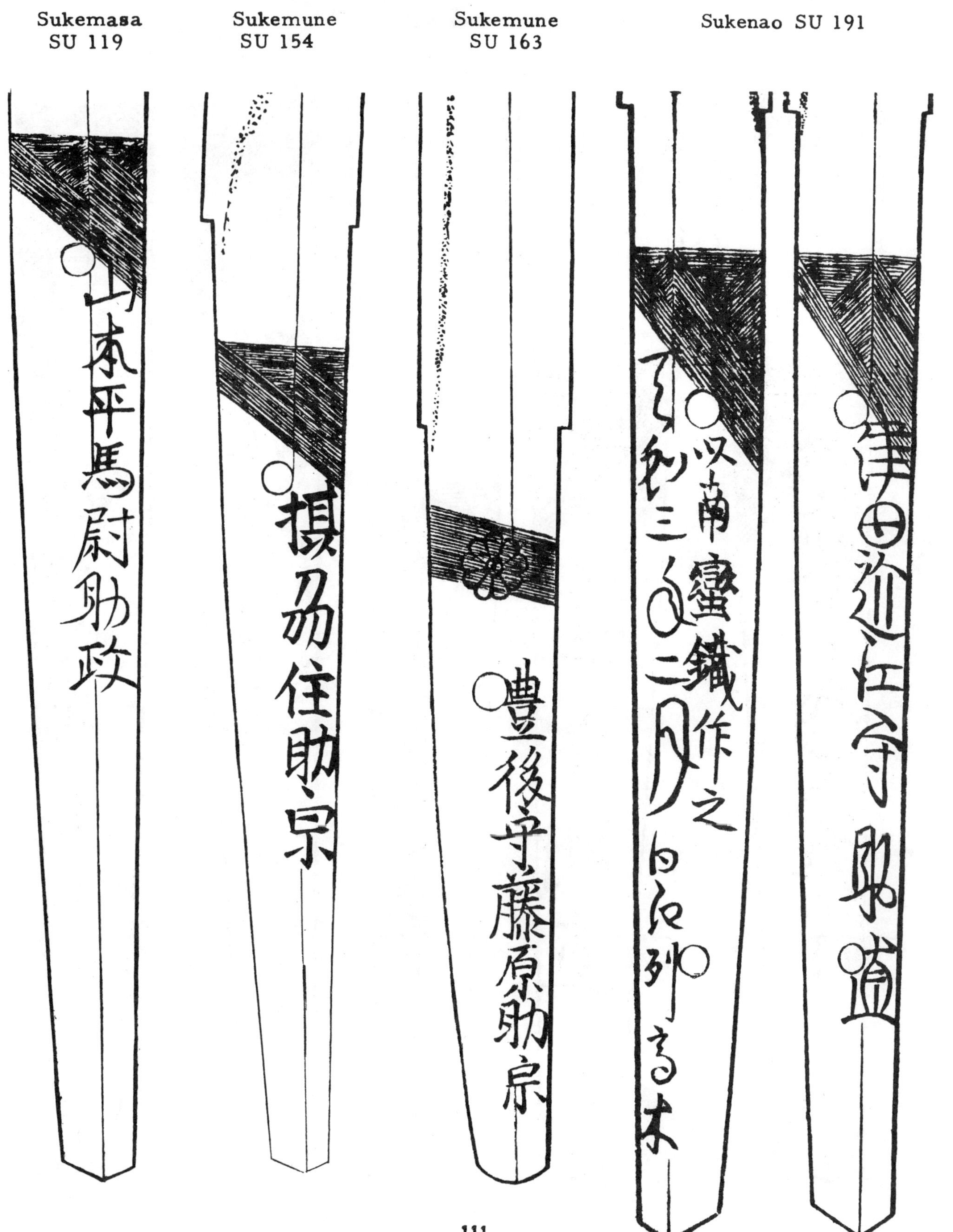

Sukemasa
SU 119
Sukemune
SU 154
Sukemune
SU 163
Sukenao SU 191
山本平馬尉助政
摂刕住助宗
豊後守藤原助宗
以南蛮鐵作之
津田近江守助直

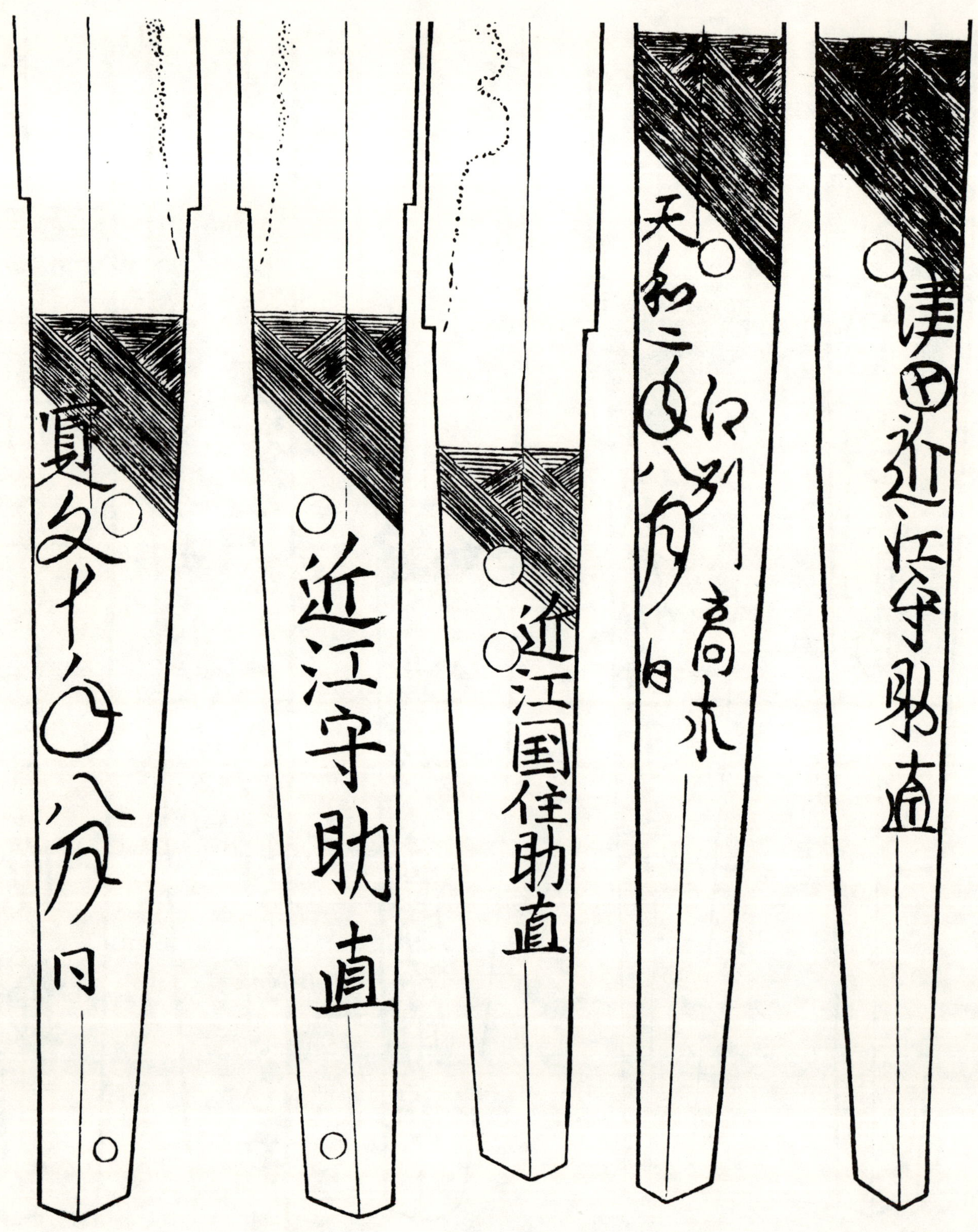

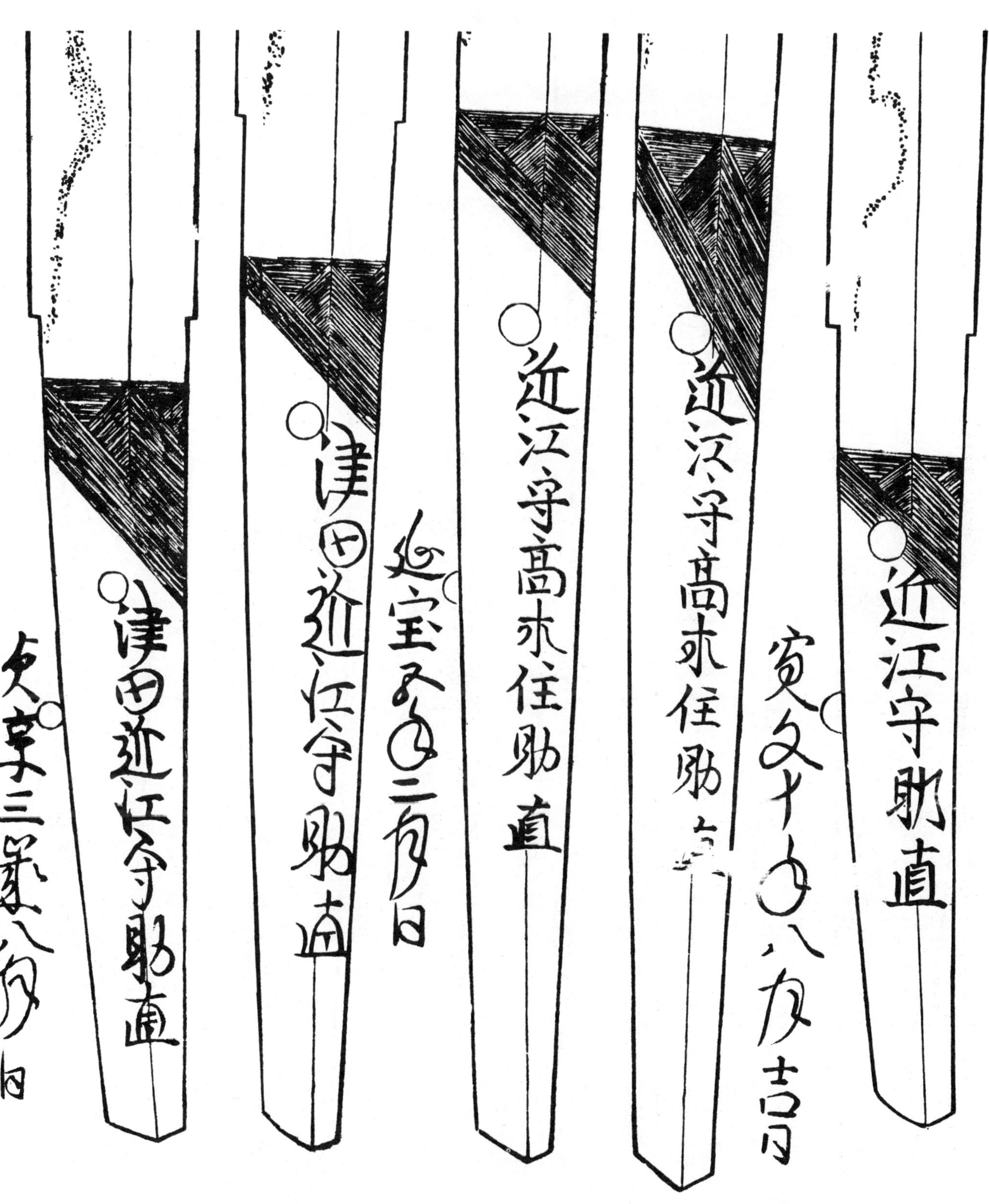

Suketaka SU 274   Suketaka SU 277   Sukekuni SU 381

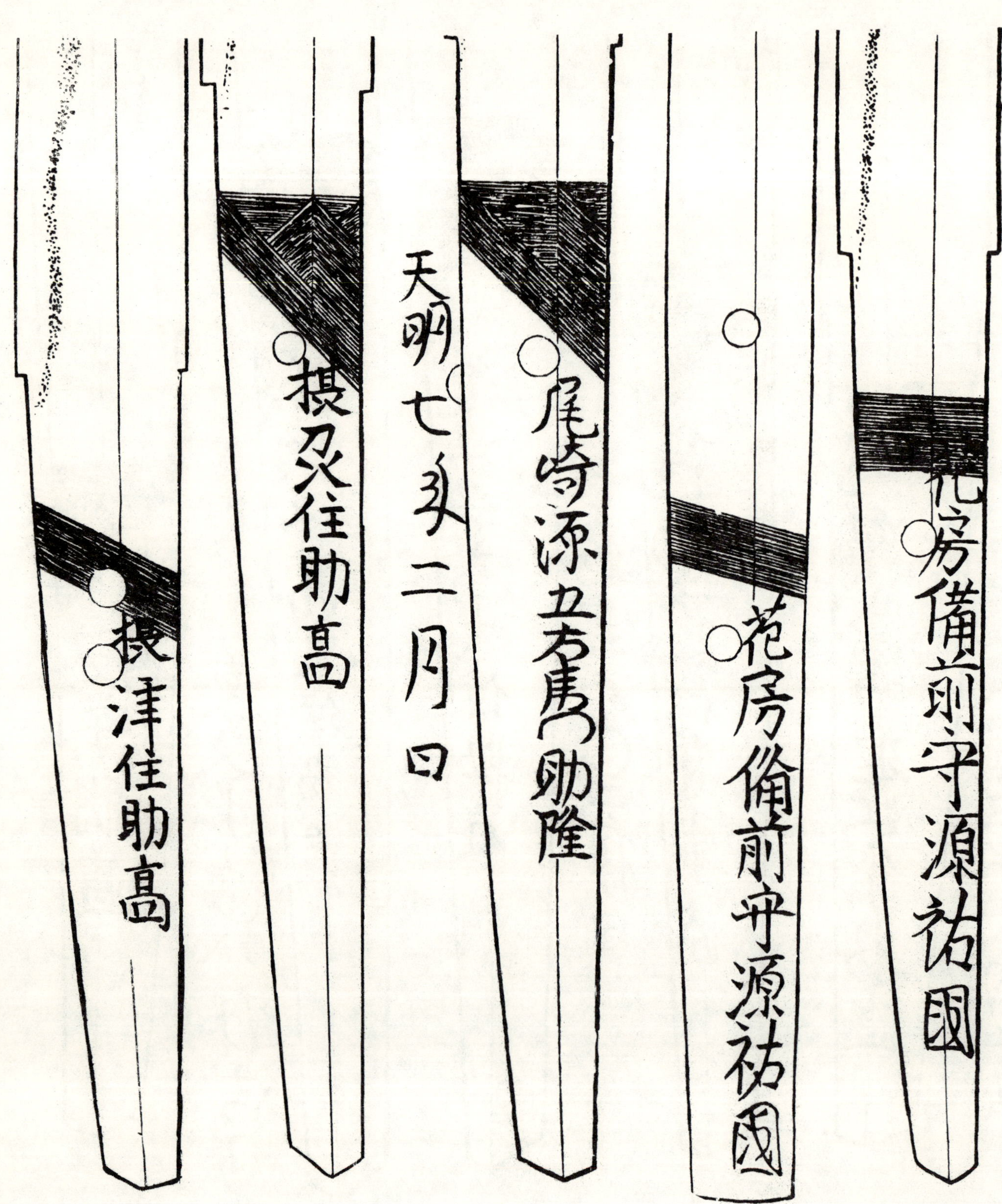

Sukesada
SU 455, SU 453, SU 456

Sukesada SU 459

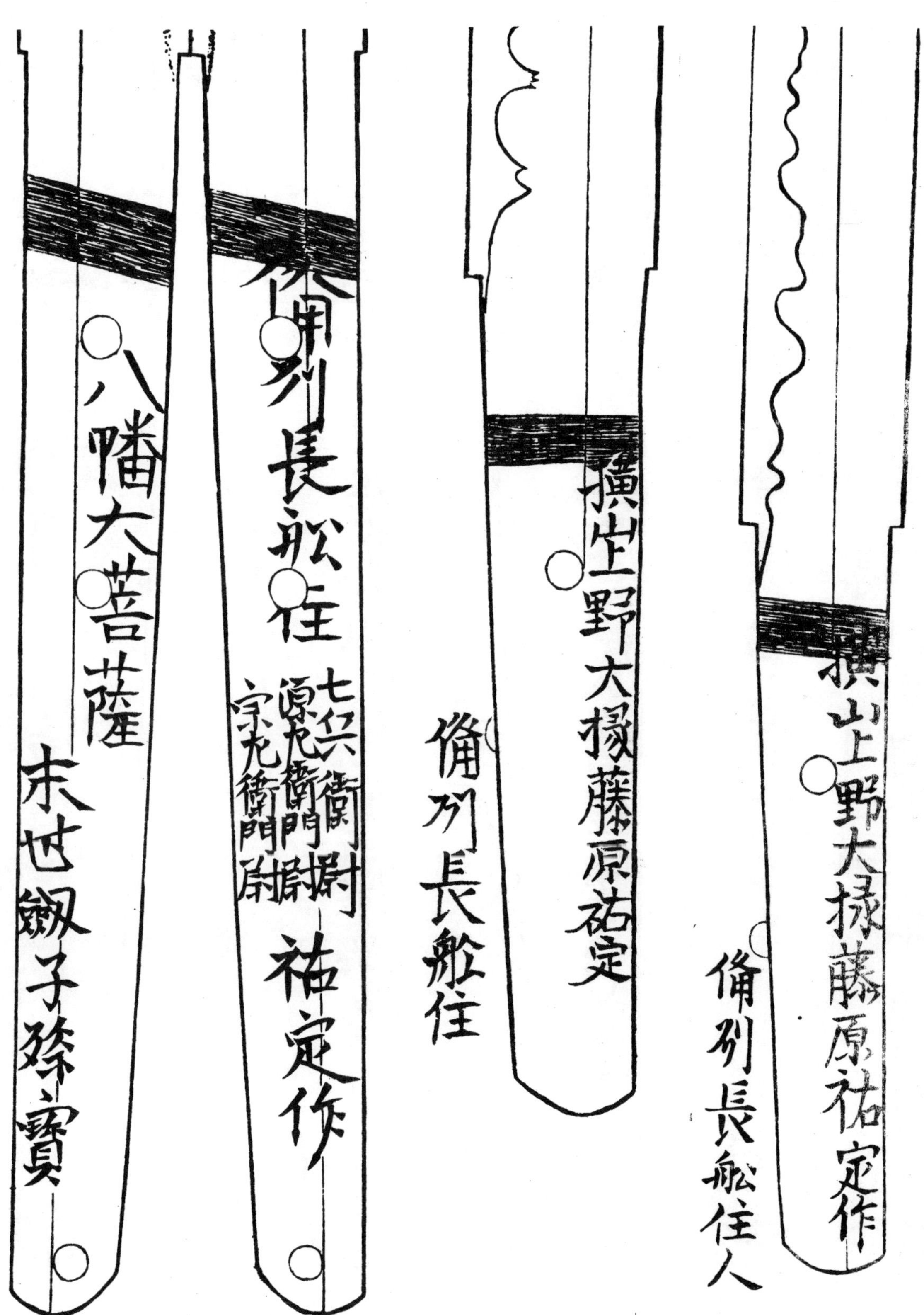

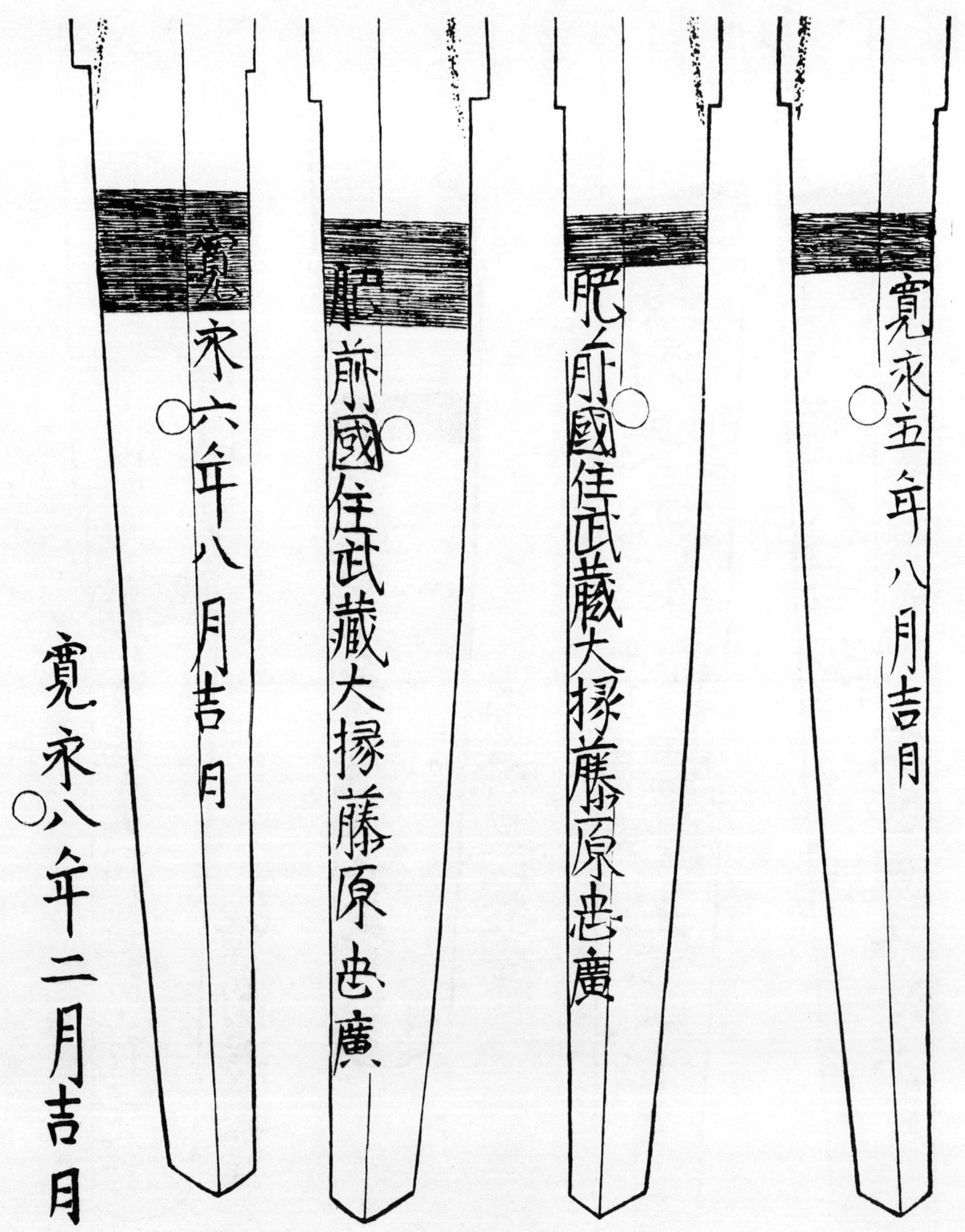
寛永五年八月吉月

肥前國住武藏大掾藤原忠廣

肥前國住武藏大掾藤原忠廣

永六年八月吉月

寛永八年二月吉月

Tadahiro TA 12   Tadayoshi & Tadahiro   Tadahiro

      TA 143   TA 12   TA 18

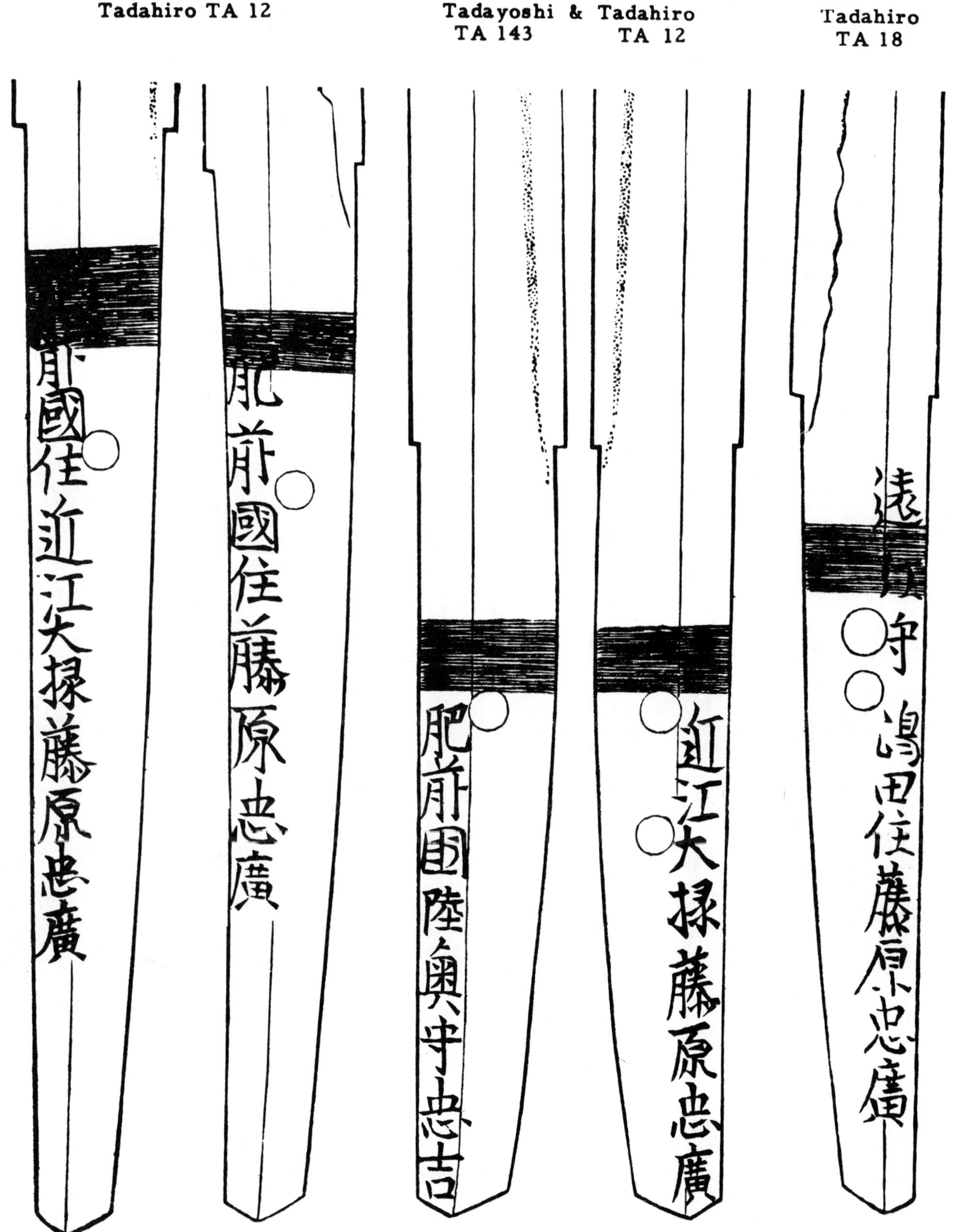

Tadakane
TA 28

Tadakuni
TA 40

Tadakuni TA 43

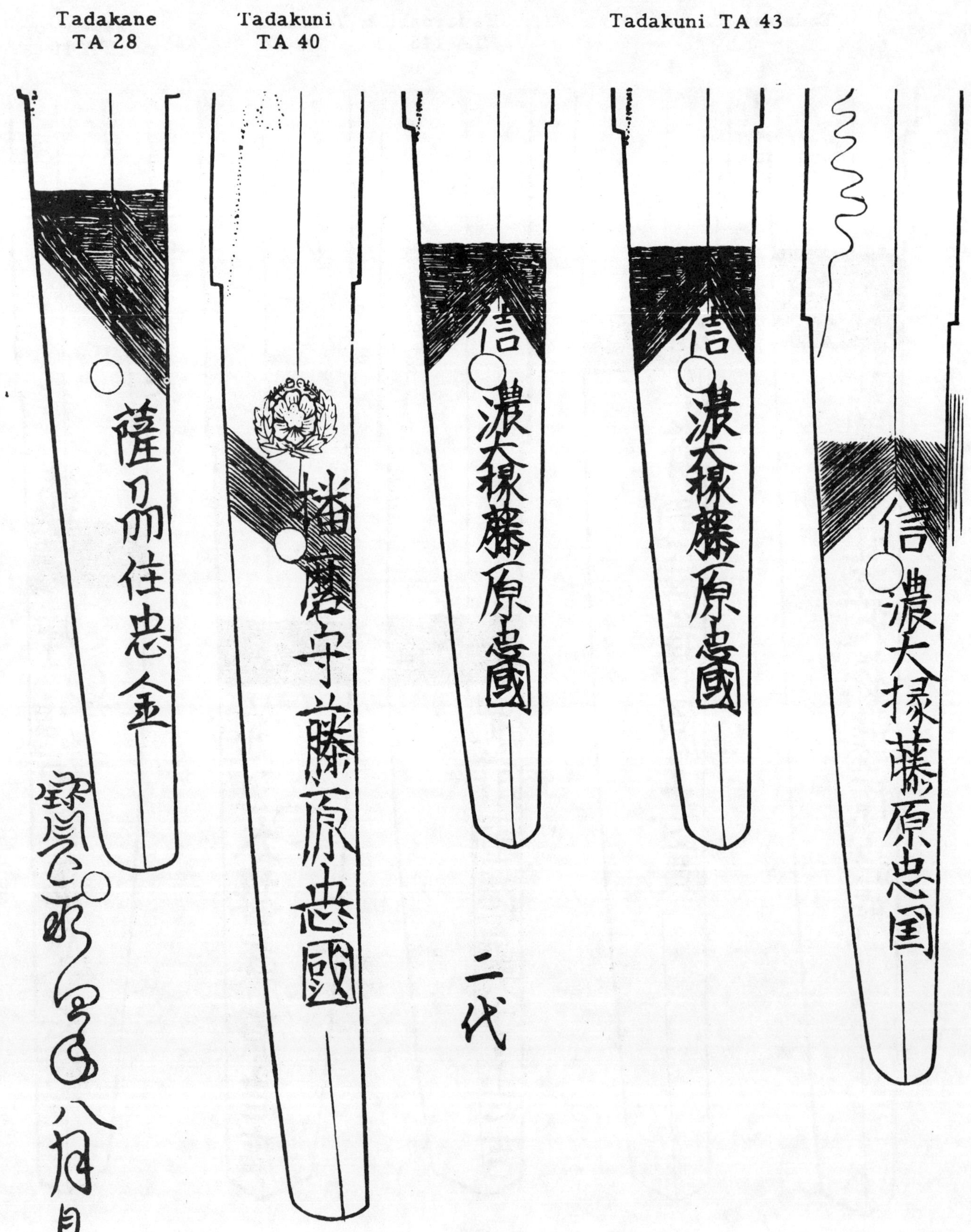

Tadakuni
TA 44

Tadakuni
TA 44a

Tadamichi
TA 60 -61

Tadamune
TA 84

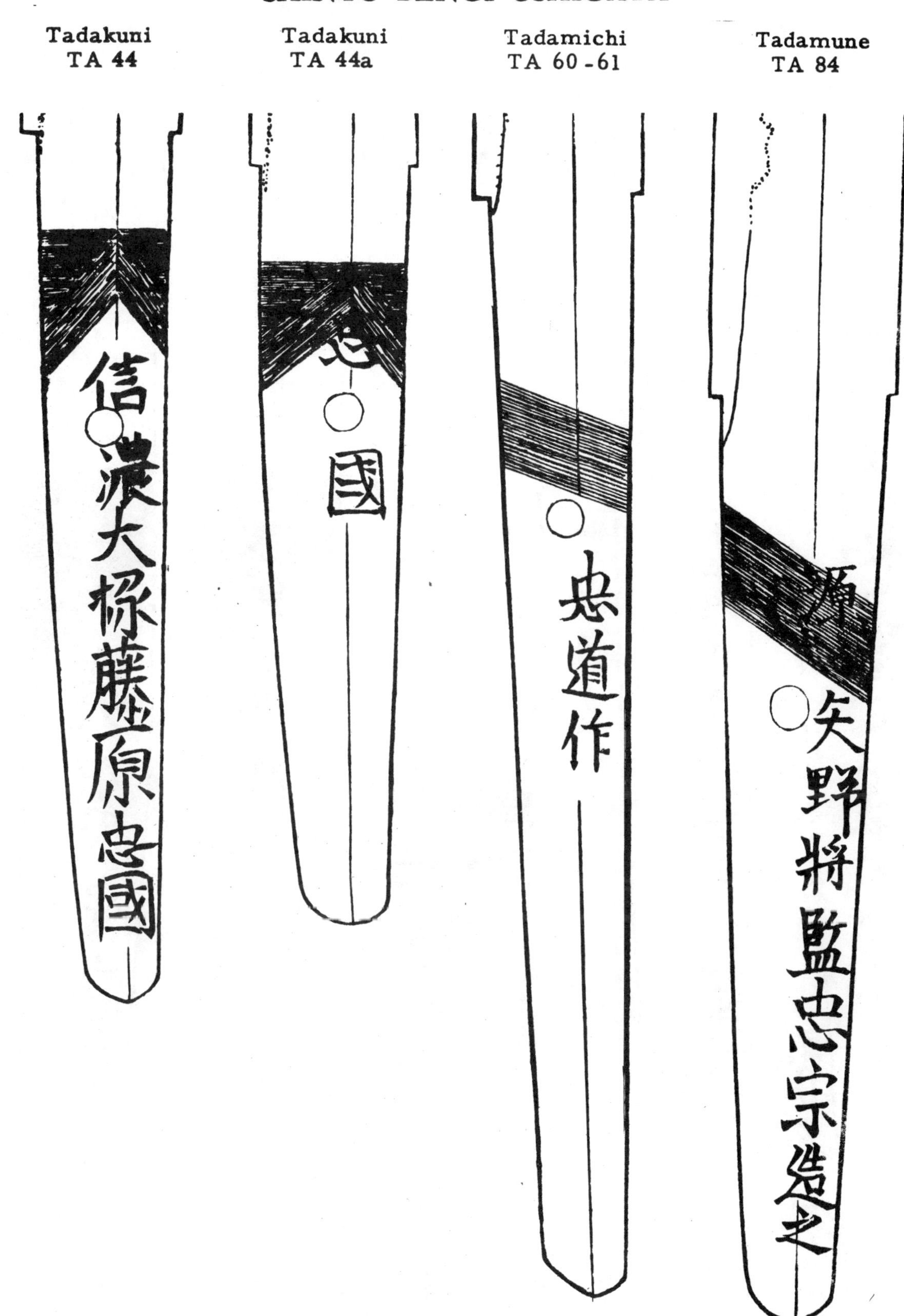

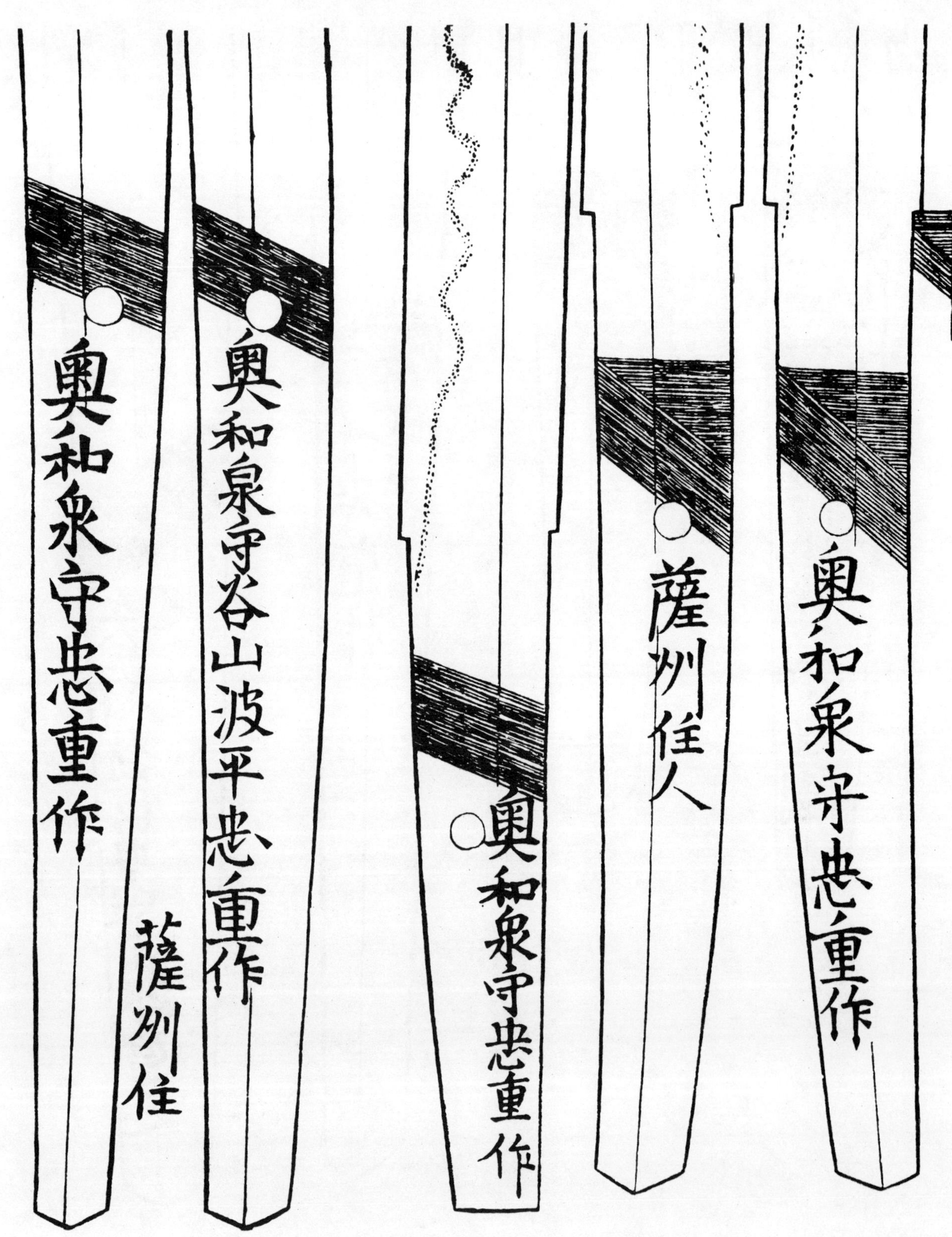

奥和泉守忠重作
奥和泉守谷山波平忠重作
薩州住
奥和泉守忠重作
薩州住人
奥和泉守忠重作

Tadatsuna
TA 128

Tadatsuna TA 129

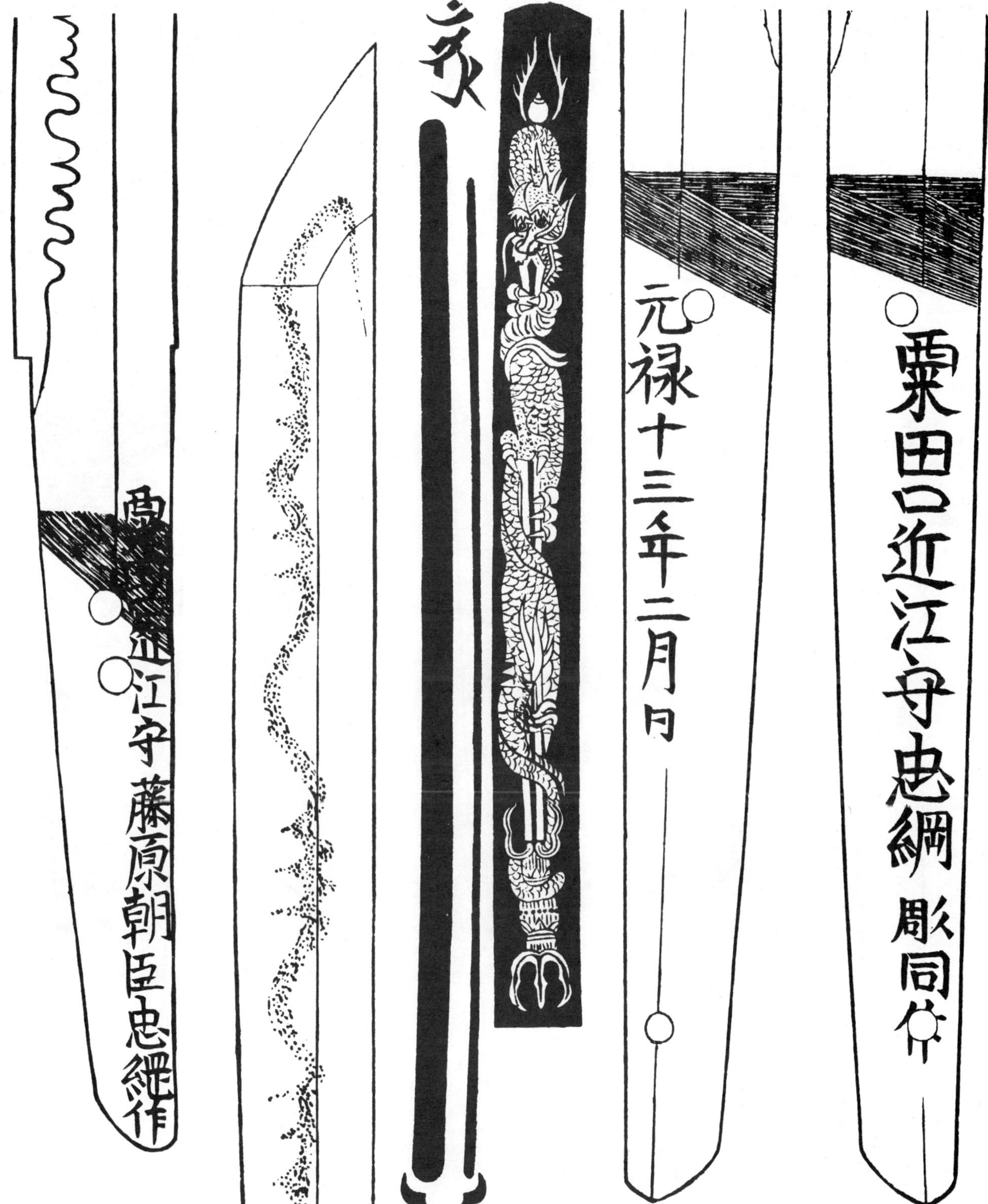

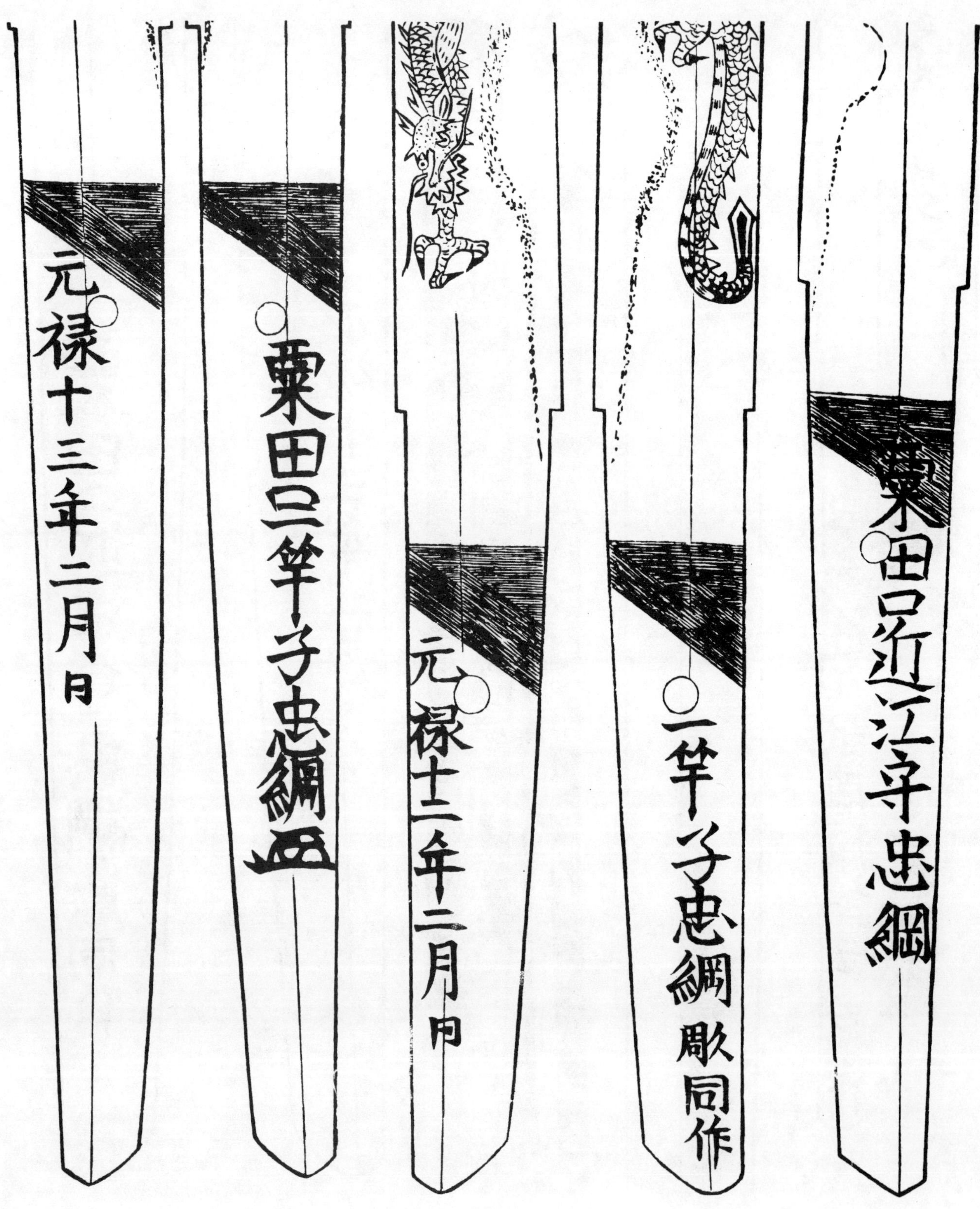
元禄十三年二月日
○粟田口一竿子忠綱画
元禄十二年二月日
○一竿子忠綱歟同作
○粟田口近江守忠綱

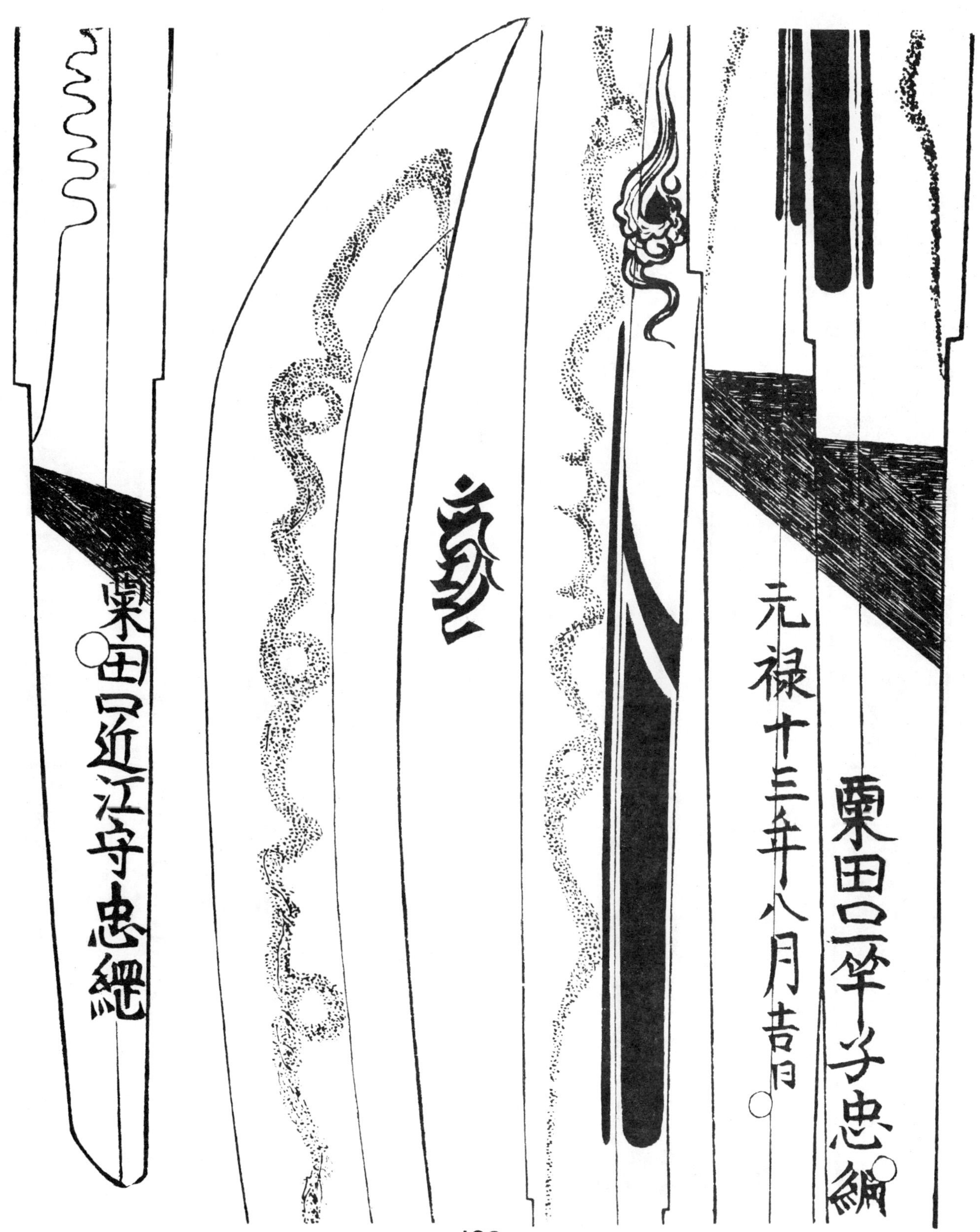
栗田口近江守忠綱
元禄十三年八月吉日
栗田口一卒子忠綱

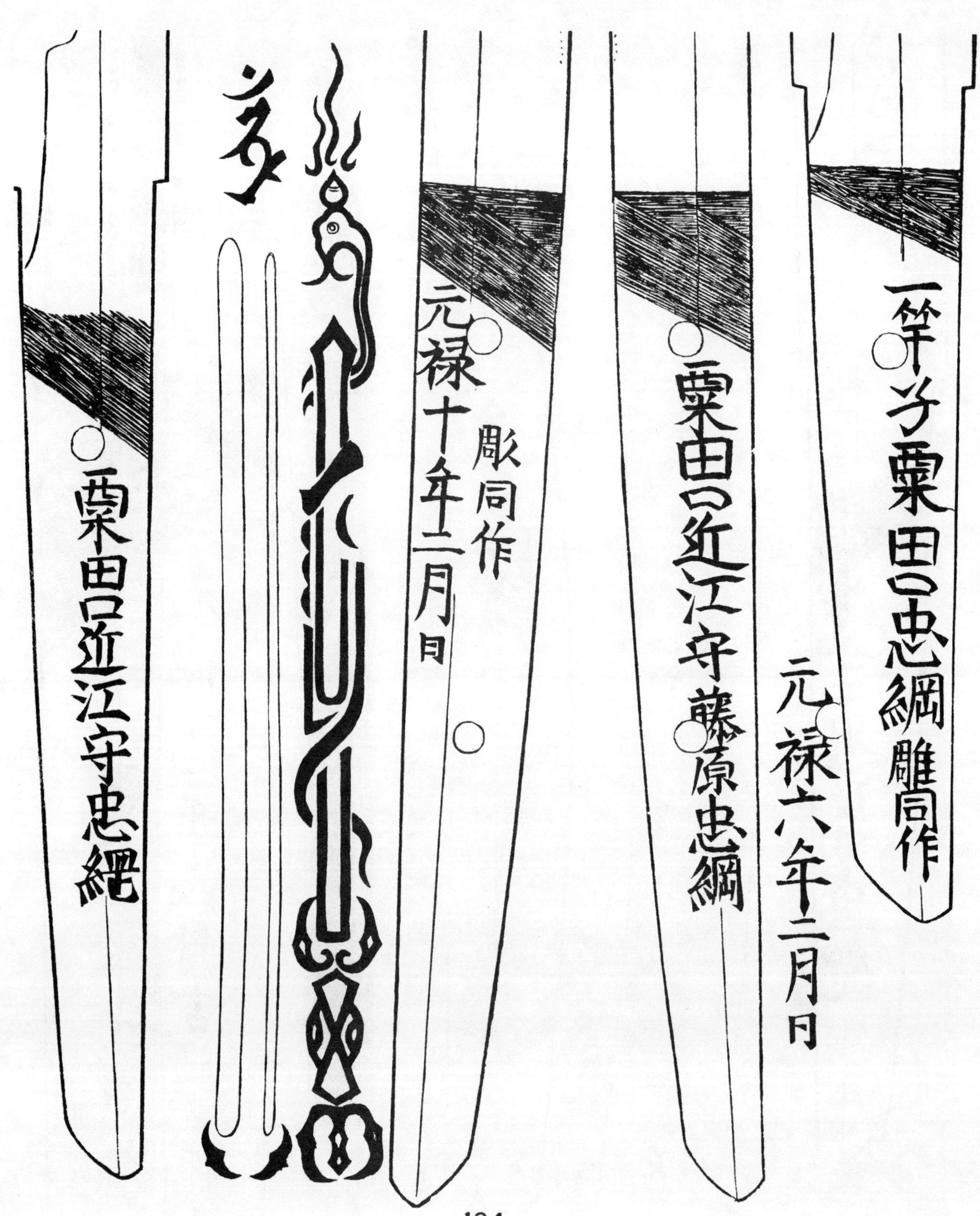

粟田口近江守忠綱
元禄十年二月日
彫同作
粟田口近江守藤原忠綱
一竿子粟田口忠綱雕同作
元禄六年二月日

Tadatsuna TA 129

Horimono by Tadatsuna

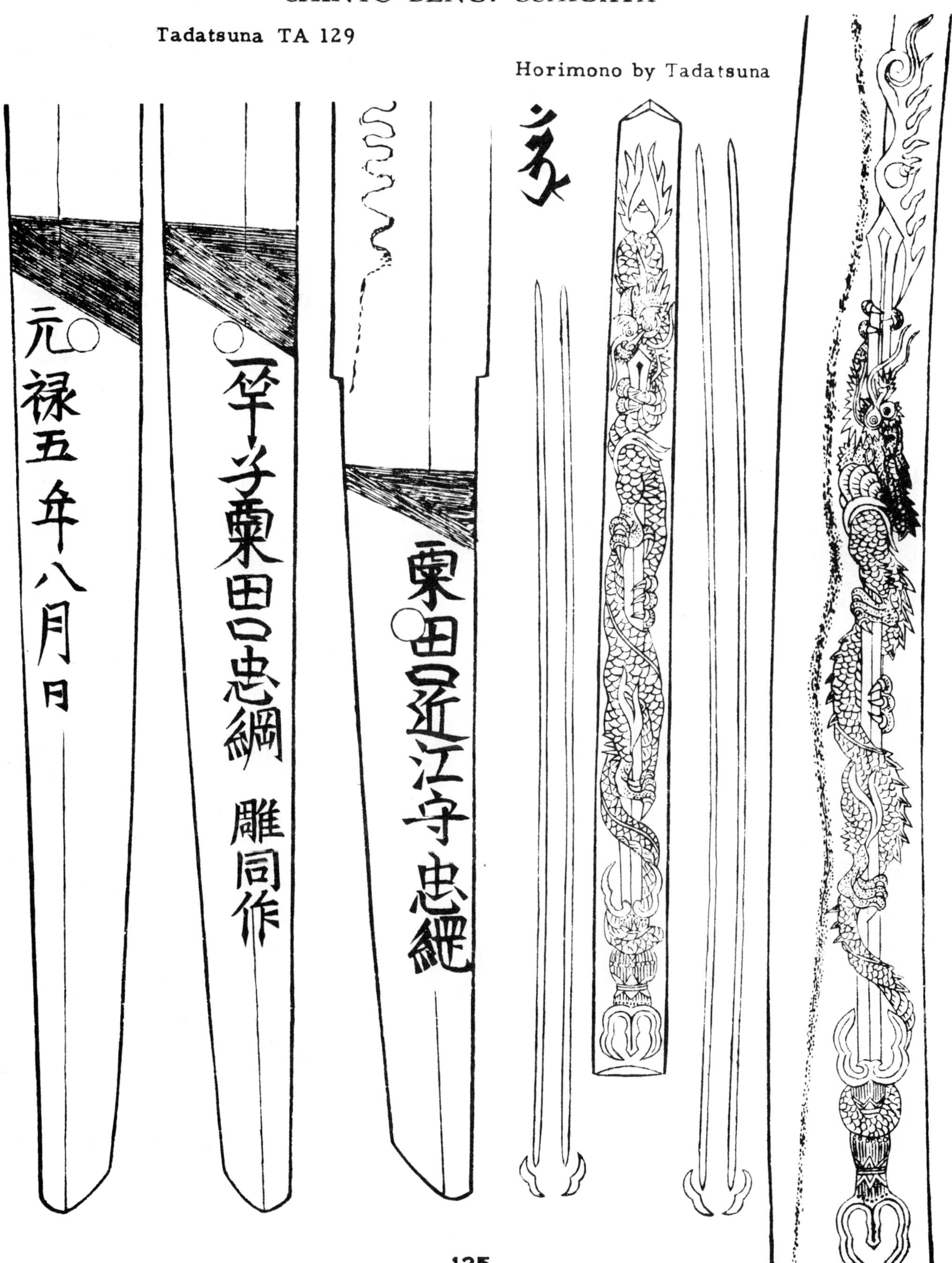

Tadayoshi
TA 146

Tadayoshi TA 140

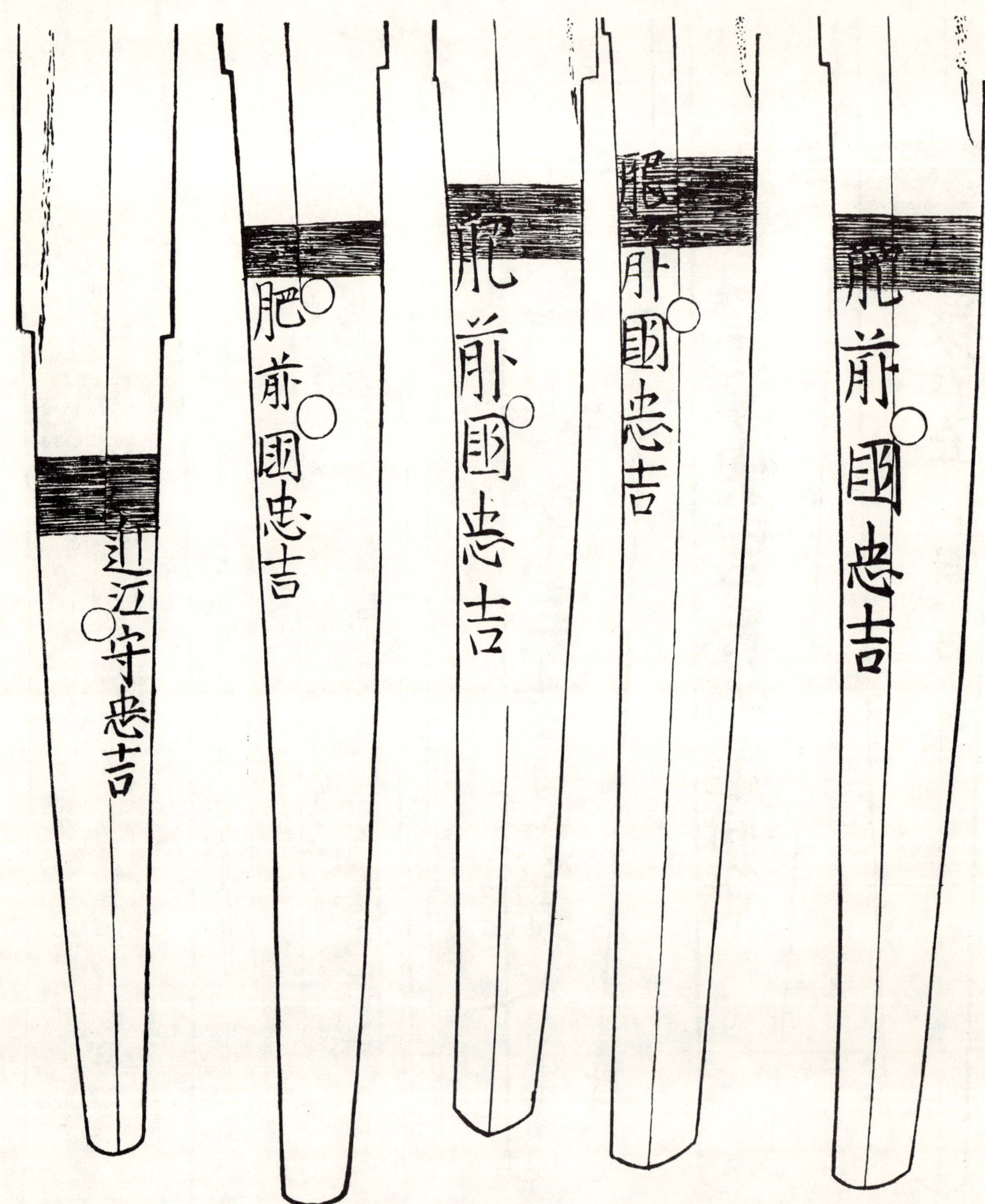

Tadayoshi
TA 140   Tadayoshi TA 143   Tadayoshi TA 144

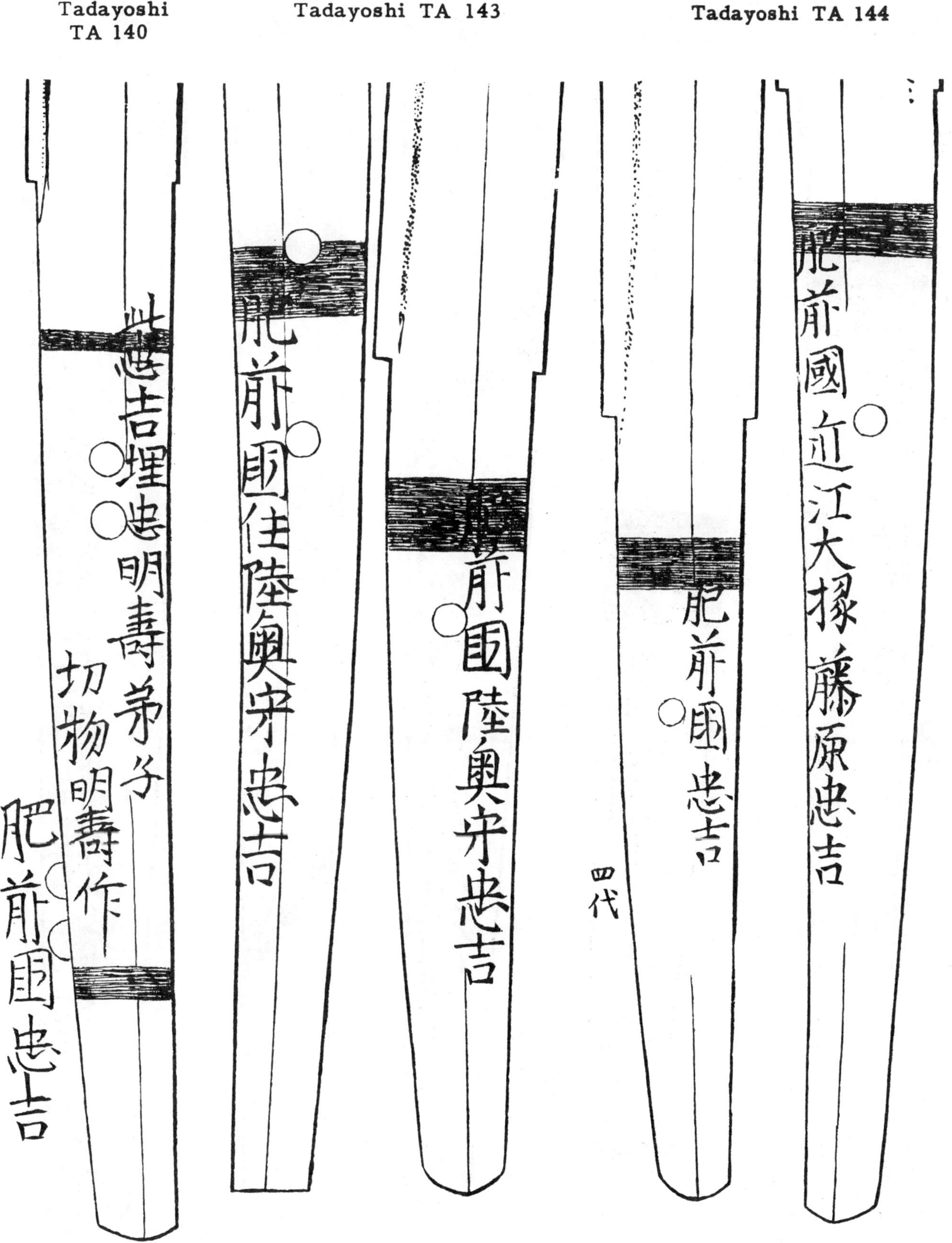

Tadayoshi
TA 146

Tadayoshi
TA 147

Tadayuki
TA 164

Tadayuki
TA 165

Tameiye
TA 334

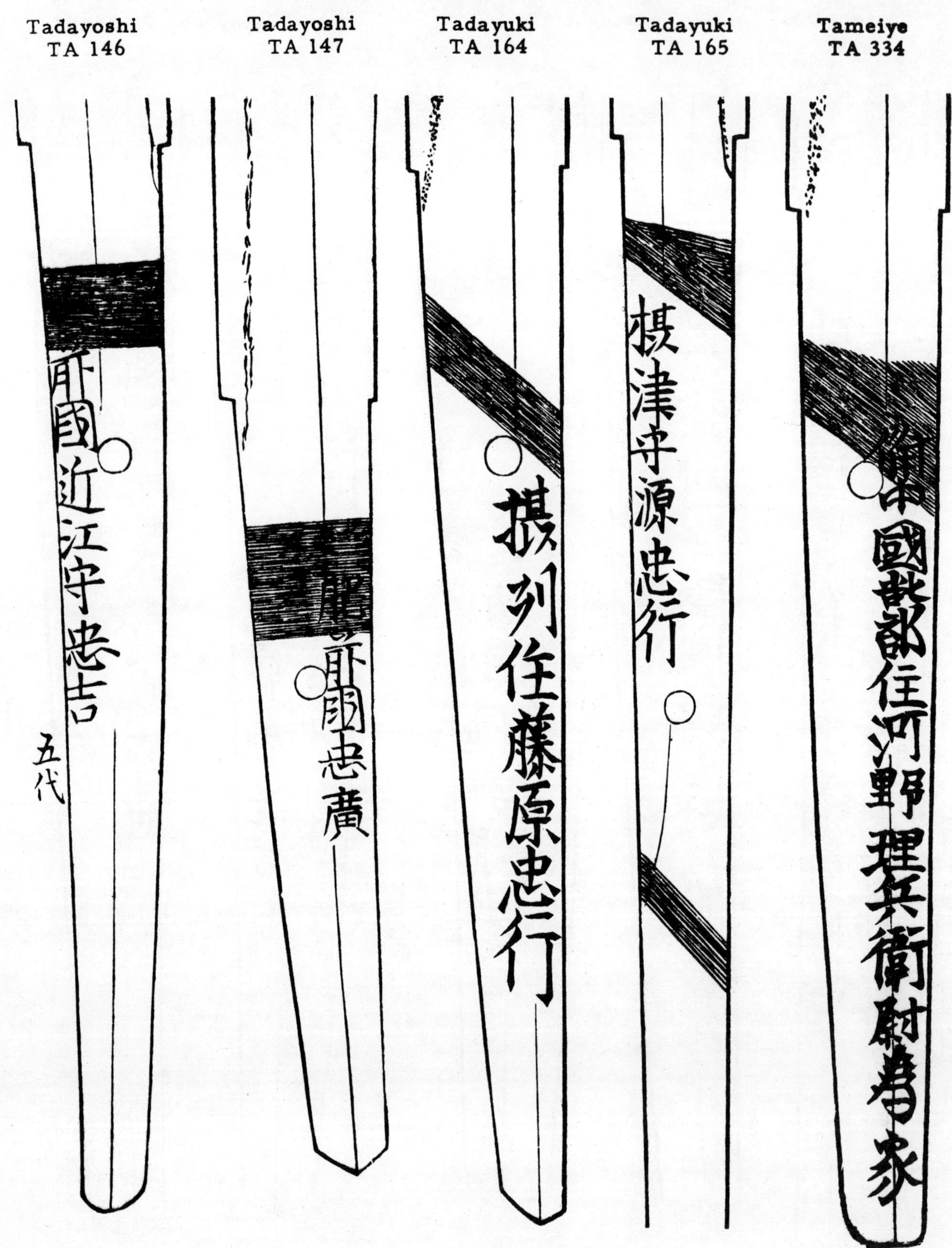

SHINTO BENGI OSHIGATA

Takahira
TA 189

Takanobu
TA 291

Takahiro
TA 195

Tameiye & Kunishige
TA 334   KU 533

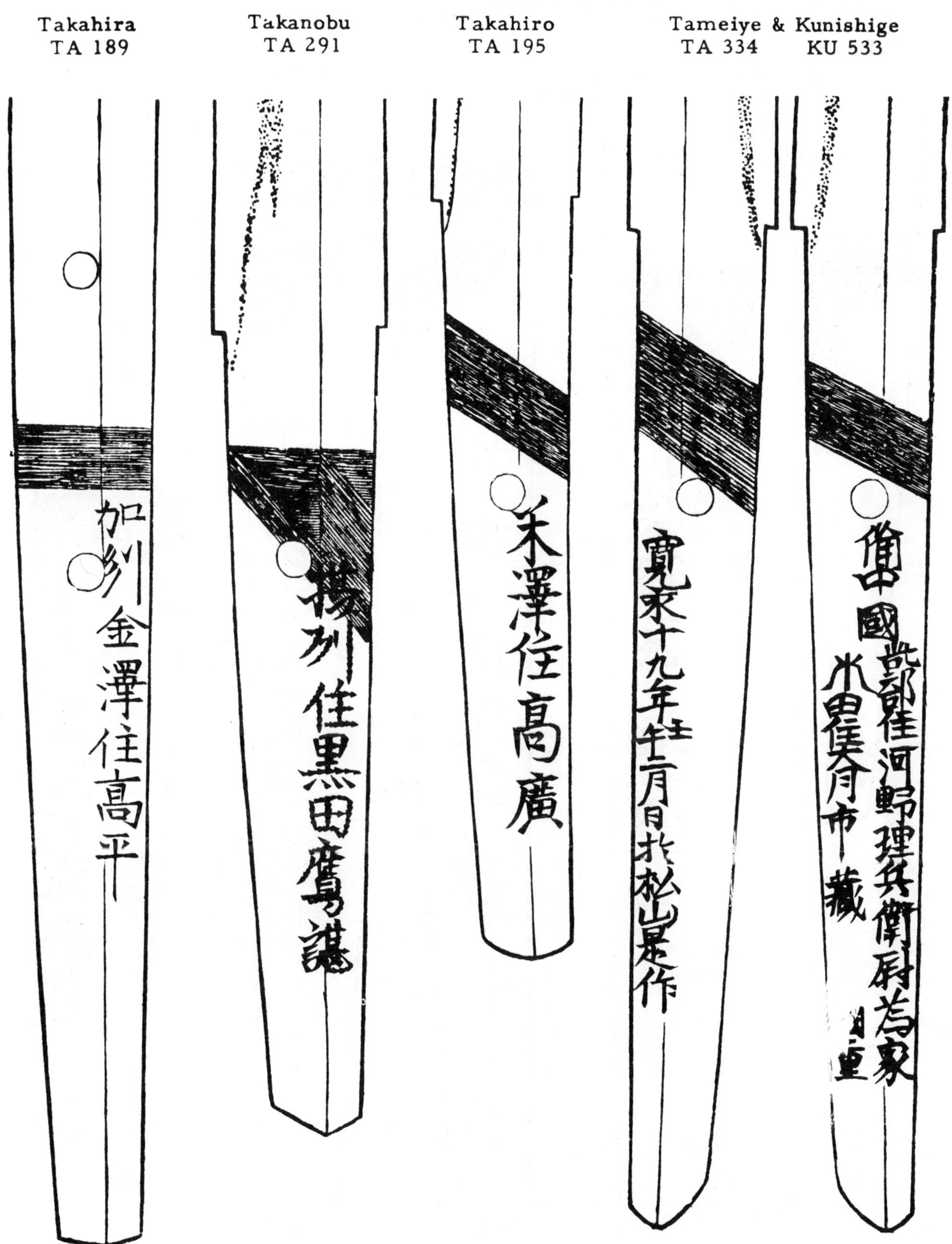

Takenaga
TA 306

Terukane TE 43

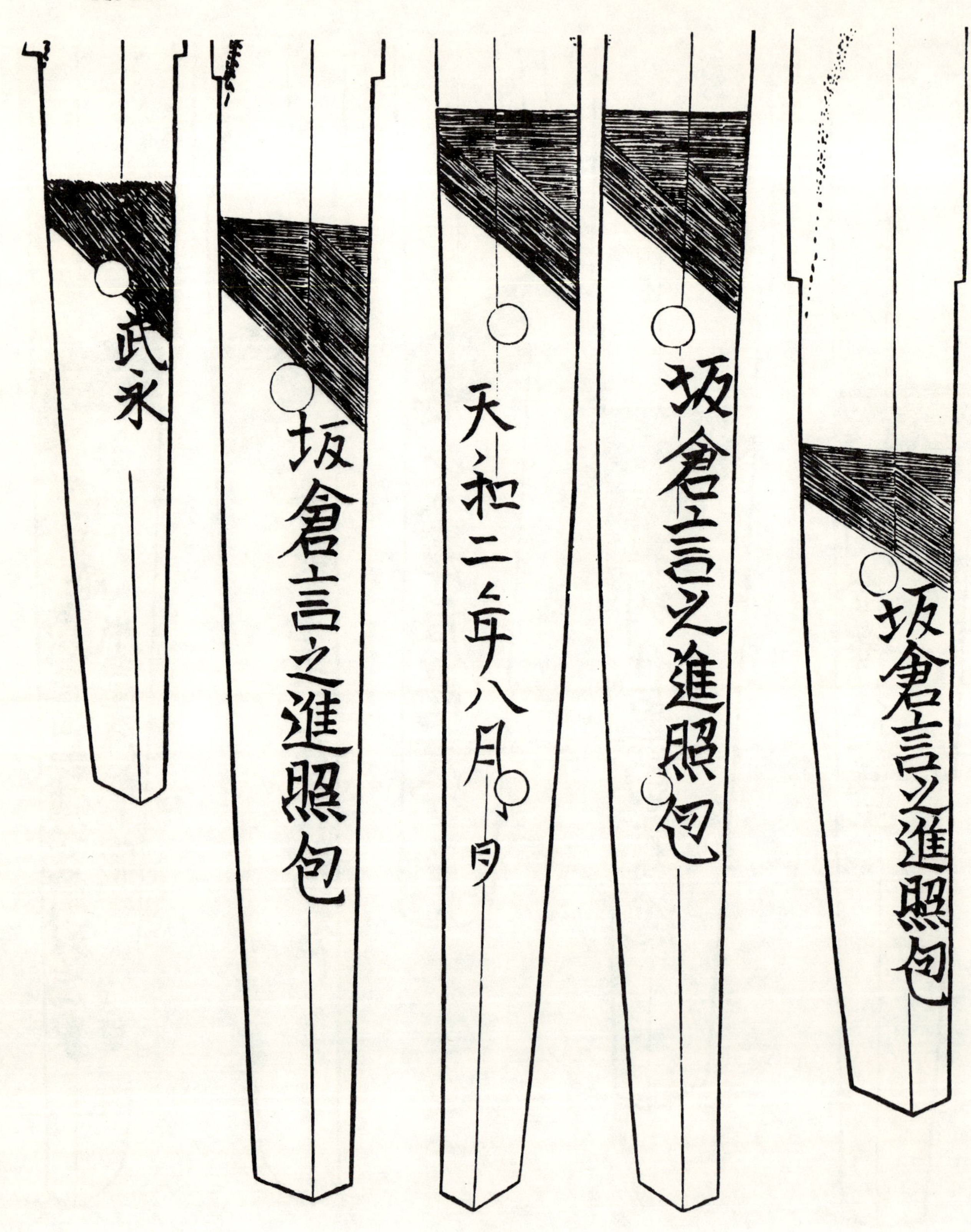

Terukane TE 43

Teruhiro
TE 64

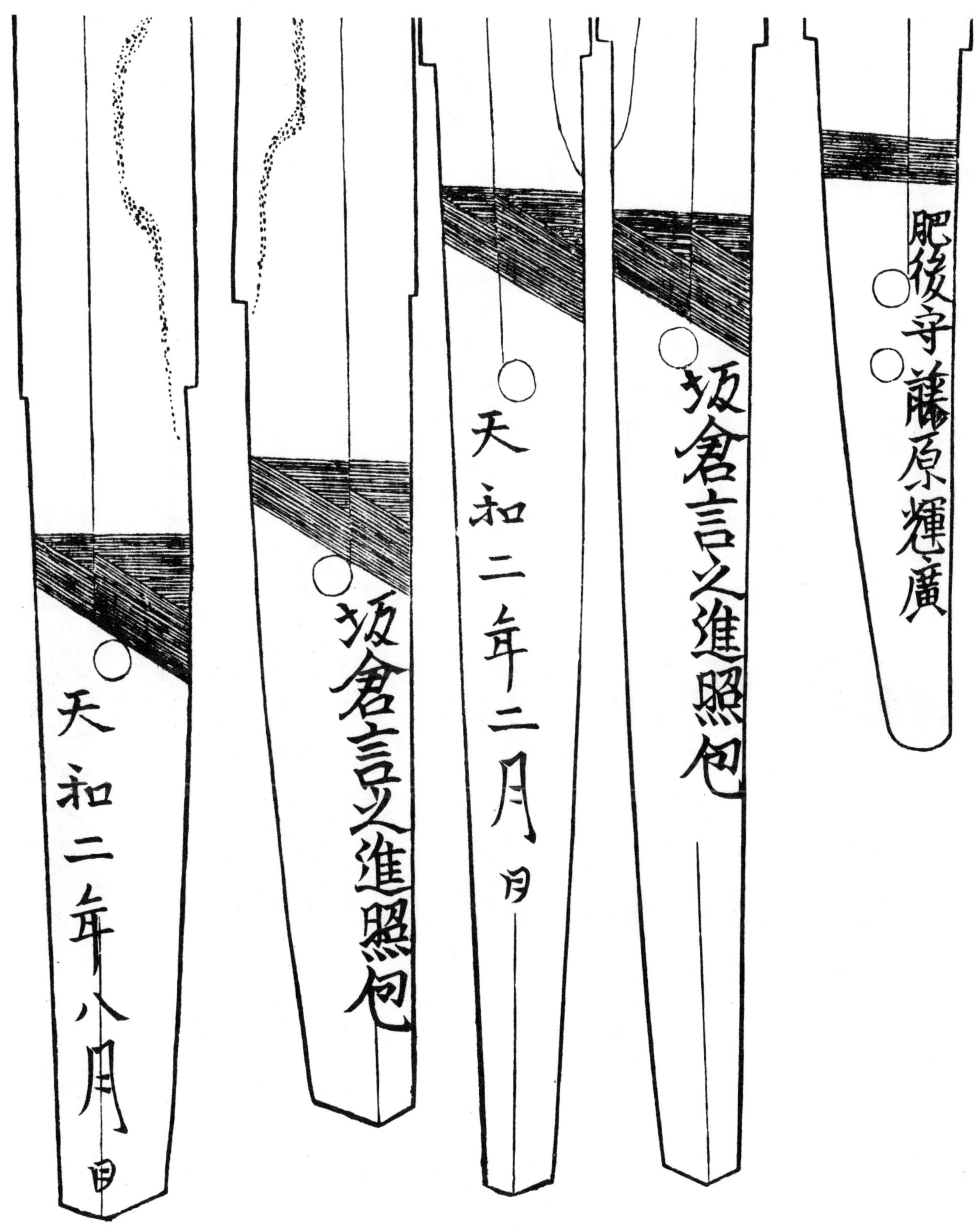

Teruhiro
TE 65

Teruhiro
TE 64

Terukane
TE 80

Terukuni TE 82

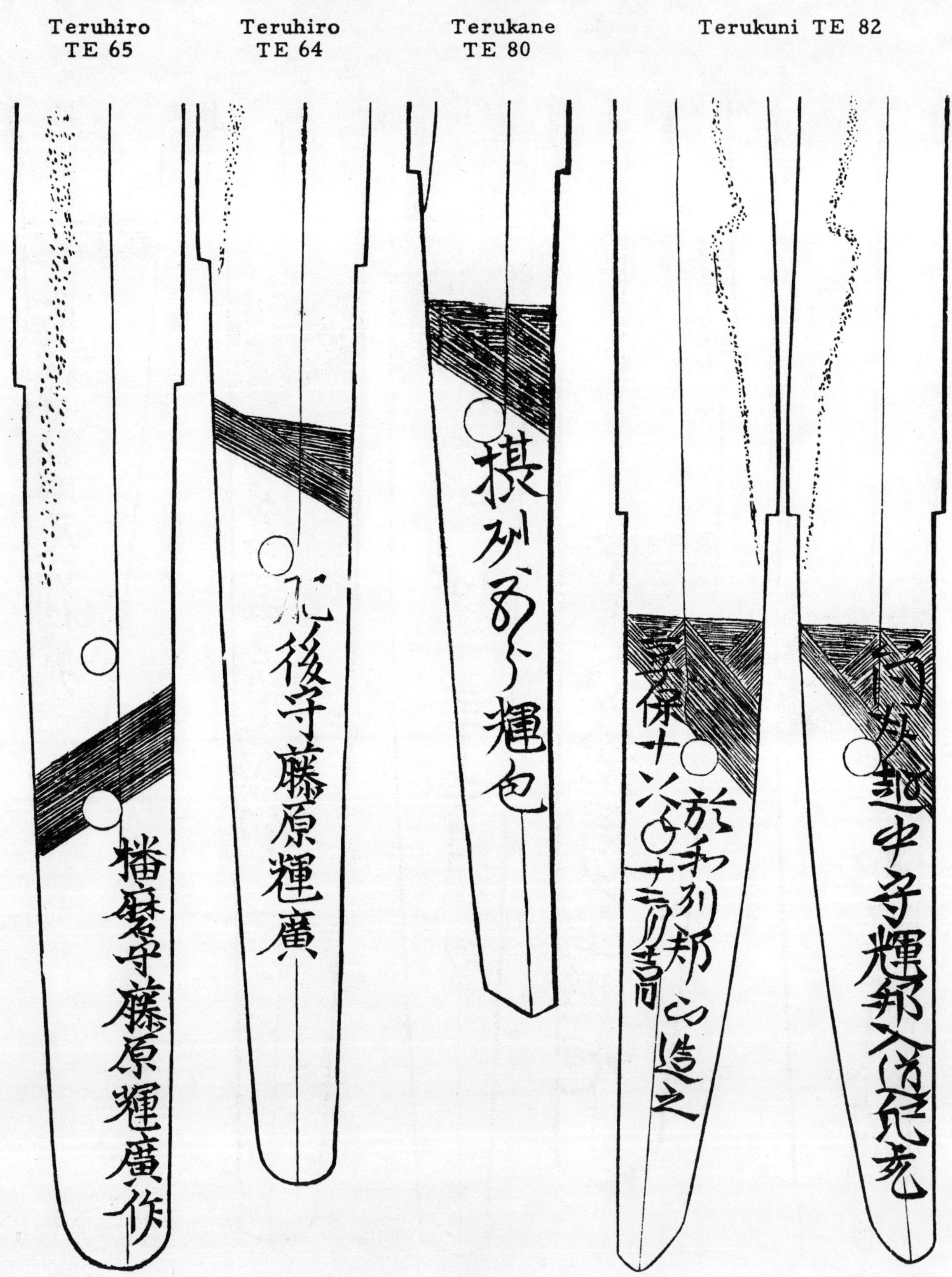

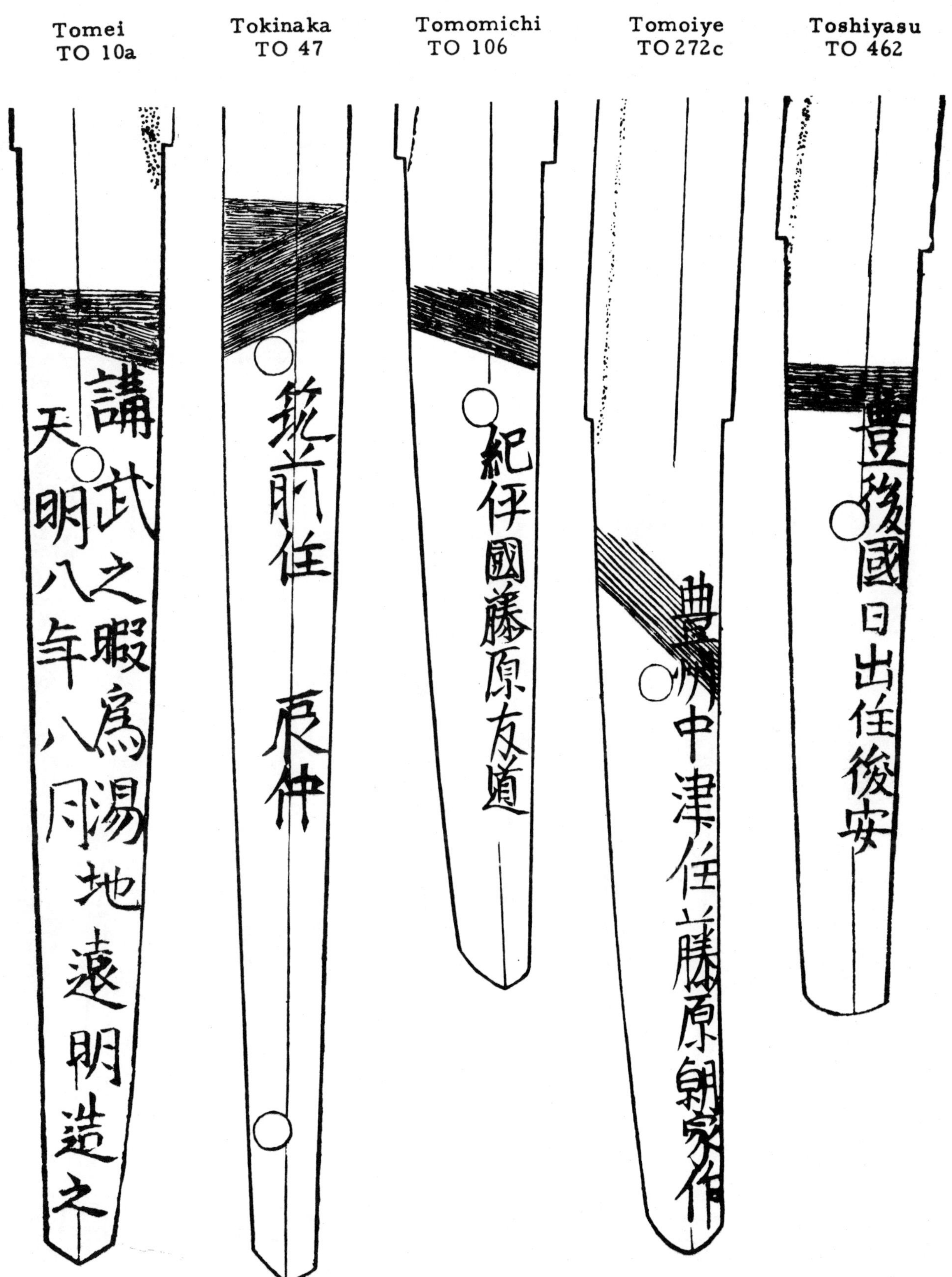

Tomei
TO 10a
Tokinaka
TO 47
Tomomichi
TO 106
Tomoiye
TO 272c
Toshiyasu
TO 462
講武之暇爲湯地遠明造之
天明八年八月
武之暇爲湯地遠明造之
肥前住忠仲
紀伊國藤原友道
豊後中津住藤原朝家作
豊後國日出住後安

Toshinaga
TO 476

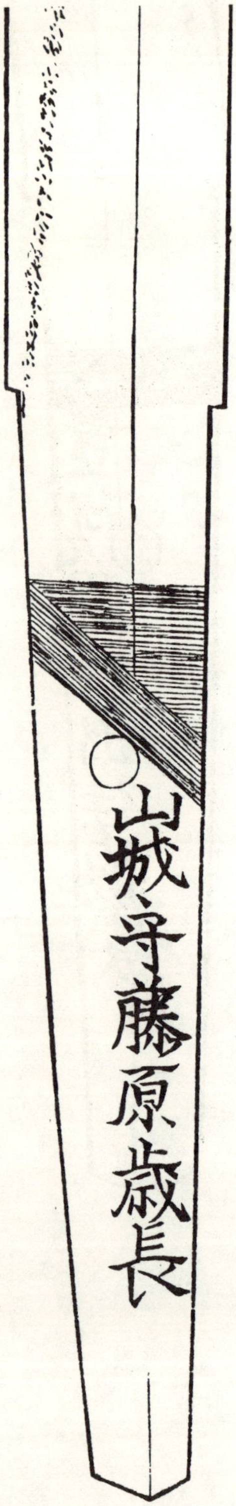

Toshinaga TO 478

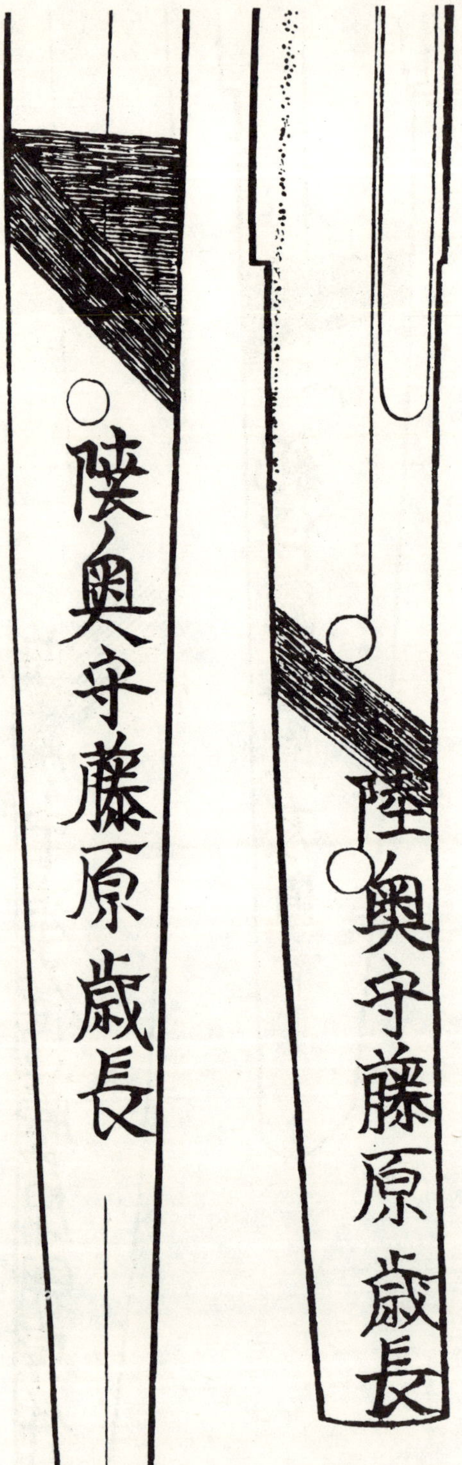

Toshinori TO 521

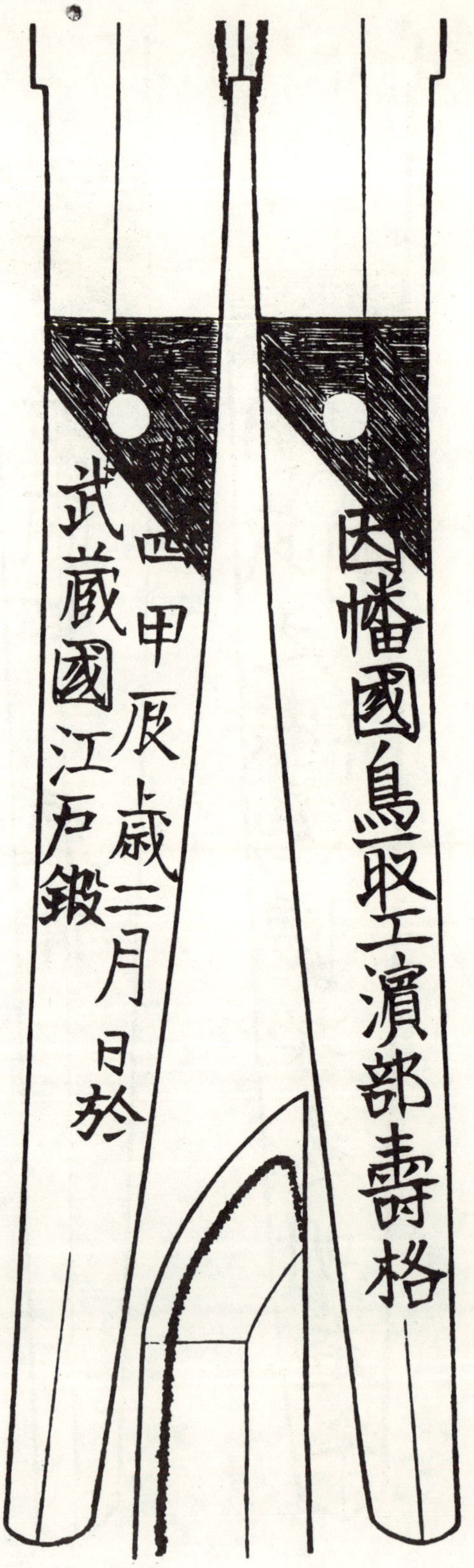

山城守藤原歳長

陸奥守藤原歳長

陸奥守藤原歳長

於日 二月歳辰甲 武蔵國江戸鍛

因幡國鳥取工濱部壽格

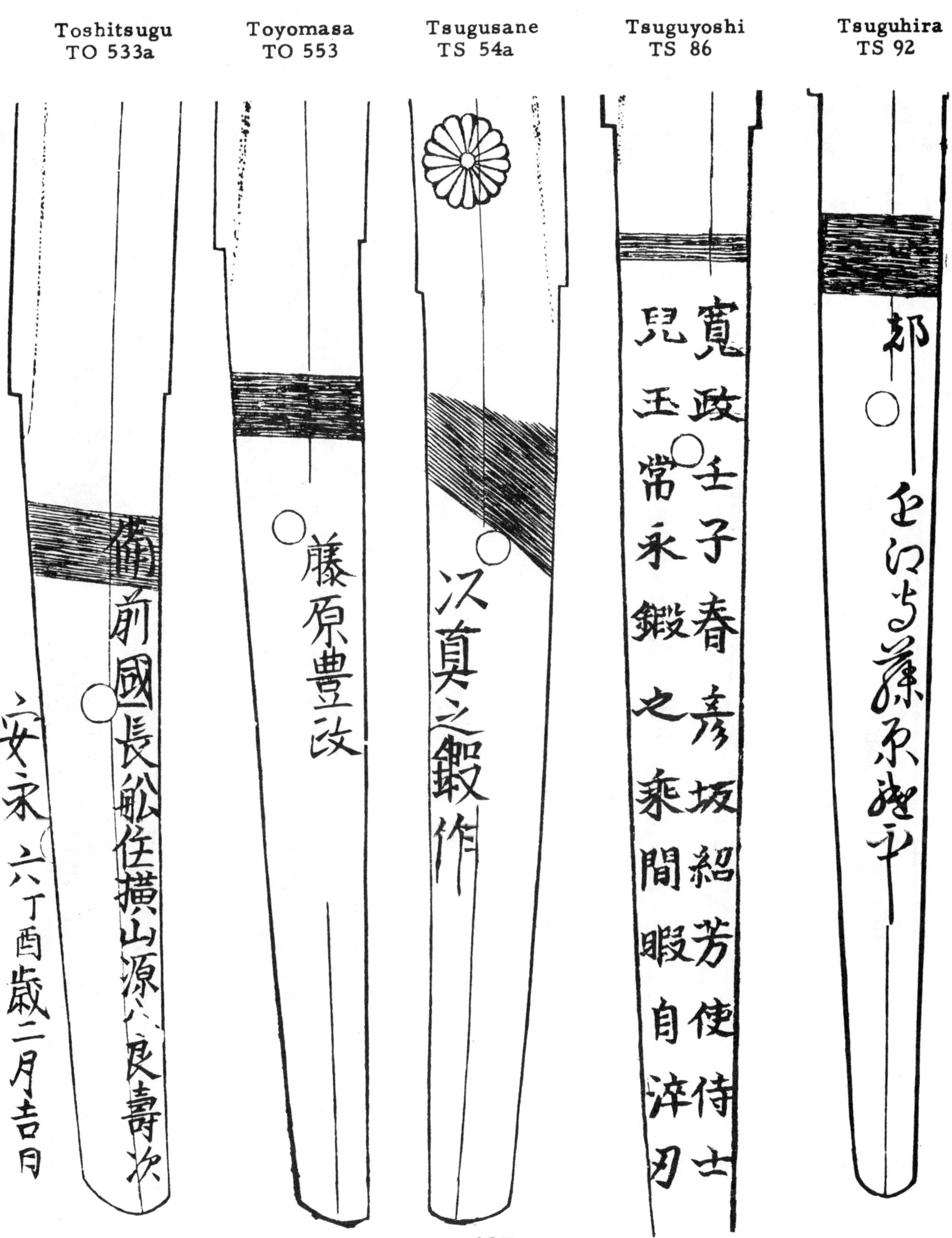

Toshitsugu
TO 533a
Toyomasa
TO 553
Tsugusane
TS 54a
Tsuguyoshi
TS 86
Tsuguhira
TS 92
備前國長船住横山源八良壽次
安永六丁酉歳二月吉月
藤原豊政
以真之鍛作
寛政壬子春彦坂紹芳使侍士
兒玉常永鍛之乗間暇自淬刃
都
藤原姓平

Tsuguhira TS 93   Tsunafusa   Tsunamune TS 162
                          TS 121

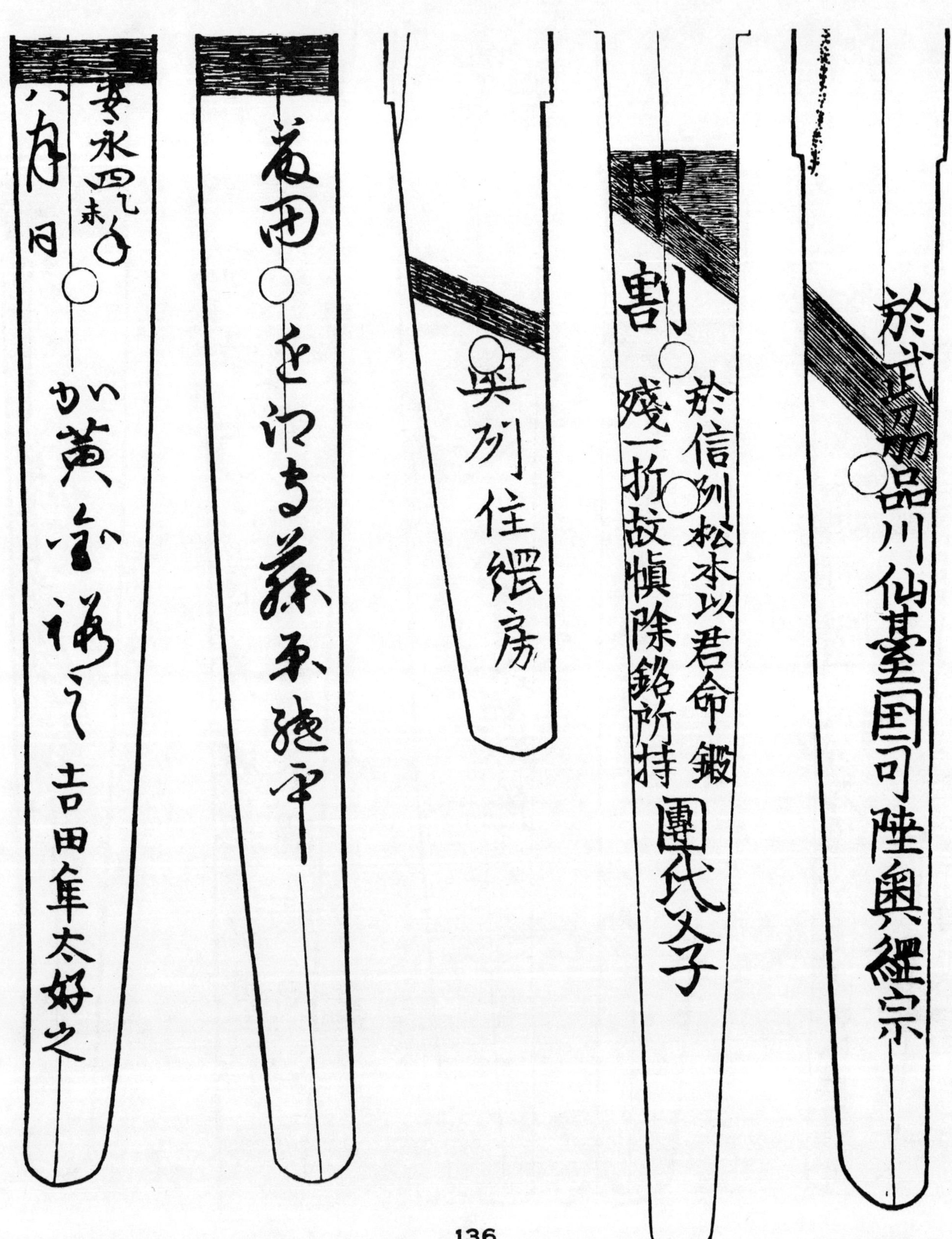

Tsunayoshi TS 193   Tsunenaga TS 266

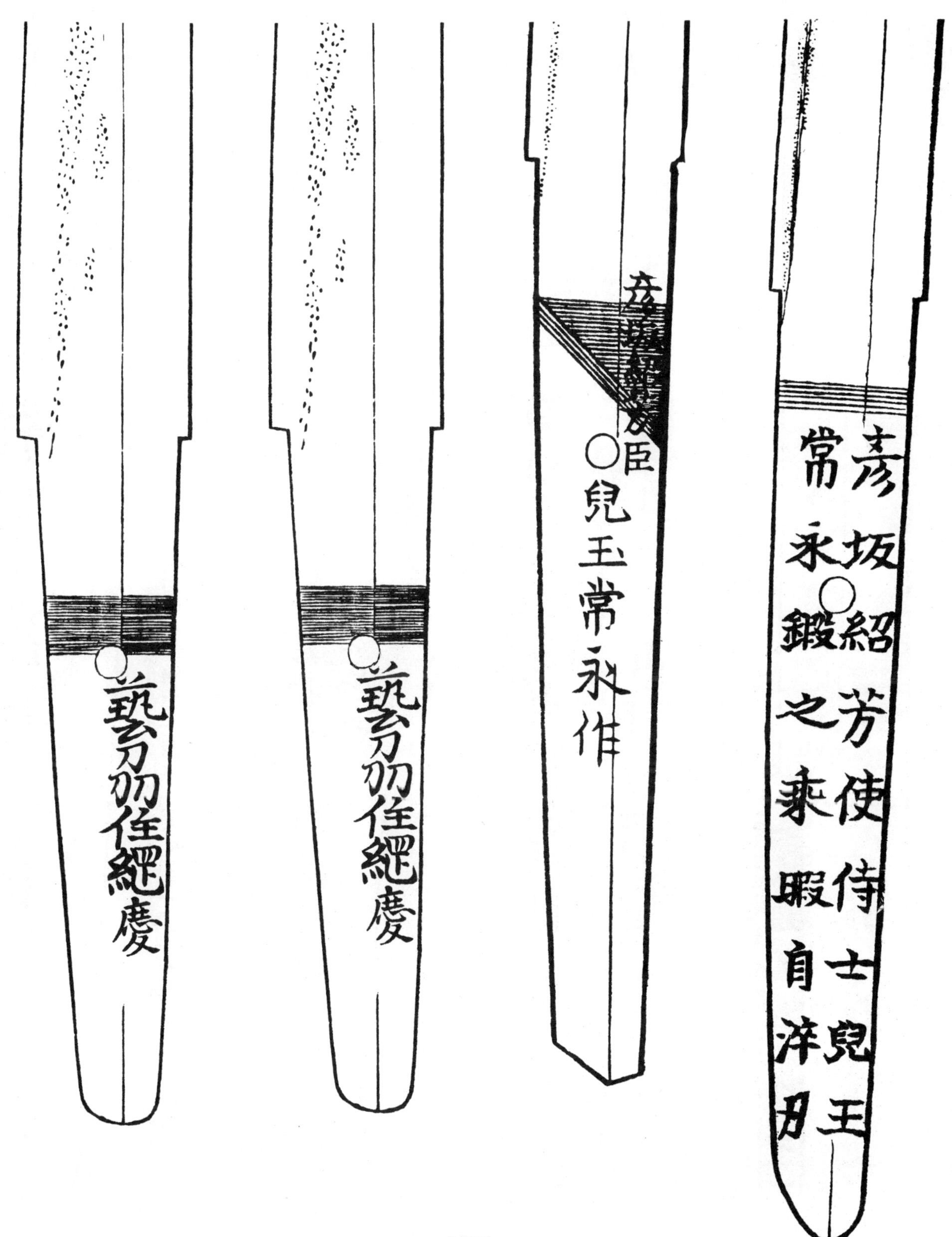

SHINTO BENGI OSHIGATA

Ujisada UJ 70 — **Ujishige UJ 88** — **Yasuaki YA 12** — **Yasuari YA 15**

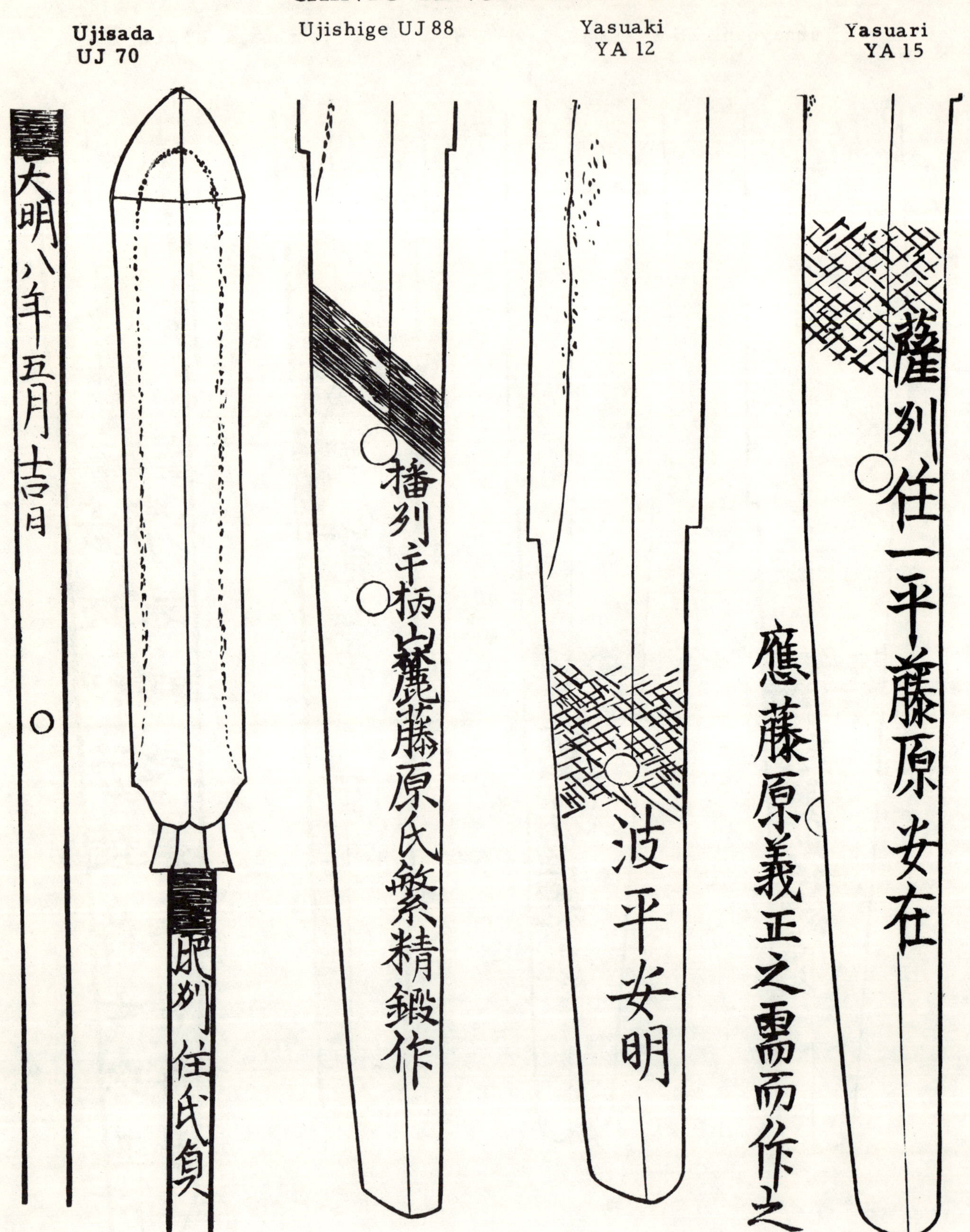

Yasuhiro	Yasukuni	Yasukuni	Yasumasa	Yasusada
YA 47	YA 80	YA 83	YA 87	YA 173

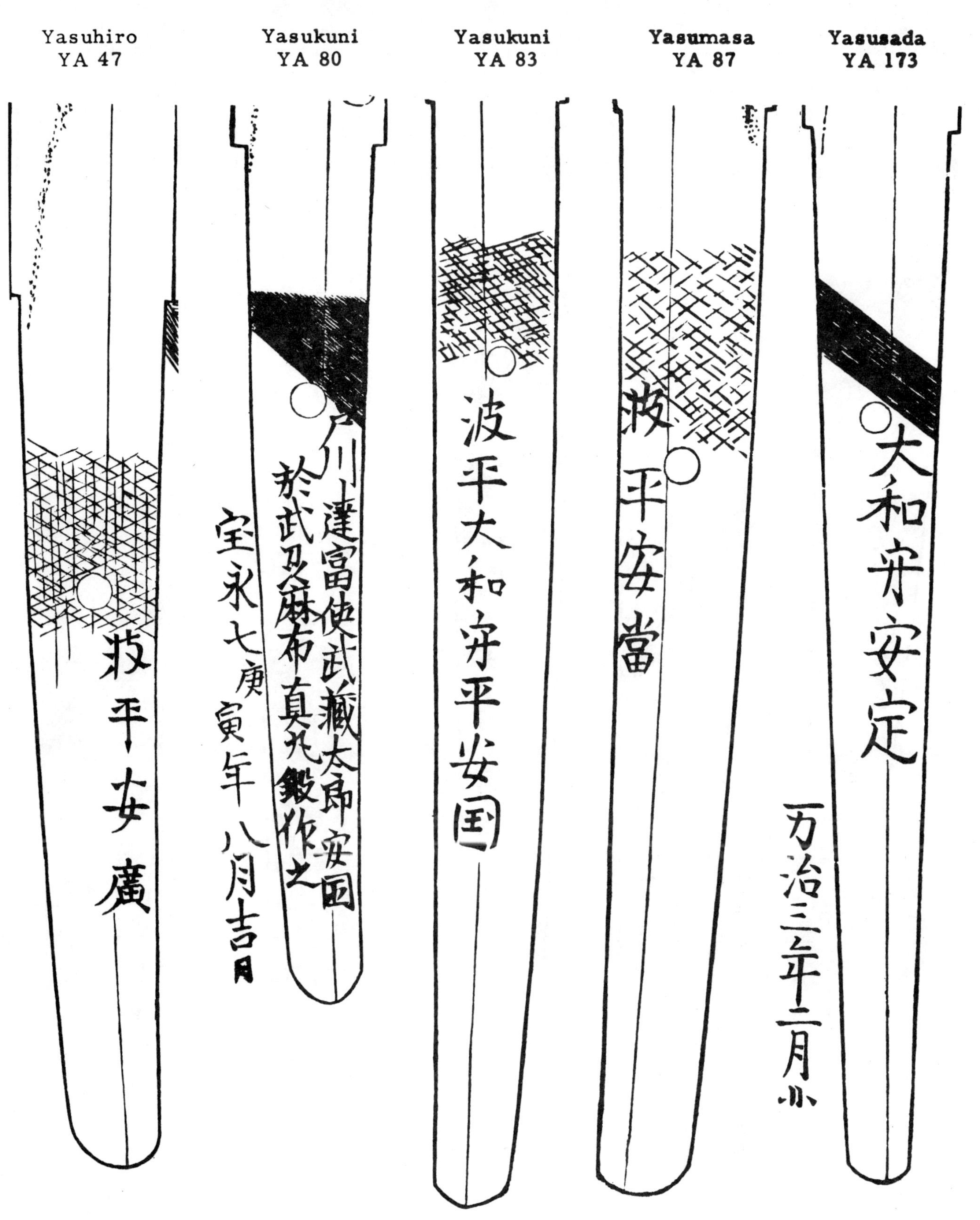

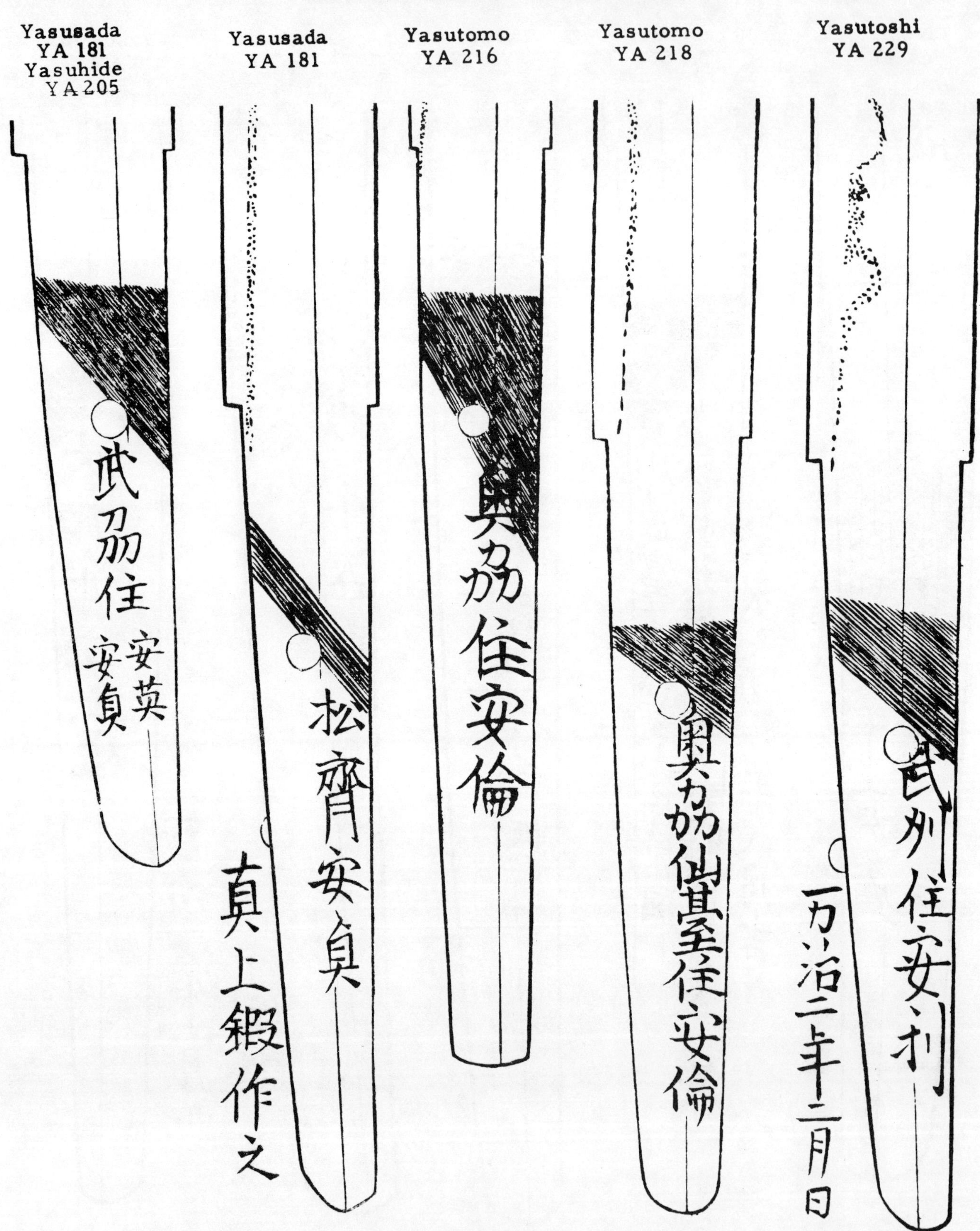

Yasusada
YA 181
Yasuhide
YA 205
Yasusada
YA 181
Yasutomo
YA 216
Yasutomo
YA 218
Yasutoshi
YA 229
武刕住安英安貞
松齊安貞
真上鍛作之
奥刕住安倫
奥刕仙臺住安倫
武刕住安利
万治二年十二月日

Yasutsugu
YA 247

Yasutsune
YA 270

Yasuyo YA 273

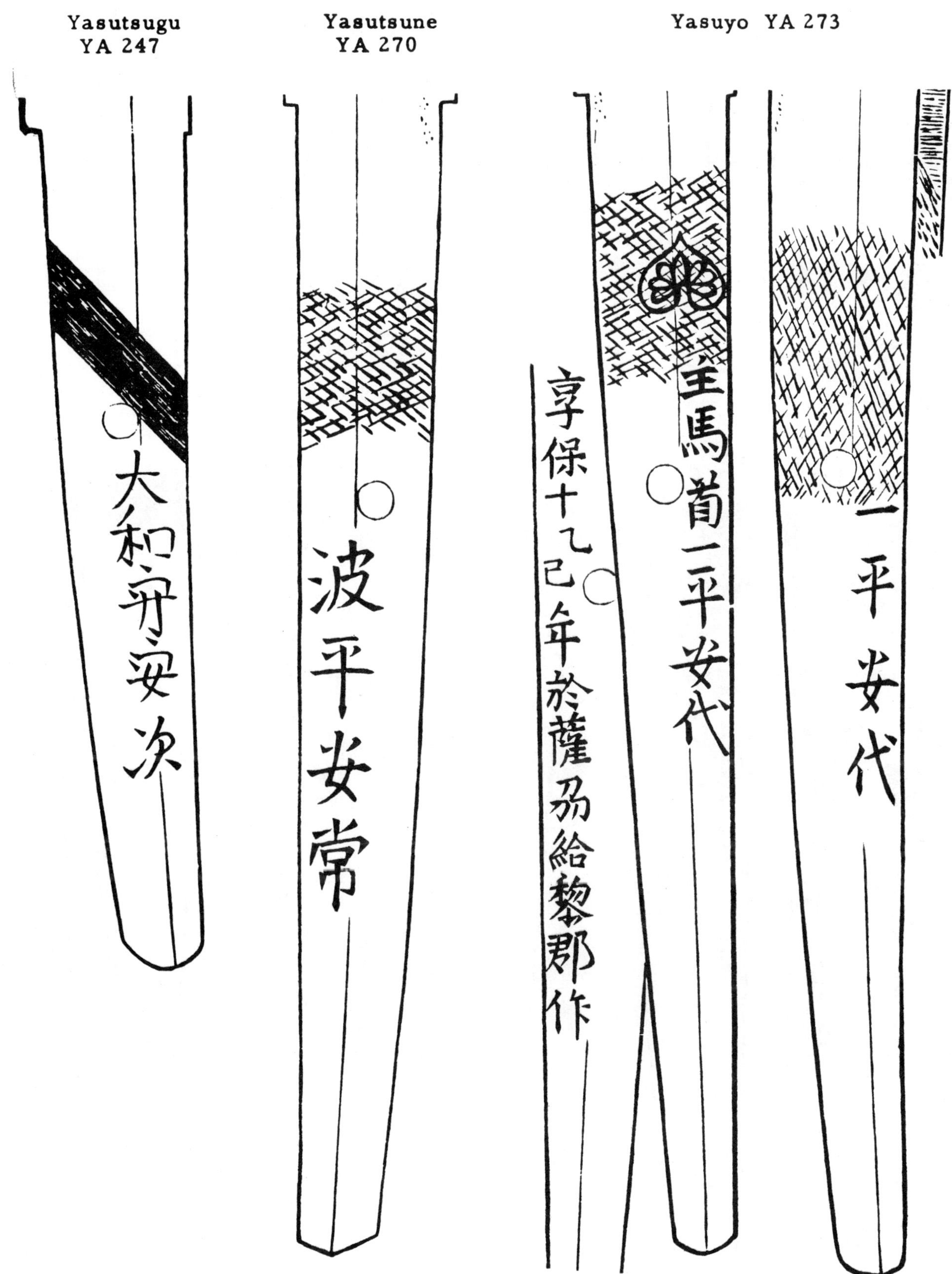

Yasuyo YA 273

Yasuyuki
YA 309 ?

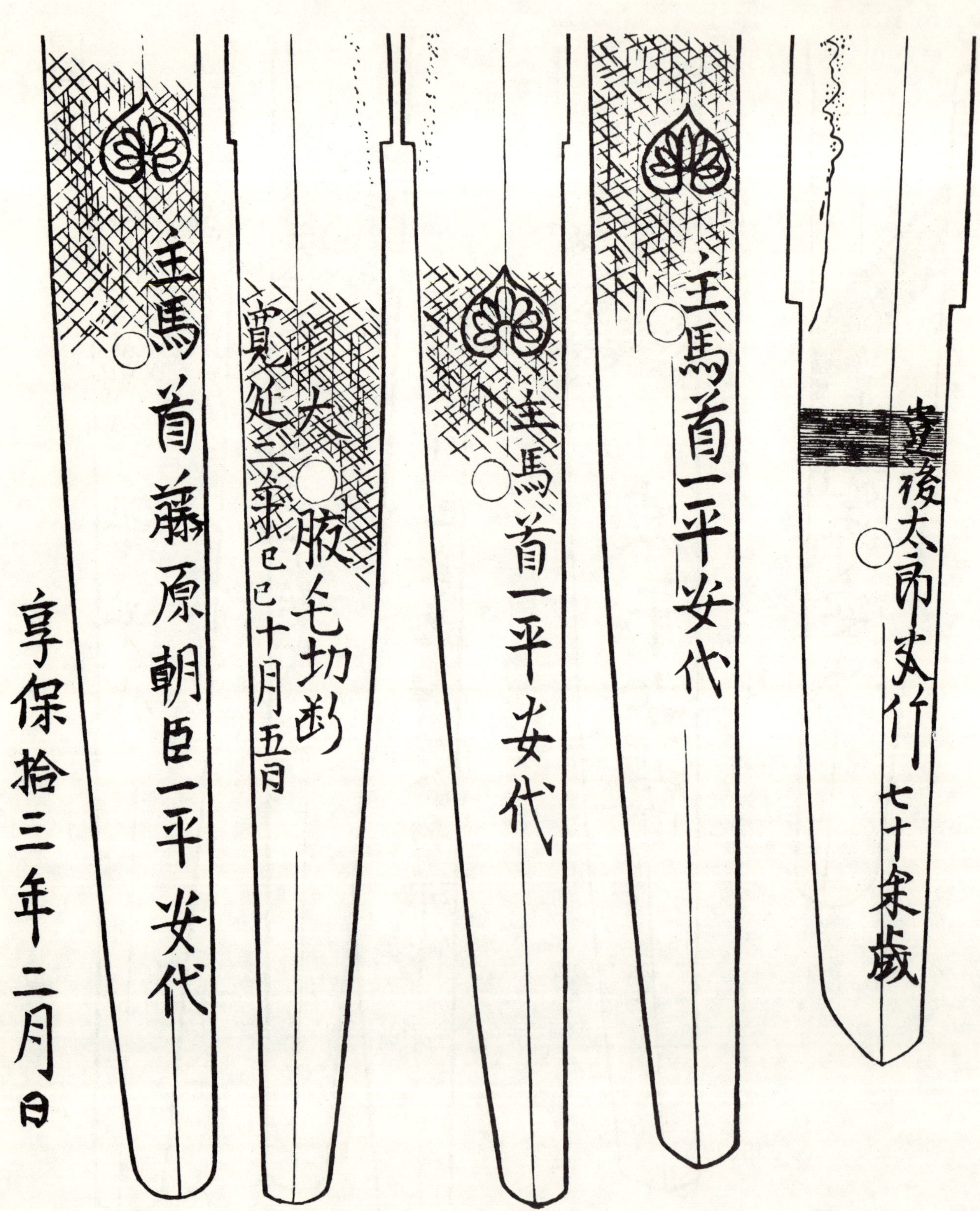

Yasunori YA 323   Yasuyuki   Yasuhiro & Tameyasu
                          YA 370   YA 381   TA 423

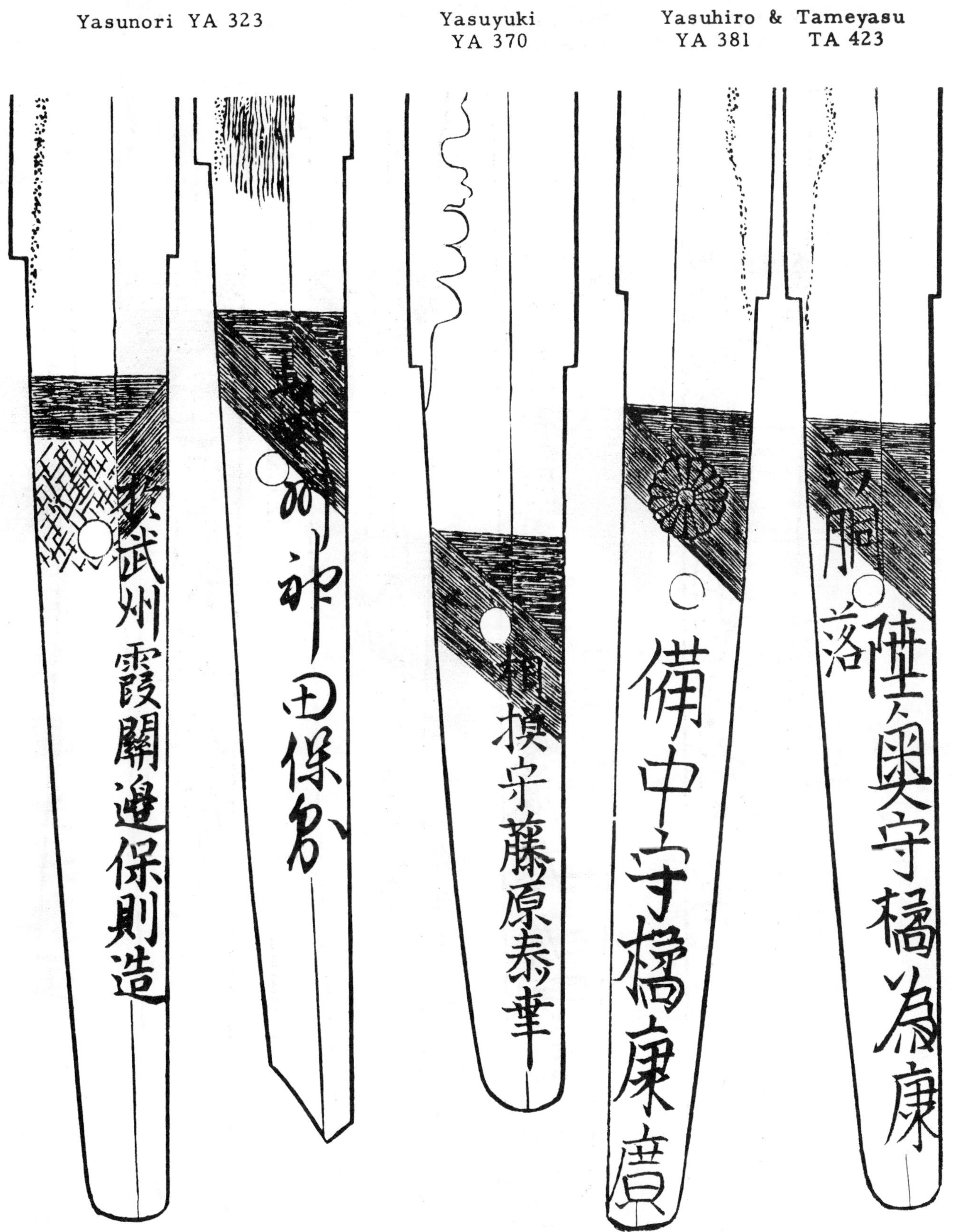

Yasumitsu
YA 410

Yasunaga
YA 417

Yasunaga YA 418

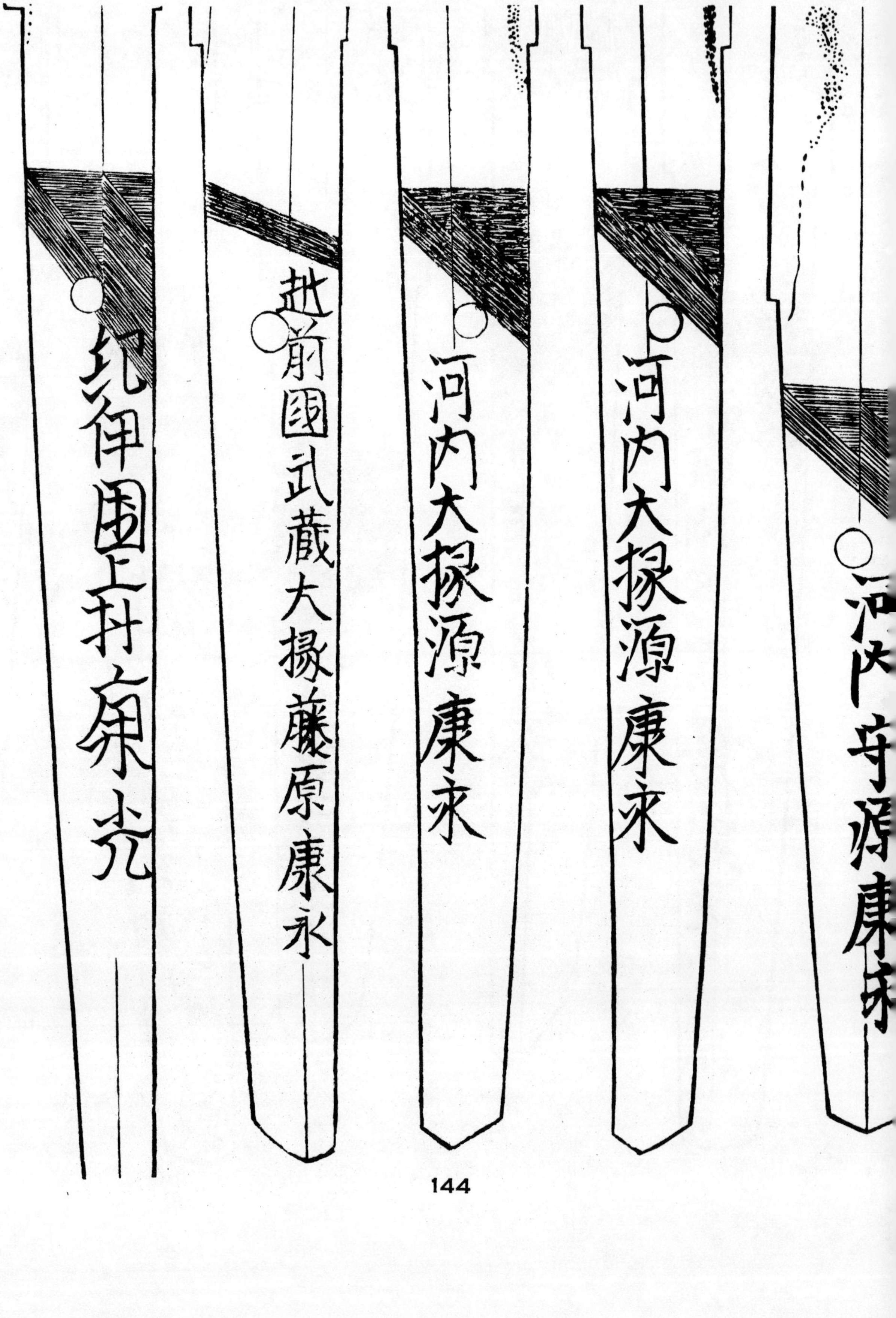

紀伊國上井康光

越前國武蔵大掾藤原康永

河内大掾源康永

河内大掾源康永

河内守源康永

Yasutsugu YA 460   Yasutsugu YA 461

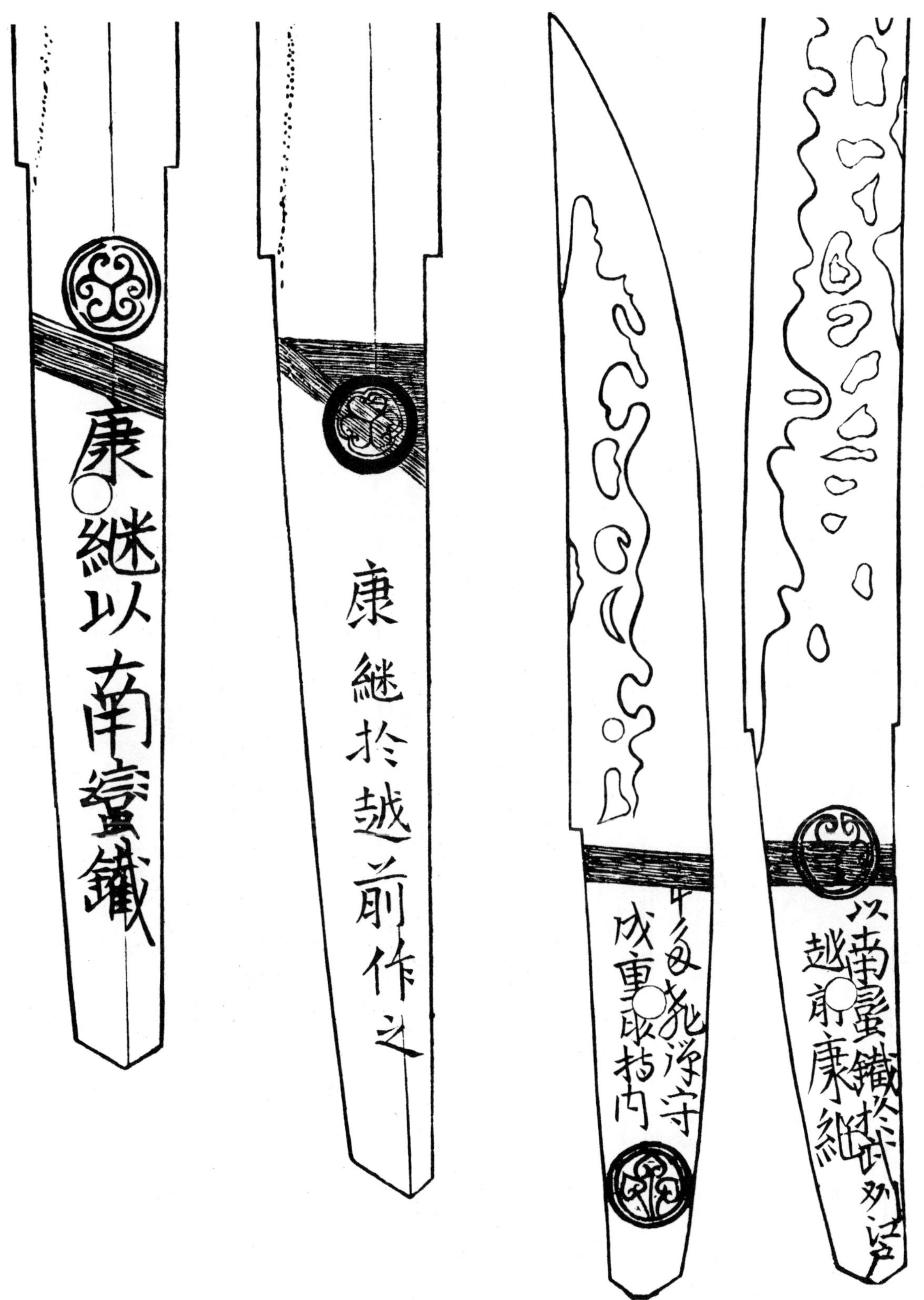

SHINTO BENGI OSHIGATA

Yasuuji
YA 486

Yorisada
YO 50

Yoshiiye
YO 176

Yoshikuni
YO 234

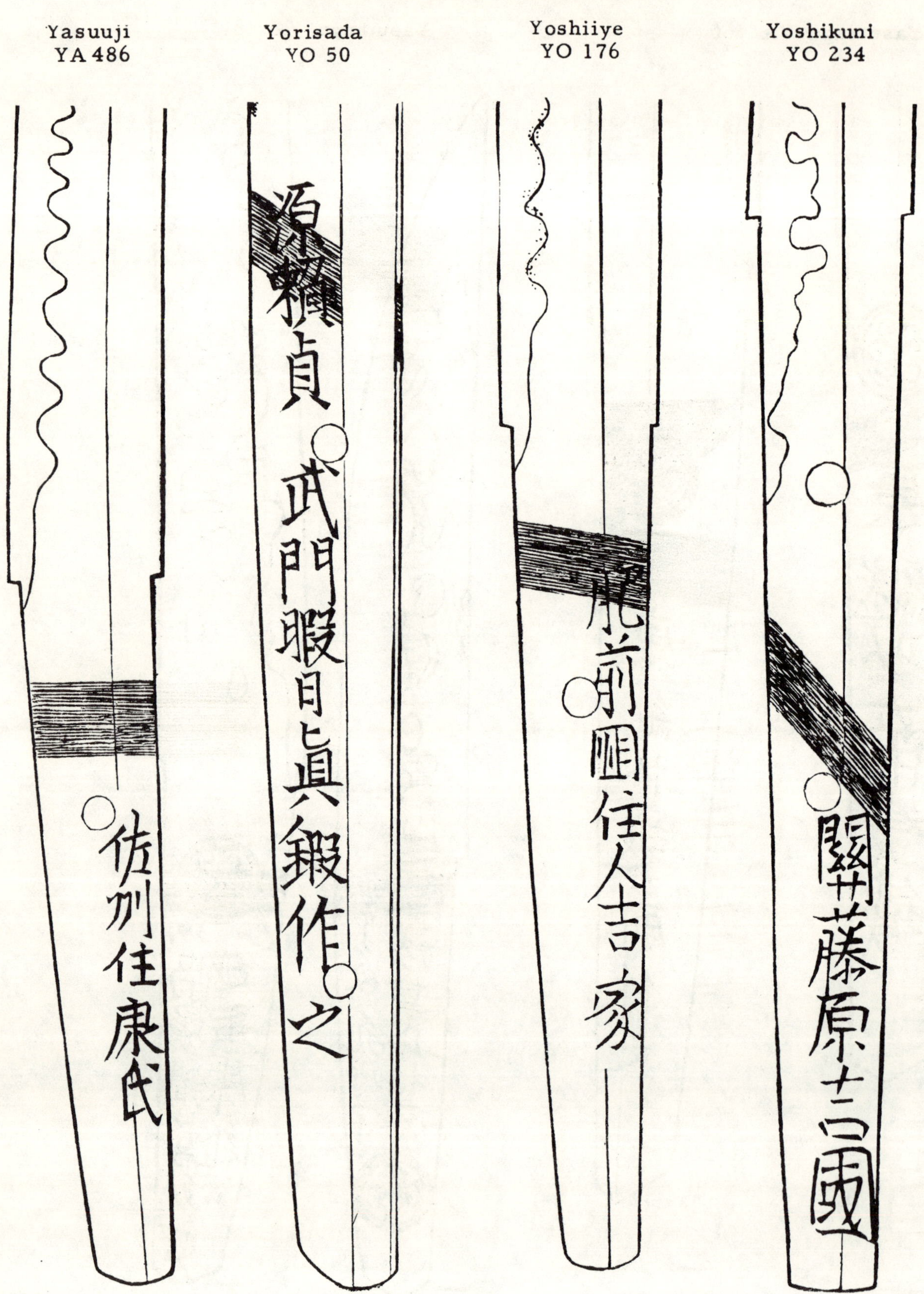

SHINTO BENGI OSHIGATA

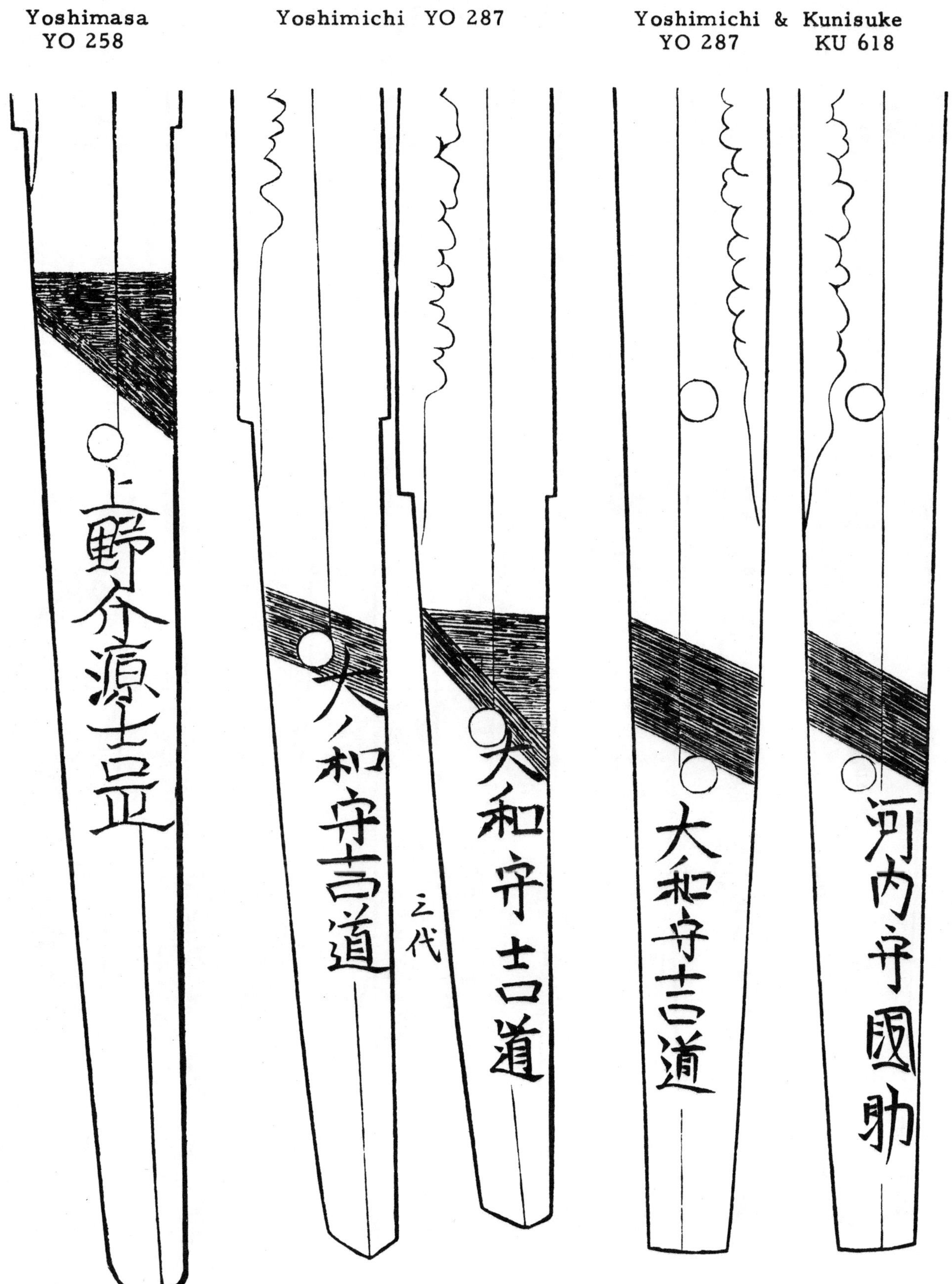

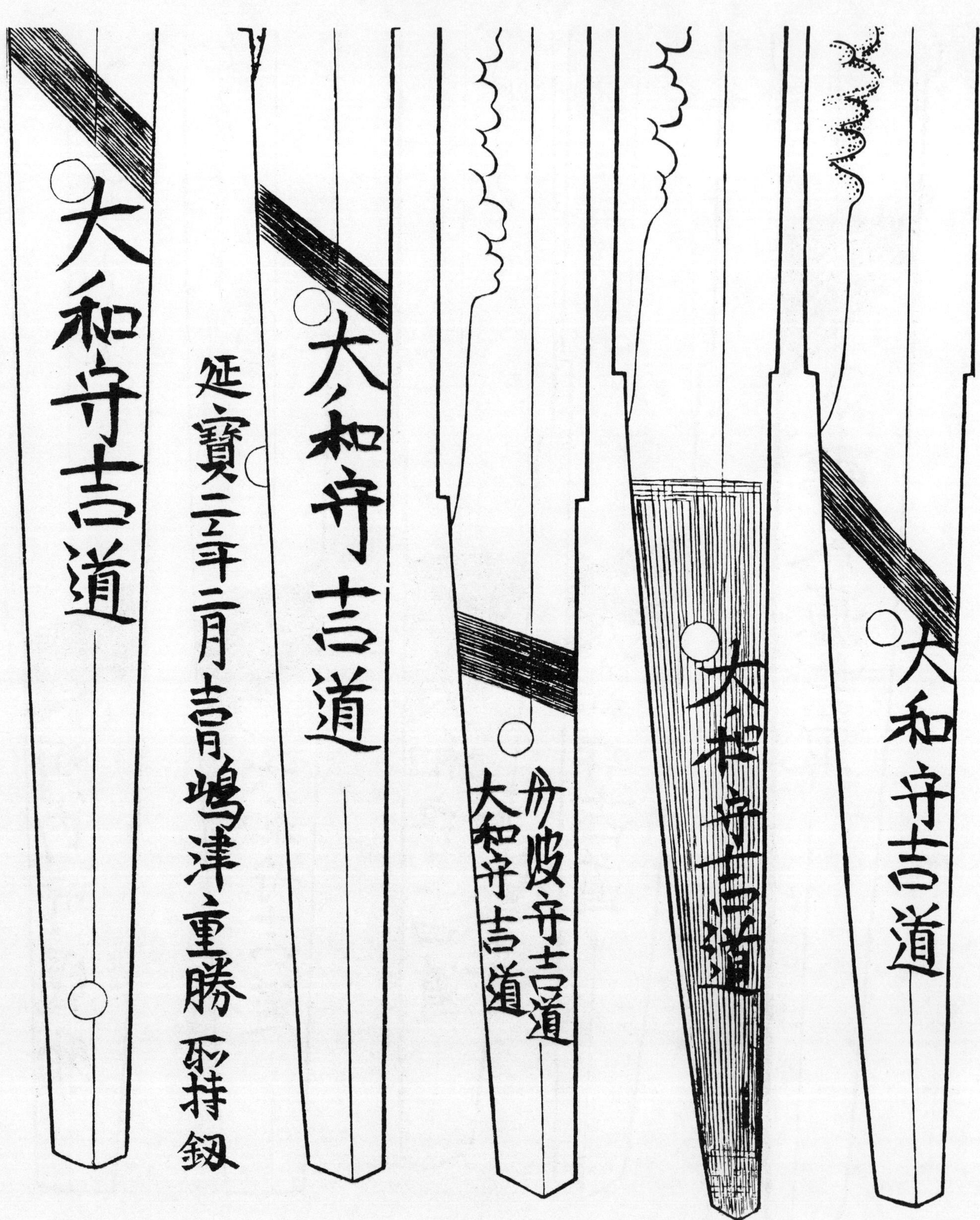

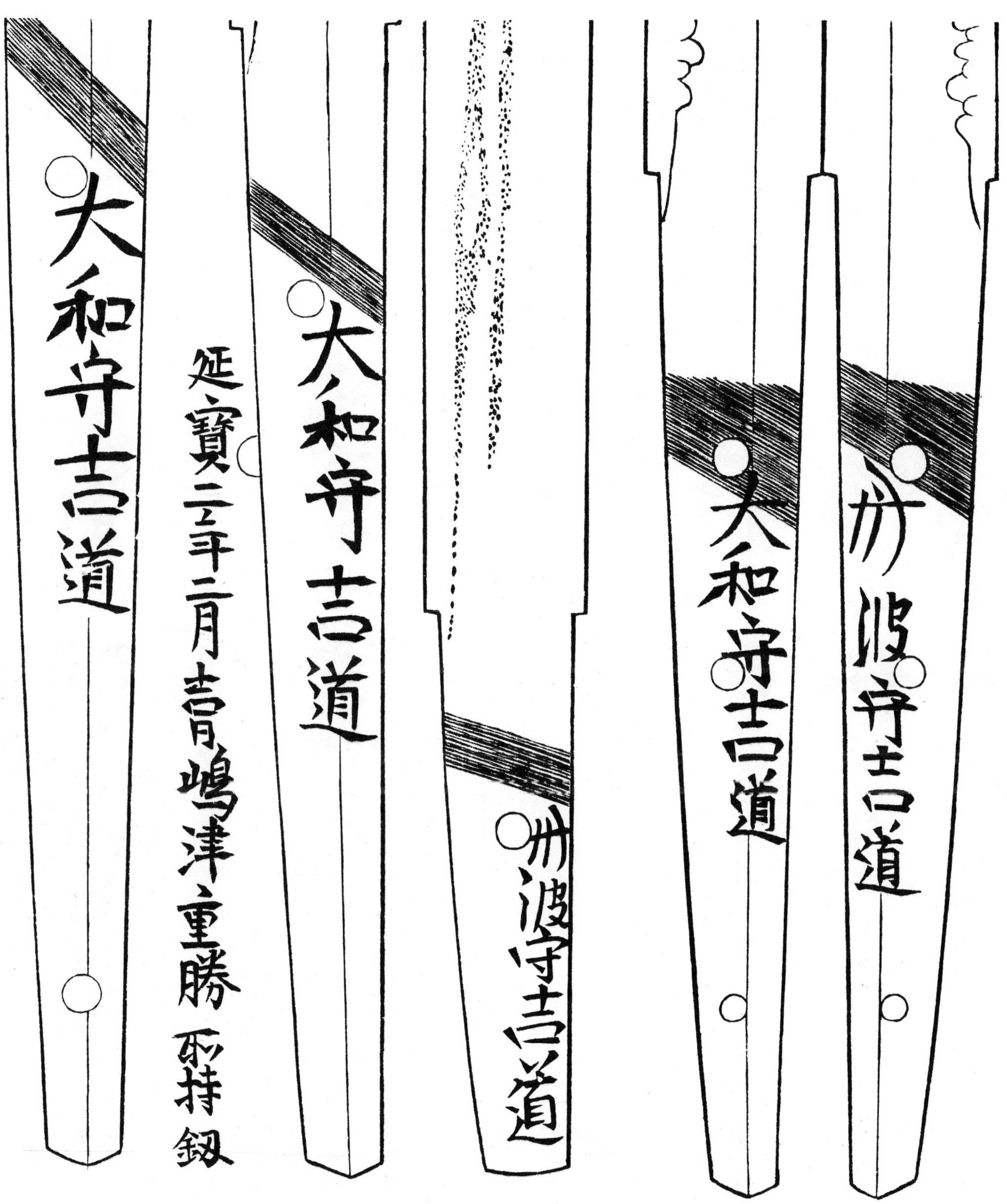
大和守吉道
延寶二二年二月吉青嶋津重勝 所持釼
大和守 吉道
波守吉道
大和守吉道
波守吉道

Yoshimichi YO 287   Yoshimichi YO 288

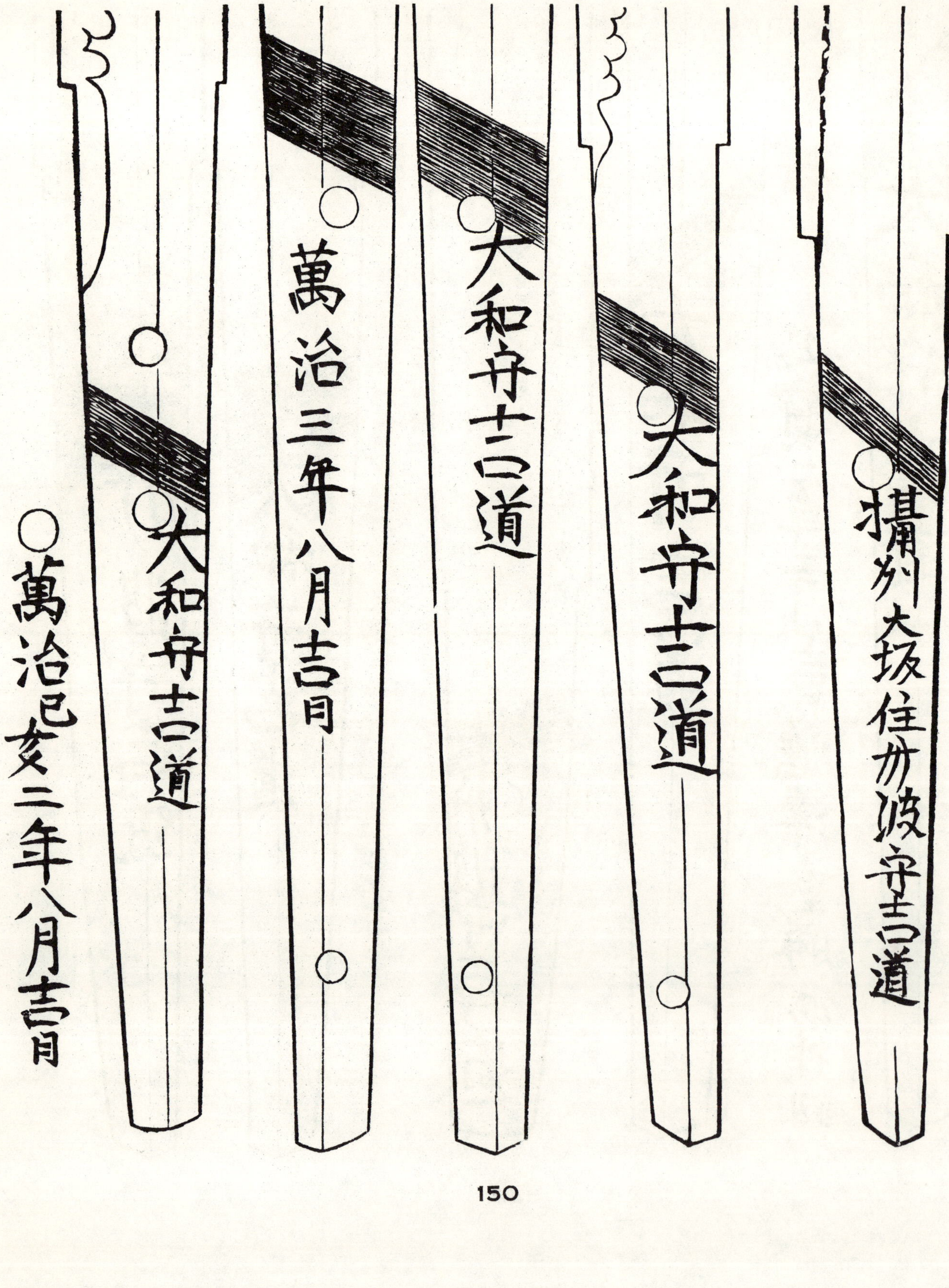

SHINTO BENGI OSHIGATA

Yoshimichi YO 288

Yoshimichi
YO 289

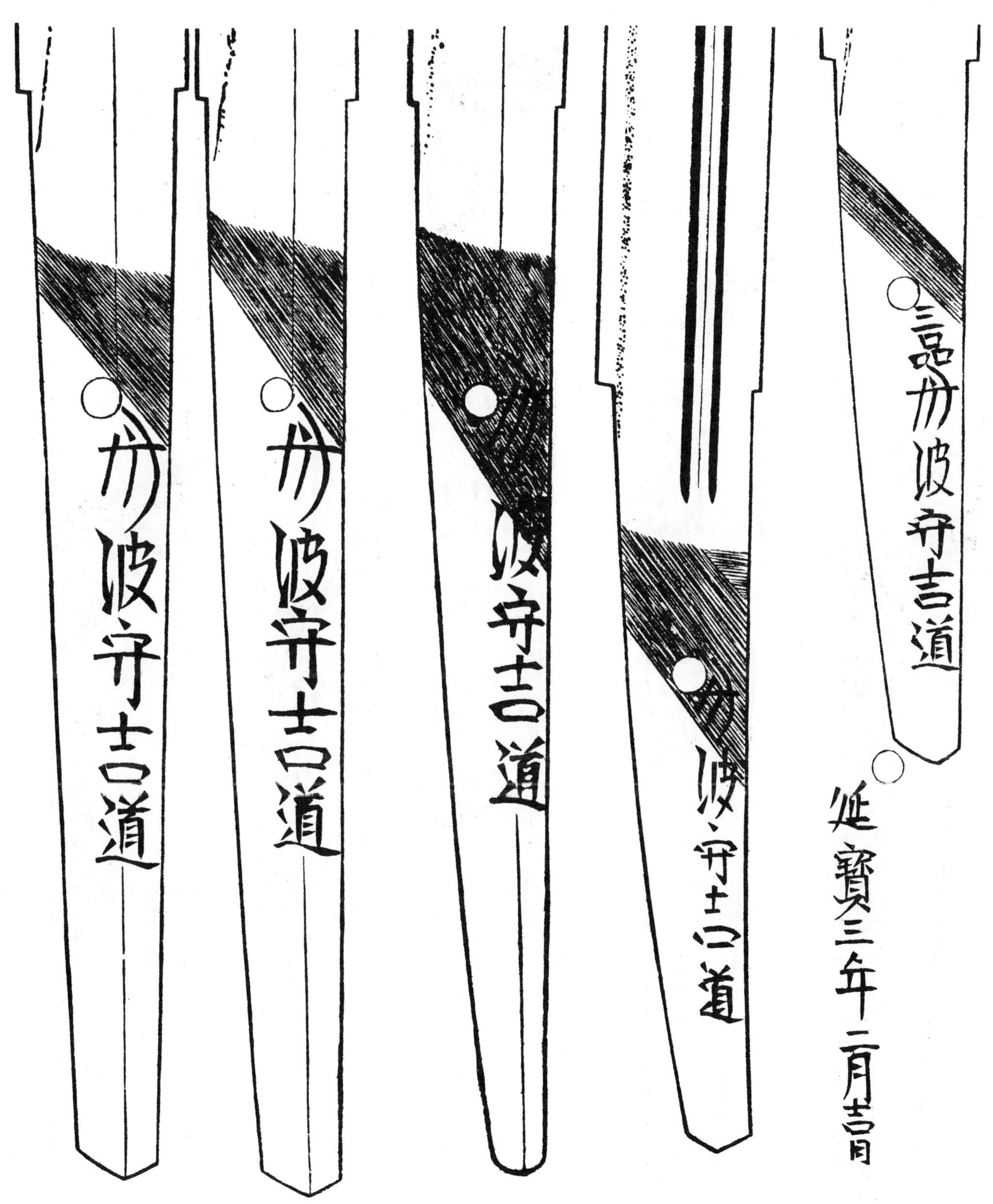

Yoshimichi YO 289   **Yoshim**ichi
YO 290

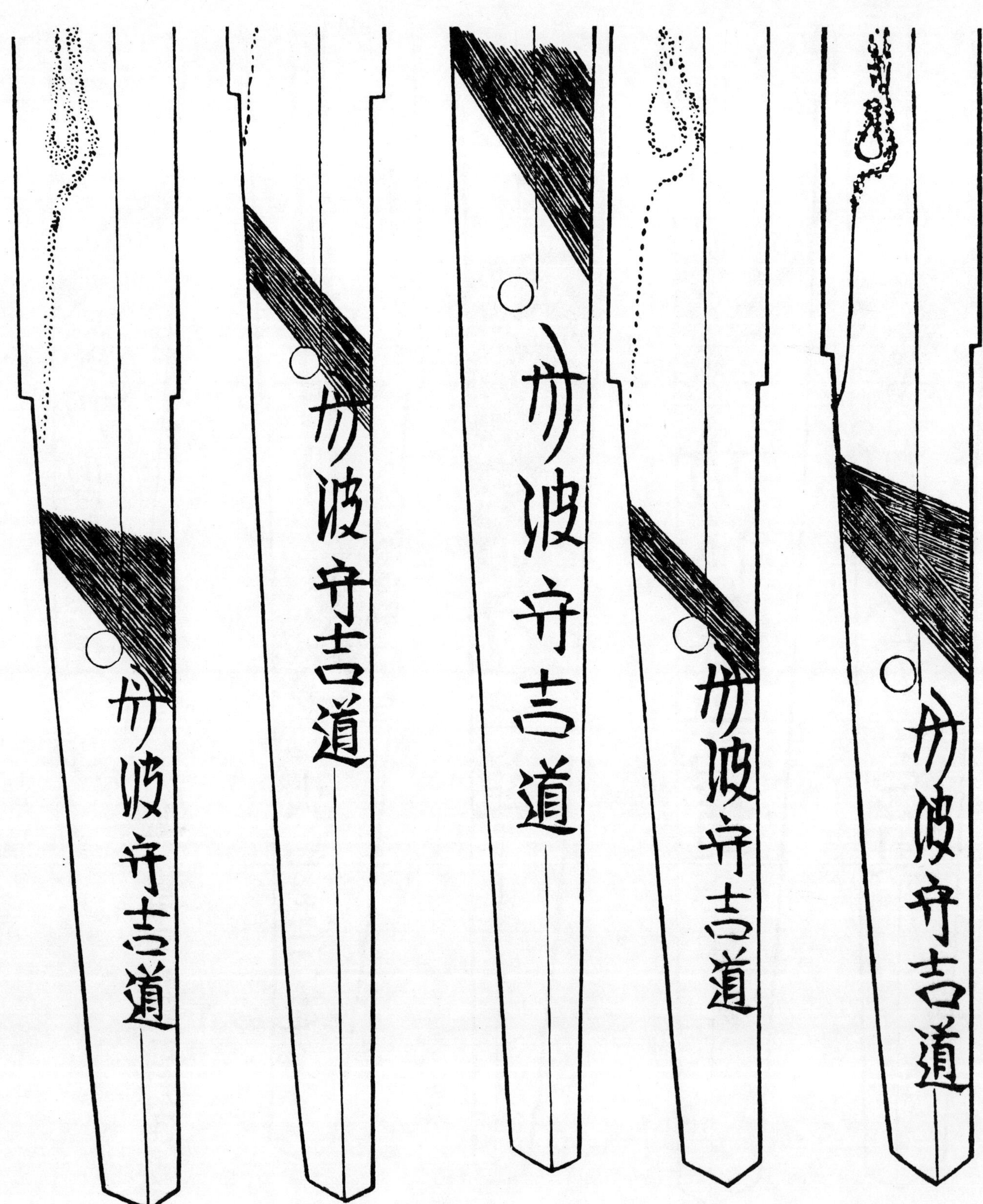

Yoshimichi YO 289   **Yoshimichi YO 291**   **Yoshimichi YO 290**

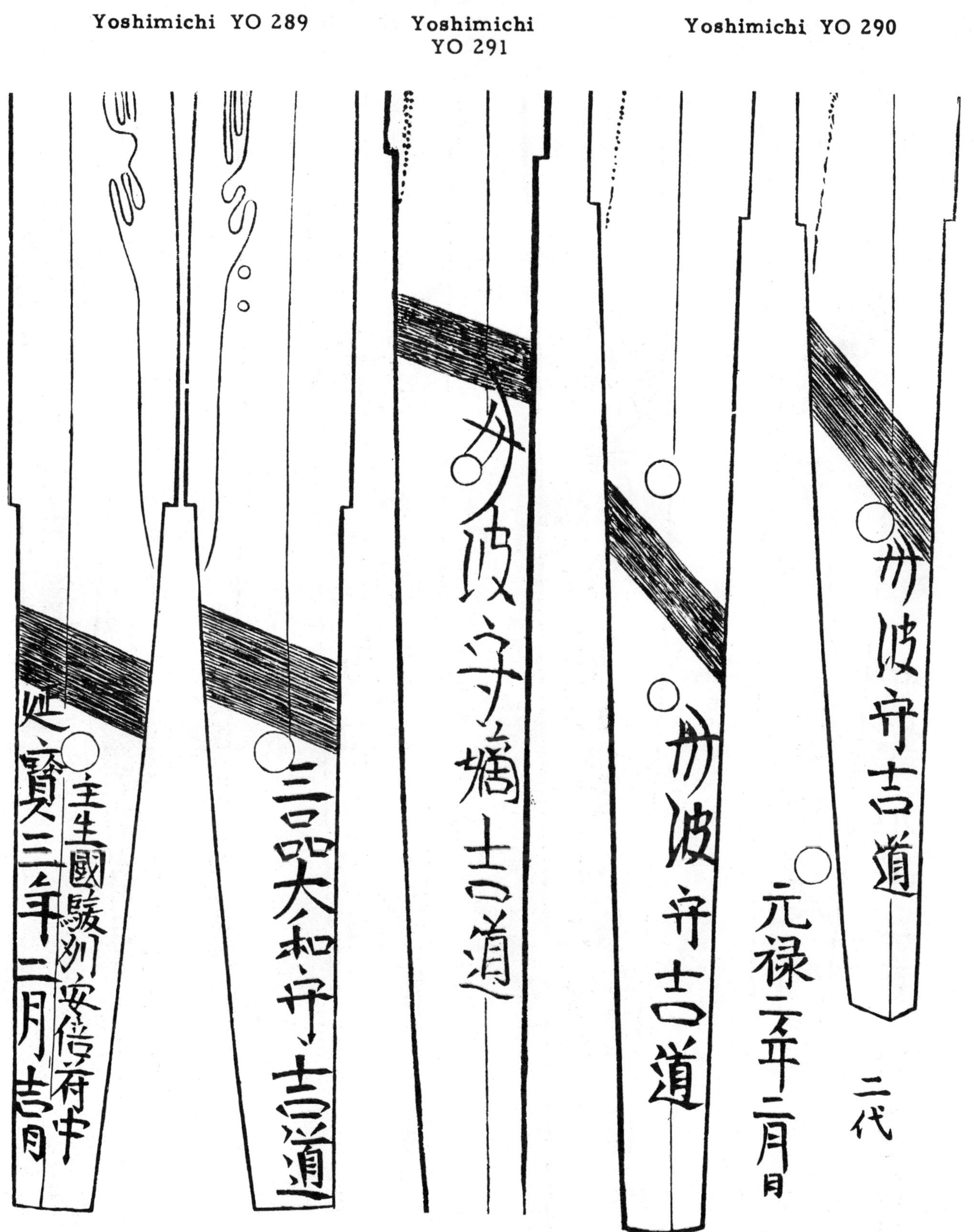

Yoshimichi
YO 293

Yoshimichi YO 294

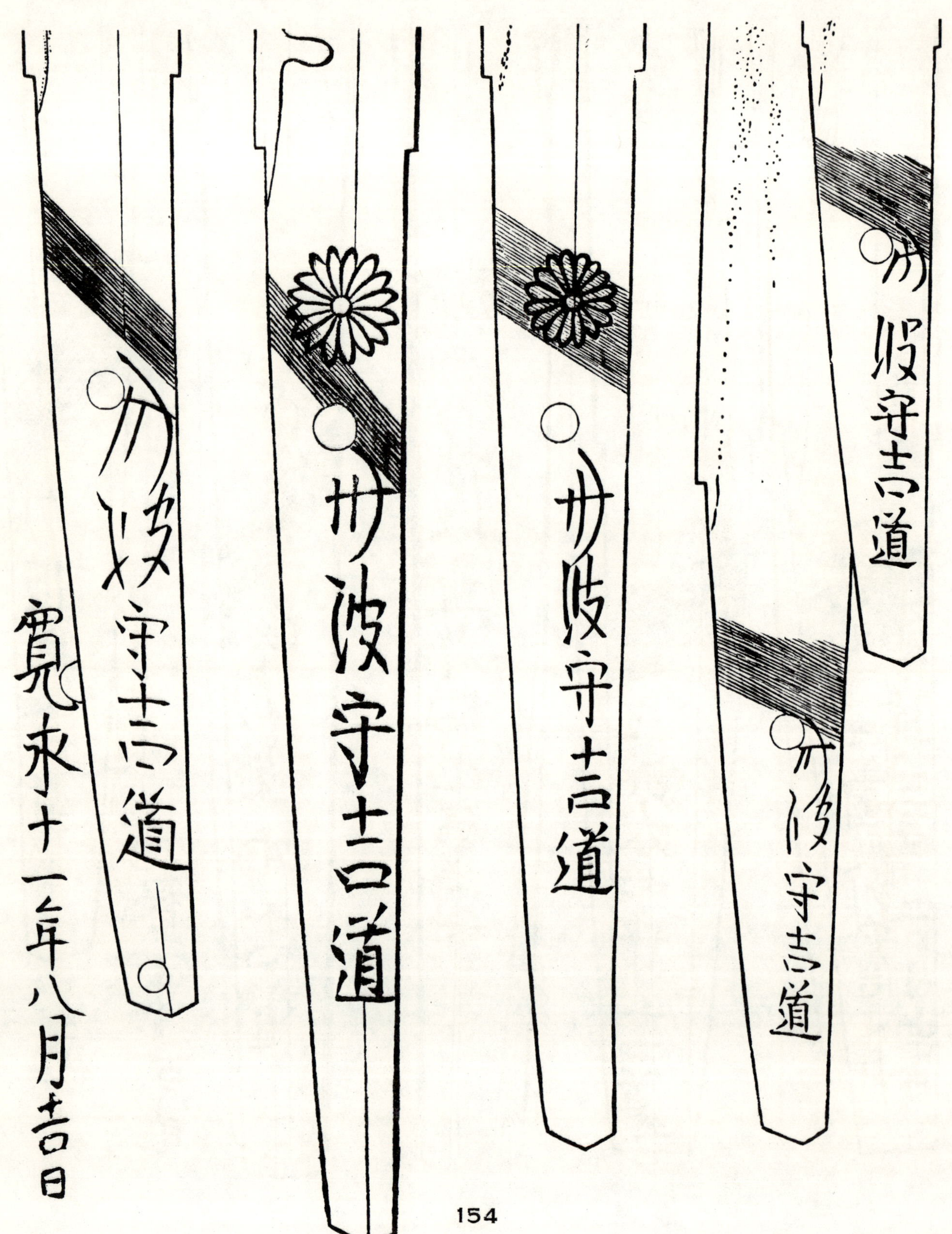

Yoshimichi YO 297

Yoshimichi
YO 299

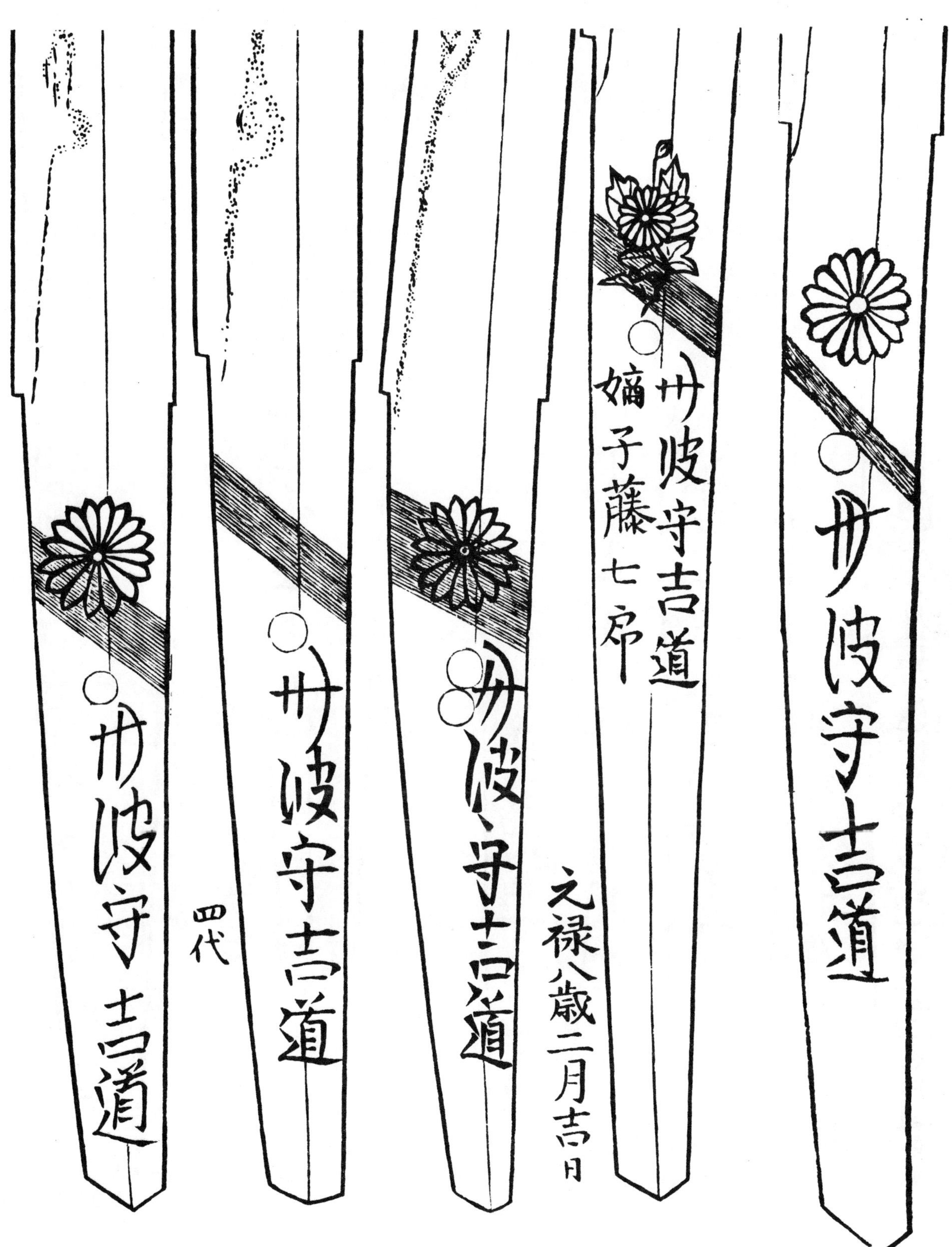

Yoshimichi YO 299 — Yoshimitsu YO 325 — Yoshimori YO 357

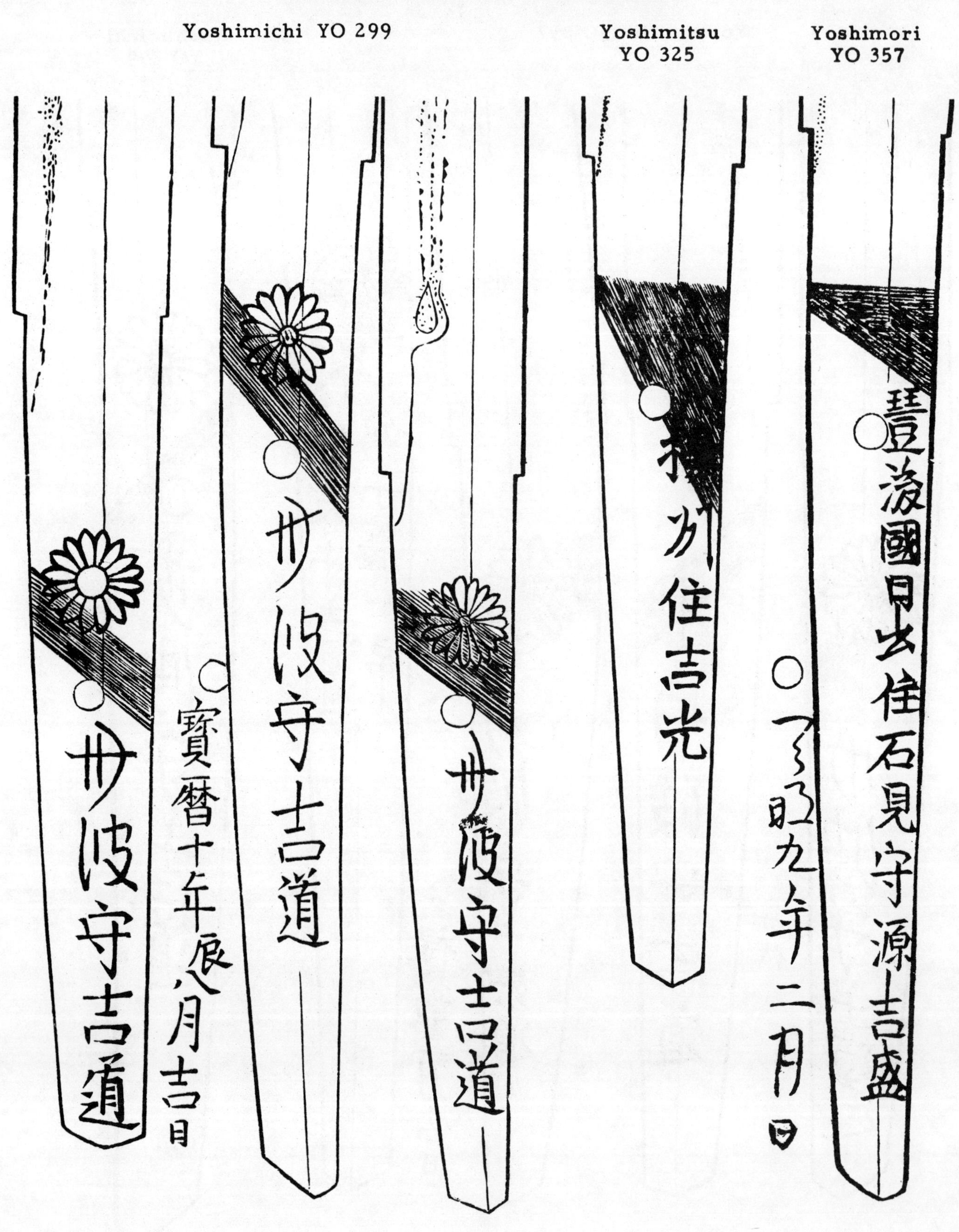

Yoshimori	Yoshinaga	Yoshinari	Yoshinobu
YO 357	YO 392	YO 430	YO 440

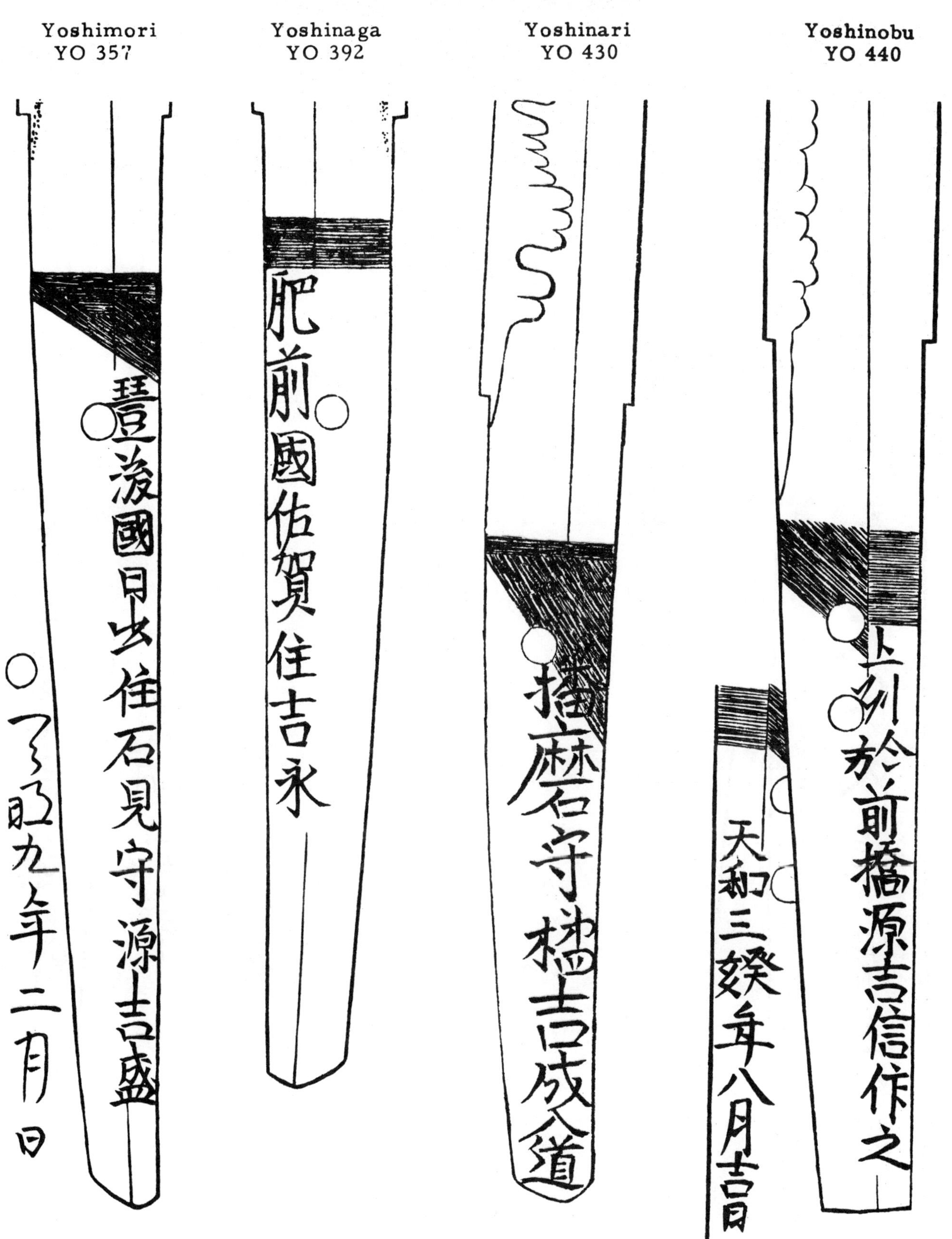

Umetada Yoshinobu YO 445 Yoshinori YO 467 Yoshitake YO 557 Yoshiaki YO 678

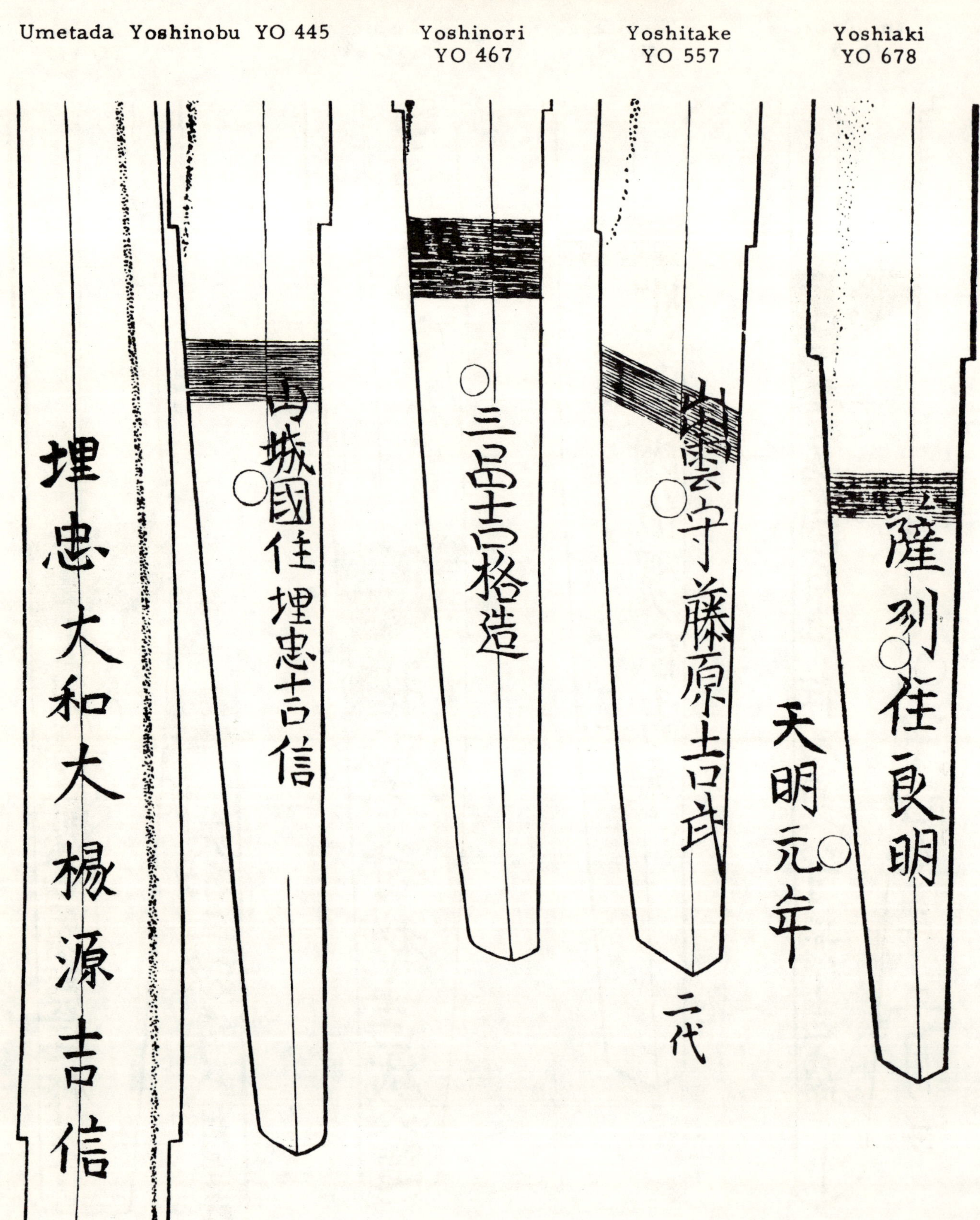

Yoshitada YO 731   Yoshitoki
YO 733   Yoshitoki
YO 733a   Yoshihira
YO 742

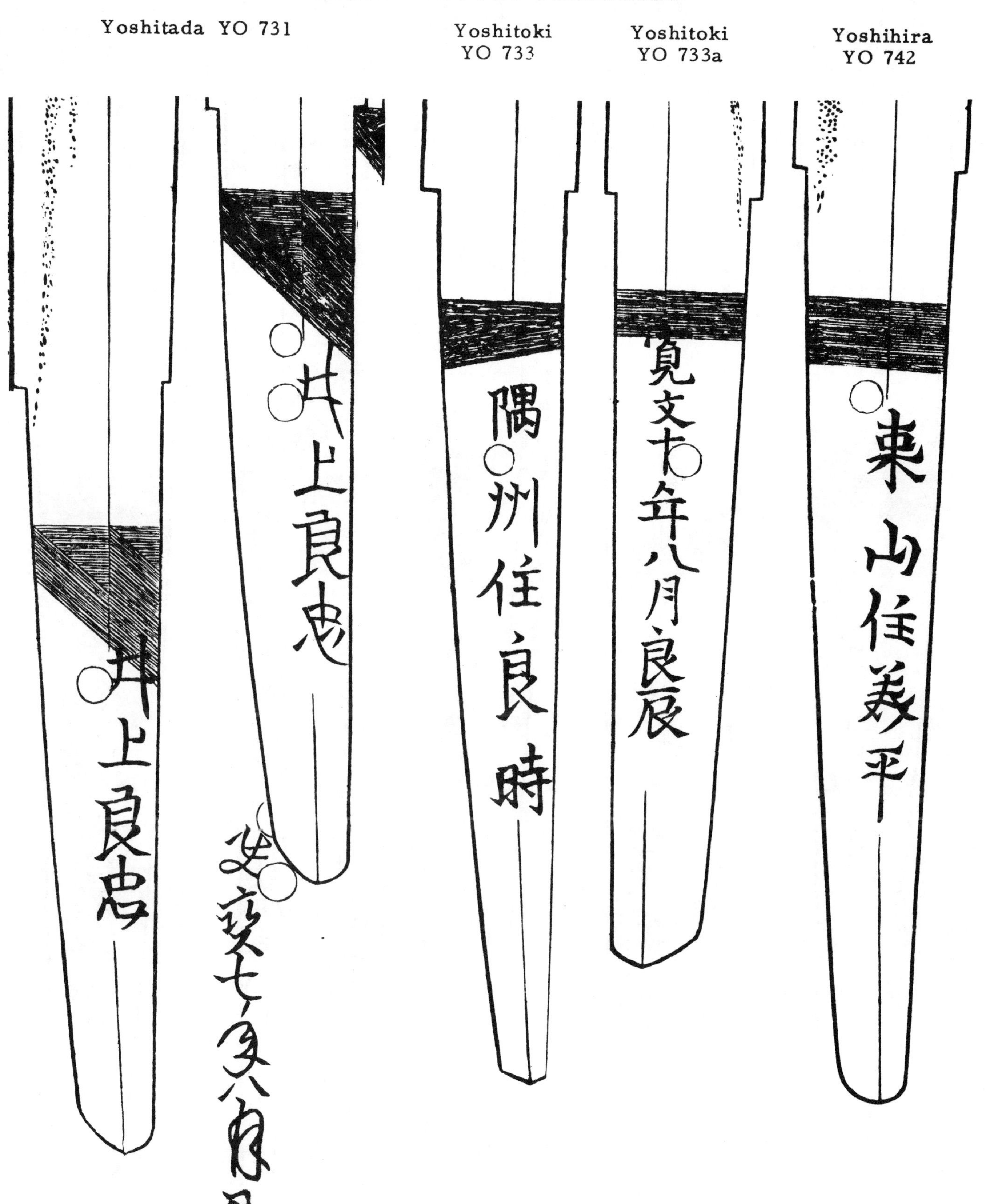

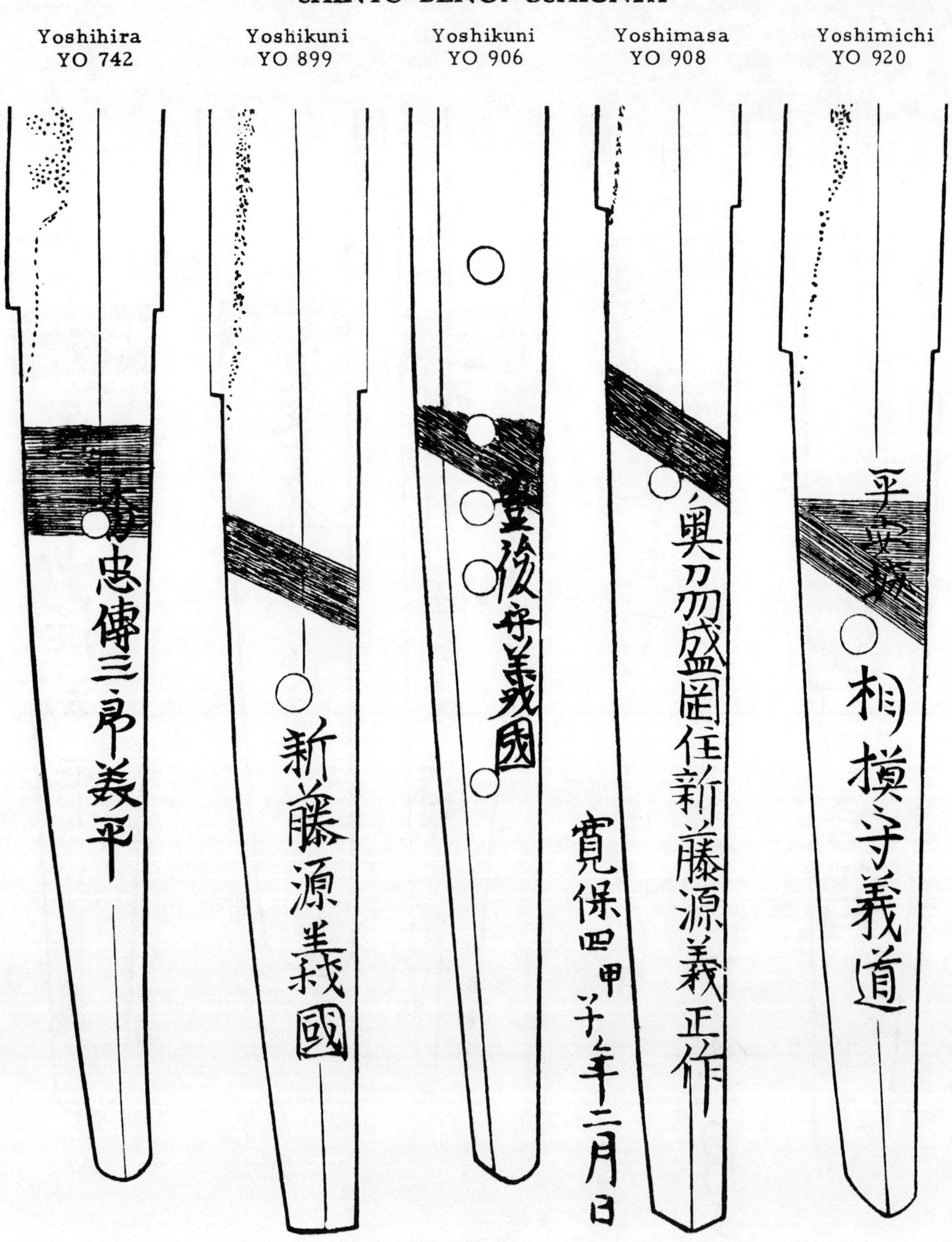
Yoshihira
YO 742

Yoshikuni
YO 899

Yoshikuni
YO 906

Yoshimasa
YO 908

Yoshimichi
YO 920

忠傳三甼義平

新藤源義國

豊後守義國

奧刀盛囶住新藤源義正作
寛保四甲子年二月日

平安城
相摸守義道

Yoshinaga YO 942	Yoshisuke YO 983	Yoshisuke YO 992	Yoshitaka YO 1054

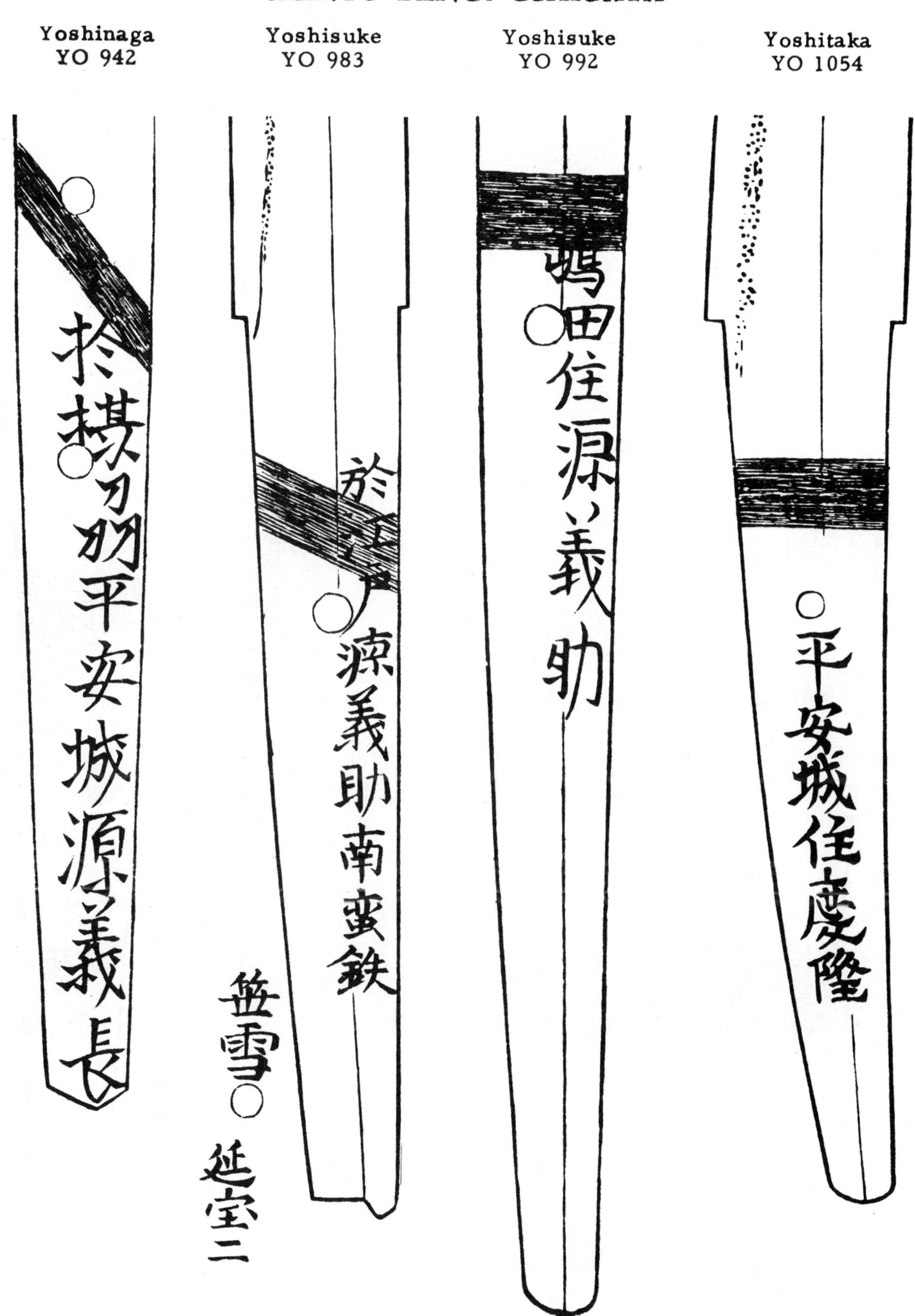

SHINTO BENGI OSHIGATA

Yoshitaka YO 1054   Yoshiyoshi   Yukihiro
                             YO 1057   YU 46

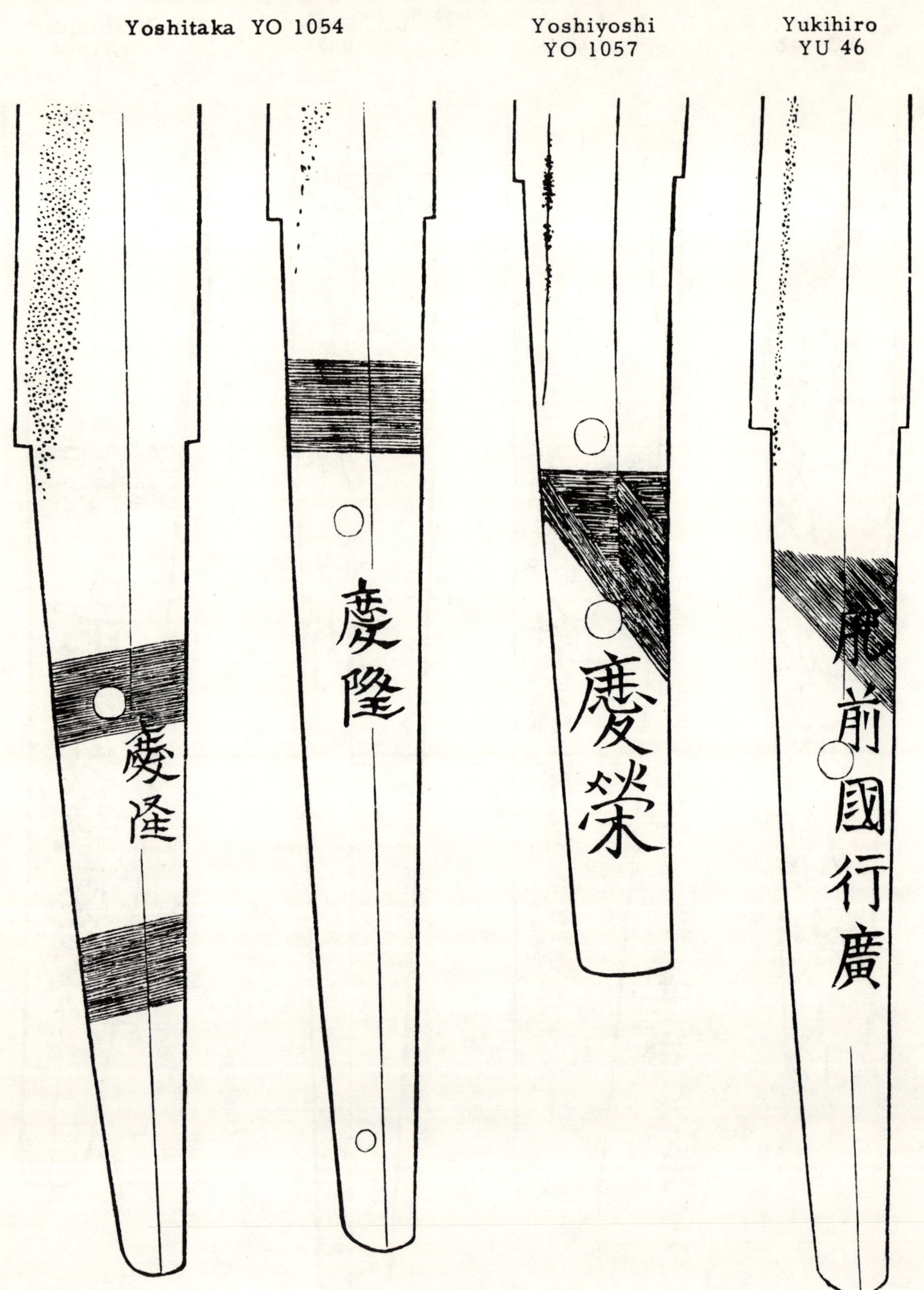

Yukihira YU 31a

Yukihiro
YU 47

Yukinaga
YU 155

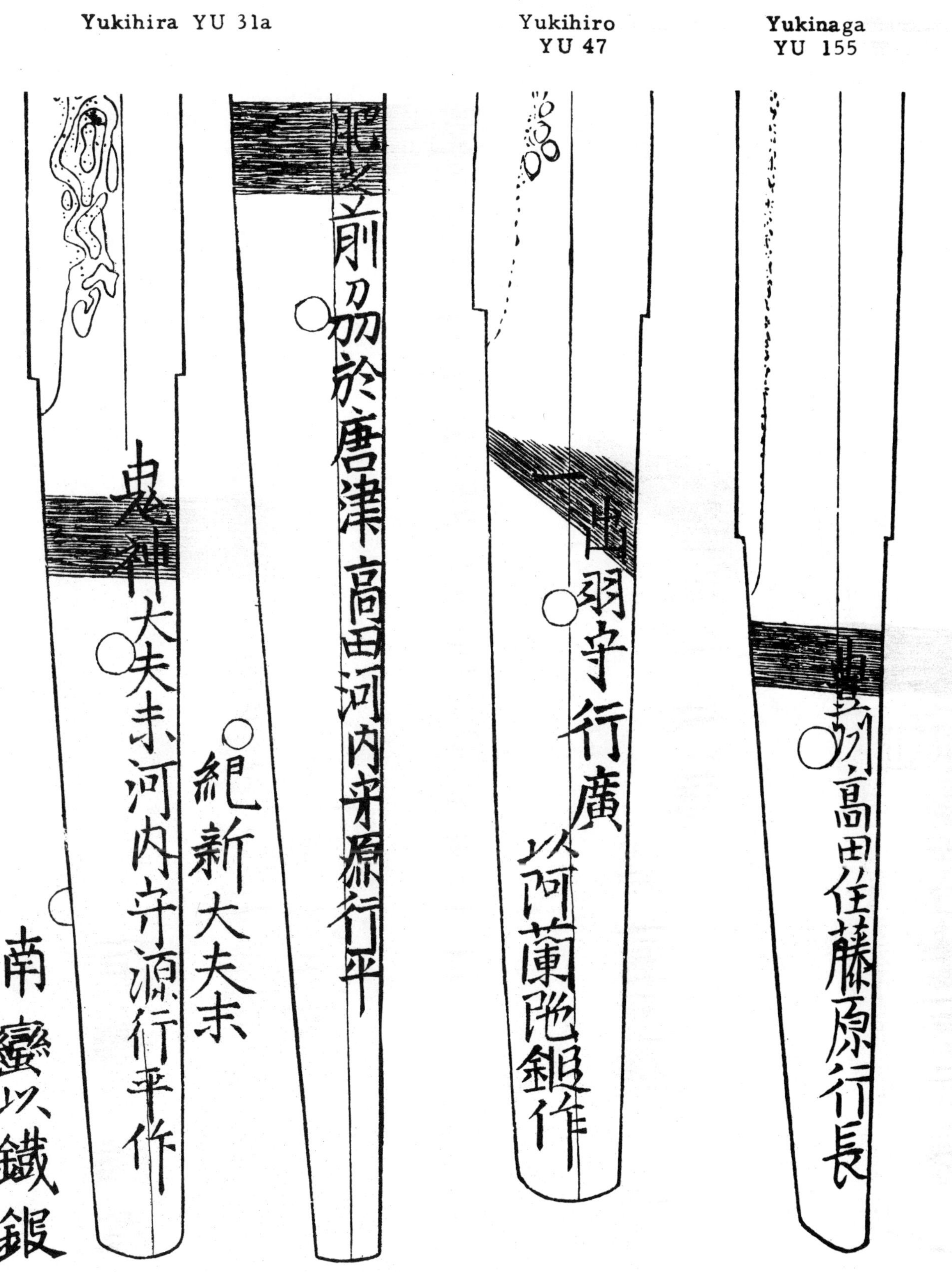

SWORD MONOGRAPHS

by W. M. HAWLEY

Each 16 pages 8 1/2" x 11" Paper-bound

JAPANESE SWORD GROUPS with fold-out Map of Japan

Lists all the main and sub-groups with their founders and most famous smiths.
The general characteristics of each group are given.

TEMPER LINES IN JAPANESE SWORDS

Shows 73 temper lines (hamon) and what groups and famous individuals used them.

LAMINATING TECHNIQUES IN JAPANESE SWORDS

Covers 38 laminating methods with drawings showing how they were made.

HONORARY TITLES USED BY SWORDSMITHS

These titles preceeding a smith's name frequently furnish a clue to the smith
when blades have been shortened enough to remove the name but leaving the title.
This list narrows down the search to the few men holding that title. Comparison
of chisel marks can identify the smith. Many blades exhibit this problem.

FALSE SIGNATURES ON SWORDS

Shows how to check signatures against known genuine examples.
Fifty true and false examples.

BUDDHIST SYMBOLS ON JAPANESE SWORDS

Bonji (priest characters) horimono carvings used to invoke the aid of Buddhas
are shown with drawings of the Buddha forms each represented plus some typical
carvings of more elaborate subjects such as swords and dragons.

FAMOUS WARRIORS OF 16th CENTURY JAPAN

Fourteen drawings by Kuniyoshi the famous print artist, from his 90 volume
Pictorial Biography of Toyotomi Hideyoshi published in a wood-block edition in the
early Meiji period. (Reprint by W. M. Hawley of over 600 battle scenes, etc. is
now available.)

The above are all available at $1.50 each except the Sword Groups with Map
at $2.00   Postage on the above 7 - .50 or .18 for 1.

Carried in stock are all Japanese books on swords, fittings, armor, that are
available. Write for list.

W. M. Hawley
8200 Gould Ave., Hollywood, California, USA